BASIC CONCEPTS IN
PATHOLOGY

Notice

Medicine is an ever-changing science. As new research and clinical experience broaden our knowledge, changes in treatment and drug therapy are required. The author and the publisher of this work have checked with sources believed to be reliable in their efforts to provide information that is complete and generally in accord with the standards accepted at the time of publication. However, in view of the possibility of human error or changes in medical sciences, neither the author nor the publisher nor any other party who has been involved in the preparation or publication of this work warrants that the information contained herein is in every respect accurate or complete, and they are not responsible for any errors or omissions or for the results obtained from use of such information. Readers are encouraged to confirm the information contained herein with other sources. For example and in particular, readers are advised to check the product information sheet included in the package of each drug they plan to administer to be certain that the information contained in this book is accurate and that changes have not been made in the recommended dose or in the contraindications for administration. This recommendation is of particular importance in connection with new or infrequently used drugs.

BASIC CONCEPTS IN
PATHOLOGY

A STUDENT'S SURVIVAL GUIDE

EARL BROWN, M.D.

Department of Pathology
James A. Quillen Medical Center
Johnson City, Tennessee

Series Editor
Hiram F. Gilbert, Ph.D.

The McGraw-Hill Companies
Health Professions Division

New York   St. Louis   San Francisco
Auckland   Bogota   Caracus   Lisbon   London   Madrid
Mexico City   Milan   Montreal   New Delhi   Paris   San Juan
Singapore   Sydney   Tokyo   Toronto

McGraw-Hill

A Division of The McGraw·Hill Companies

BASIC CONCEPTS IN PATHOLOGY:
A STUDENT'S SURVIVAL GUIDE

1 2 3 4 5 6 7 8 9 0 DOC DOC 9 9 8 7

ISBN: 0-07-008321-5

This book was set in Times Roman by Better Graphics, Inc. The editors were James Morgan and Pamela Touboul; the series editor was Hiram F. Gilbert, Ph.D.; the production supervisor was Richard Ruzycka; the project was managed by Hockett Editorial Services; the cover designer was Marsha Cohen.

R. R. Donnelley & Sons Company was printer and binder.

This book is printed on acid-free paper.

Library of Congress Cataloging-in-Publication Data

Brown, Earl J., 1956–
    Basic concepts on pathology : a student's survival guide / Earl J. Brown.—1st ed.
       p.   cm.
    Includes index.
    ISBN 0-07-008321-5
    1. Physiology, Pathological. 2. Pathology. I. Title.
    [DNLM: 1. Pathology. 2. Cells—physiology. 3. Abnormalities.
    4. Genetics. 5. Immune System—physiology. QZ 4 B877b 1998]
    RB113.B76   1998
    616.07   cc21
    DNLM/DLC
    for Library of Congress   97-35643

· C O N T E N T S ·

CHAPTER 4   CELL DEPOSITS
   AND ACCUMULATIONS   **29**

CHAPTER 5   CELL ADAPTATIONS   67

CHAPTER 6   CELL SIGNALING   88

CHAPTER 7   CELL GROWTH   112

CHAPTER 8   CELL DEGENERATIONS   124

CHAPTER 9   DEVELOPMENTAL
ABNORMALITIES   139

CHAPTER 10   GENETICS   155

CHAPTER 11   INFLAMMATION—PART ONE   183

CHAPTER 12 INFLAMMATION—PART TWO 206

CHAPTER 13   REPAIR AND REGENERATION   236

CHAPTER 14   FLUIDS AND HEMODYNAMICS   255

CHAPTER 15   HEMOSTATSIS AND INFARCTION   271

CHAPTER 16   IMMUNOLOGY—PART ONE: CELLS OF THE IMMUNE SYSTEM   301

CHAPTER 17   IMMUNOLOGY—PART TWO: HYPERSENSITIVITY REACTIONS   321

CHAPTER 18   IMMUNOLOGY—PART THREE: AUTOIMMUNE AND IMMUNODEFICIENCY DISEASE   347

CHAPTER 19 NEOPLASIA—PART ONE: BENIGN AND MALIGNANT TUMORS 362

CHAPTER 20 NEOPLASIA—PART TWO: CARCINOGENESIS 386

· A C K N O W L E D G M E N T S ·

I would like to express my appreciation to my colleagues in the Department of Pathology for their support and help over the past decade that I have been director of our sophomore pathology course. I would like to especially thank Dr. Philip S. Coogan, the chairman of our department, who has supported my efforts over the years and has enabled me to progress as a teacher. It is because of Dr. Coogan's support and effort that our department has entered the new age of computer-based instruction. This book is due in large part to that evolution of teaching. I cannot express my deeply felt thanks to all of my many students who over the years have inspired me with their spirit, their comon sense, and their enthusiasm. They have showed me time and time again different and better ways to explain concepts and organize material. They have taught me much. Finally, I would like to thank my family, my wife, Janet, and my two children, Kevin and Heather, who have supported me through way too many late night and weekend typing sessions. Without them this book would never have been written.

· C H A P T E R · 1 ·

HOW TO USE THIS BOOK

·

- **Organization of the Chapters of This Book**
- **Organization of Pathology**
- **Purpose of This Book**
- **How to Use This Book**

· · · · · · · · · · · ·

ORGANIZATION OF THE CHAPTERS OF THIS BOOK

- Summary boxes
- Text
- Schematics and diagrams

The basic organization of the chapters in this book is rather simple. Each chapter begins with an index of the sections within that chapter. Each section begins with a box that provides a short summary of the key points for that section. Sometimes the summary box contains an outline of that section. The text for each section further explains the key points and basic concepts for that section. The text is supplemented by schematics and diagrams, which help to illustrate the organization and interrelationships of the basic concepts. Finally, the glossary provides a few key definitions.

ORGANIZATION OF PATHOLOGY

- General pathology
- Systemic pathology

1

The basic organization of pathology is also rather simple. Pathology is the study of disease and is divided into general pathology and systemic pathology. General pathology refers to the study of the general mechanisms of disease, while systemic pathology refers to the study of individual organ systems, such as the heart, lungs, or kidneys. The first half of most pathology textbooks covers general pathology, and the second half usually covers systemic pathology. General pathology with its numerous mechanisms tends to be much more difficult to master than systemic pathology.

PURPOSE OF THIS BOOK

- Basic concepts of general pathology
- Integration of organ system diseases

The purpose of this book is to make the study of general pathology more interesting by integrating into it the concepts of systemic pathology and diseases that are usually covered during the study of organ systems. The chapters are organized according to the basic concepts of general pathology and cover all of the basic mechanisms of general pathology. These chapters are augmented, however, by in-depth discussions of diseases that result from these basic abnormalities.

HOW TO USE THIS BOOK

- Preview
- Integration
- Review

This book can be used in several ways. First, you can use it while studying general pathology to get a more in-depth preview of the diseases that result from the general mechanisms of disease. Second, you can use it while studying systemic pathology to supplement the study of organ disease and obtain a greater understanding of how these diseases result from the mechanisms of general pathology. Third, you can use the summary boxes for a general review of pathology before board examinations. These summary boxes contain the same information that is found in general board review books. In contrast to those books, however, in this book if you do not understand the basic points in the boxes you can find more information in the text that follows.

CELL INJURY

·

· · · · · · · · · · · ·

CAUSE OF DISEASE
- Injury to cells
- Damage to cell membranes

3

CAUSES OF CELL MEMBRANE INJURY

Direct cell injury

- Free radicals

Indirect cell injury

1. Toxins
2. Decreased energy production
   - Hypoglycemia
   - Hypoxia

Pathology is the study of disease. Even though there seems to be an infinite number of diseases, they all have one basic abnormality in common. All pathologic processes that produce disease are the result of injury to cells. It is cellular injury and the body's reaction to cellular injury that produce disease.

How do these pathologic processes lead to cell injury? The basic concept is that all cell injury results in damage to cell membranes (Fig. 2-1). How can cell

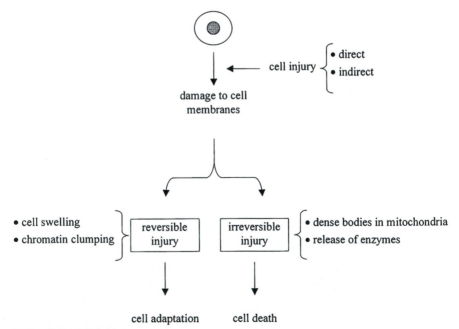

Figure 2-1 Cell Injury
Damage to cell membranes can result from direct or indirect mechanisms. Damaged cells are either reversibly or irreversibly injured.

membranes be damaged? Cells can be damaged directly or indirectly. Free radicals can damage cells directly. Toxins or processes that decrease the energy production of the cells damage cells indirectly.

FREE RADICALS

- Single unpaired electron in outer orbit
- Unstable, highly reactive (catalytic) molecules
- Direct damage to cell membranes
- Carbon tetrachloride liver damage: the model for free radical damage
- Superoxide, hydroxyl radical, and carbon tetrachloride

MECHANISMS TO CLEAR AND CONTROL FREE RADICALS

Enzymes

- Superoxide dismutase (SOD): $O_2^{\cdot} \rightarrow H_2O$
- Catalase (peroxisomes): $H_2O_2 \rightarrow O_2 + H_2O$
- Glutathione peroxidase: $GSH + OH^{\cdot} \rightarrow GSSG + H_2O$

Antioxidants

- Vitamin C
- Vitamin E

Free radicals have a single, unpaired electron in their outer orbit. They are very unstable and react with nearby molecules. Examples of free radicals include superoxide, the hydroxyl radical, and carbon tetrachloride. Because free radicals are very reactive, they can react with cell membranes and damage them. In fact, free radicals are used by certain cells of the body for protection against bacteria. (Because they are so reactive, the body has several mechanisms to clear and control free radicals.)

Cell membranes are composed of abundant lipid. Oxygen-derived free radicals react with the lipid in cell membranes. This process, called lipid peroxidation, leads to cell damage. Another free radical, carbon tetrachloride, is the model for free radical damage. Carbon tetrachloride damages the liver by the actions of the free radical $CCl_3^{\cdot}$. Carbon tetrachloride is converted to $CCl_3^{\cdot}$ by cytochrome P-450. $CCl_3^{\cdot}$ causes lipid peroxidation of phospholipids in membranes, such as the rough endoplasmic reticulum (RER) and the plasma membrane. Damage to the RER of hepatocytes causes decreased synthesis of lipoproteins and leads to accumulation of fat.

BACTERIAL TOXINS
Endotoxins

- Lipopolysaccharide (lipid A)
- Gram-negative rods and cocci
- Part of outer cell membrane of cell wall

Exotoxins

1. *Bacillus anthracis*
   - Adenylate cyclase edema factor, protective antigen, and lethal factor
2. *Bordetella pertussis*
   - Stimulates ADP-ribosylation
   - Inhibits Gi proteins ("off switch off")
   - Increases cAMP
3. *Clostridium botulinum*
   - Inhibits presynaptic release of acetylcholine
4. *Clostridium tetani*
   - Inhibits release of glycine (inhibitory neurotransmitter) in brain
5. *Corynebacterium diphtheria*
   - Stimulates ADP-ribosylation
   - Inhibits elongation factor 2 (EF-2)
6. *Escherichia coli*
   - Heat-labile toxin → similar to cholera toxin
   - Heat-stable toxin → stimulates guanylate cyclase
   - Verotoxin → inhibits protein synthesis
7. *Pseudomonas species*
   - Exotoxin A → similar to *diphtheria* toxin
8. *Staphylococcus aureus*
   - Coagulase → stimulates formation of fibrin clot
   - Protein A → inhibits phagocytosis and binding of complement
   - TSST → toxic shock syndrome
9. *Streptococcus pyogenes*
   - Streptolysin O → hemolysin
10. *Vibrio cholera*
    - Stimulates ADP-riboxylation
    - Inhibits deactivation of Gs proteins ("on switch on")
    - Increases cAMP

Cell membranes can be damaged indirectly by toxins or processes that cause decreased energy production by cells. Among the most important toxins are those produced by bacteria. These bacterial toxins are classified as endotoxins or exotoxins. The toxins can be further classified based on their mechanisms of action.

IMPAIRED ENERGY PRODUCTION

1. Hypoglycemia
2. Hypoxia
    • Impaired absorption of oxygen
    • Decreased blood flow
    • Diseases of blood or blood vessels

Impaired energy production by the cell is an important cause of cell injury. It can be the result of several different abnormalities, such as decreased glucose (hypoglycemia) or decreased oxygen (hypoxia). *Hypoxia*, a very important pathologic process, serves as a model for cell injury. Hypoxia may be the result of disease processes that affect the normal transport of oxygen from the lungs to the tissue. Examples of these abnormalities include decreased blood flow (*ischemia*), diseases of the lungs, diseases of the blood vessels (atherosclerosis), or diseases of the blood itself (anemia).

RESULTS OF DECREASED ENERGY PRODUCTION

• Decreased ATP production by mitochondria
• Decreased functioning of membrane ion pumps
• Abnormal intracellular ion concentrations
• Excess water into cells
• Damage to cell organelles

How does decreased energy production damage cell membranes? The decreased oxygen delivery to the cell leads to decreased oxidative phosphorylation within mitochondria, and this decreases the production of ATP. Cells rely on an ATPase-dependent sodium-potassium membrane pump to maintain the proper concentration of ions inside and outside of the cell. Decreased ATP production by the mitochondria decreases the pumping of sodium out of the cell and potassium into the cell. Since normally three sodium ions are pumped out of the cell by the sodium-potassium membrane pump for every two potassium ions pumped into the cell, decreased functioning of this pump results in a greater number of sodium ions entering the cell than potassium ions leaving the cell. This increased number of solutes causes excess water to enter the cell, leading to swelling of the cell. This pathologic change, called *hydropic degeneration*, is an important sign of cellular injury. Histologically this change is seen as enlarged cells with abundant pale cytoplasm.

REVERSIBLE CELL INJURY

- Swelling of cell and cell organelles
- Ribosomes dissociate from endoplasmic reticulum
- Decreased energy production by mitochondria
- Increased glycolysis $\rightarrow$ decreased pH $\rightarrow$ nuclear chromatin clumping

---

To recap, cells are injured by damage to cell membranes. Take a look again at Figure 2-1. Cell injury may be reversible, in which case the cells live and adapt, or it may be irreversible, in which case the cells die. In either case, the influx of water causes the injured cells to swell. In reversibly injured cells the influx of water also causes the organelles within the cells to swell. Swelling of the endoplasmic reticulum impairs protein synthesis, causes ribosomes to detach from the rough endoplasmic reticulum, and causes mitochondria to swell. As energy production from aerobic mechanisms decreases as the mitochondria swell, cells begin to obtain energy instead from anaerobic mechanisms (glycolysis). Unfortunately, glycolysis increases the production of lactic acid within cells and decreases the intracellular pH. This in turn causes clumping of the chromatin in the nucleus. All of these are signs of reversible injury.

IRREVERSIBLE CELL INJURY

- Dense bodies within mitochondria (flocculent densities in heart)
- Release of cellular enzymes
- Nuclear degeneration
- Cell death

Continued cell injury eventually reaches a point where the cellular changes are irreversible, and the injured cell will die. The exact point or change that determines whether a cell will die or survive is unknown. One of the most reliable signs of irreversible cellular injury is the formation of dense bodies within mitochondria (Fig. 2-1). These dense bodies are the result of calcium influx into the mitochondria. In the heart they are called *flocculent densities* and are a very early sign of cell death following a myocardial infarction.

Continued membrane injury causes enzymes stored within lysosomes to be released into the cytoplasm. These enzymes, such as acid hydrolases, damage the proteins within the cytoplasm. Damage to ribonucleoprotein results in increased basophilia (blue color) of the cytoplasm. Damage to the membrane of the cell causes enzymes normally stored within the cytoplasm of the cell to be released. An example is the release of cardiac enzymes, such as CPK and LDH, from myocardial cells in patients with a myocardial infarction.

CELL DEATH

1. Results from irreversible cell injury
2. Basic patterns
    *   Apoptosis
    *   Necrosis

APOPTOSIS

*   Physiologic or pathologic processes
*   Involves single cells
*   Cells shrink and form apoptotic bodies
*   Condensation of chromatin
*   Gene activation forms endonucleases
*   Lack of inflammatory response

Irreversibly injured cells eventually die. This cell death is due to one of two basic mechanisms: apoptosis or necrosis. It is important to understand the differences between these two types of cell death. *Apoptosis* is a form of cell death in which individual cells literally destroy themselves. It is sometimes referred to as "programmed" cell death or cell "suicide." Apoptosis usually involves the death of single cells or small clusters of cells. Apoptosis is an active process in which certain genes are turned on and form new enzymes, such as endonucleases. These newly formed enzymes then destroy the cell that made them. This destruction increases the eosinophilia (red color) of the cytoplasm and causes condensation of the chromatin of the nucleus. Together these changes form characteristic shrunken cells called apoptotic bodies. It is important to realize that apoptosis is not associated with the influx of inflammatory cells, and this lack of inflammation is characteristic. Apoptotic bodies, however, may be phagocytized (eaten) by individual cells, such as macrophages.

EXAMPLES OF APOPTOSIS

Physiologic apoptosis

- Involution of the thymus
- Cell death within germinal centers of lymph nodes
- Fragmentation of endometrium during menses
- Lactating breast during weaning

Pathologic apoptosis

- Viral hepatitis
- Cytotoxic T cell–mediated immune destruction

Apoptosis can be a normal process that is associated with growth, or it can be an abnormal process that is associated with abnormal cell death. Apoptosis is a normal process during embryonic development. Apoptosis is also found in some normal hormonal physiologic processes, such as the fragmentation of endometrial glands during menses. An important normal site for apoptosis is within the germinal centers of lymph nodes. Within these germinal centers B lymphocytes are activated in response to certain antigens and develop into plasma cells. Some of the developing B lymphocytes undergo apoptosis and are phagocytized by macrophages. (Macrophages within germinal centers that have phagocytized cellular debris are called *tingible-body macrophages*.) Activation of a certain gene, *bcl-2*, inhibits the B lymphocytes from undergoing apoptosis. These abnormal B lymphocytes become immortal and produce a form of non-Hodgkin's lymphoma (follicular lymphoma).

An example of pathologic apoptosis is the death of hepatocytes in patients with viral hepatitis. These individually dying cells form apoptotic bodies, which are called Councilman bodies.

NECROSIS

- Involves many cells or clusters of cells
- Cells swell
- Several patterns of necrosis
- Hypoxia or cellular toxins
- Destruction due to irreversible injury
- Inflammatory response present

In contrast to apoptosis, *necrosis* involves the death of large sheets of cells, such as portions of organs. In addition, numerous inflammatory cells are usually present. The early microscopic changes of necrotic cells involve both the cytoplasm and the nucleus. The cytoplasm of necrotic cells becomes acidophilic (red). This color change is due to the denaturation of proteins within the cytoplasm and the breakup of ribosomes. Normally ribosomes are responsible for the normal basophilic color of the cytoplasm of cells.

In contrast to the cytoplasm, the chromatin of the nucleus of necrotic cells clumps together, and the nucleus shrinks and becomes markedly basophilic (blue). This processes is called pyknosis (Fig. 2-2). Pyknotic nuclei then either break up into multiple small fragments (karyorrhexis) or literally fade away (karyolysis).

PATTERNS OF CELLULAR NECROSIS

- Coagulative necrosis → ischemia (except the brain)
- Liquefactive necrosis → bacterial infection
- Fat necrosis → pancreatitis and trauma to the breast
- Caseous necrosis → tuberculosis
- Fibrinoid necrosis → autoimmune disease
- Gangrene → ischemia to extremities

The two most basic patterns of cellular necrosis that you need to understand and be able to differentiate are coagulative necrosis and liquefactive necrosis. These processes are the result of either denaturation of proteins (coagulative necrosis) or enzymatic digestion of cells (liquefactive necrosis).

In *coagulative necrosis* the dead cells lose their nuclei, but the cytoplasmic outline of the dead cells remains intact. This type of necrosis is called coagulative because the cytoplasm remains as a coagulated mass. The "ghost" of these dead cells remains intact, and histologically the type of tissue can still be determined. We will examine coagulative necrosis in more detail in the chapter dealing with hemostasis and infarction, because the main cause of coagulative necrosis is decreased blood supply. Infarction of tissue results from decreased blood supply and as a general rule produces coagulative necrosis. For example, a classic example of coagulative necrosis is myocardial infarction. Important exceptions to this general rule, however, are infarctions of the brain. Rather than coagulative necrosis, brain infarcts result in liquefactive necrosis.

Liquefactive necrosis differs from coagulative necrosis in that the tissue is totally digested and nothing remains, except for a liquid composed of inflammatory cells, commonly called pus. We will look at liquefactive necrosis in more

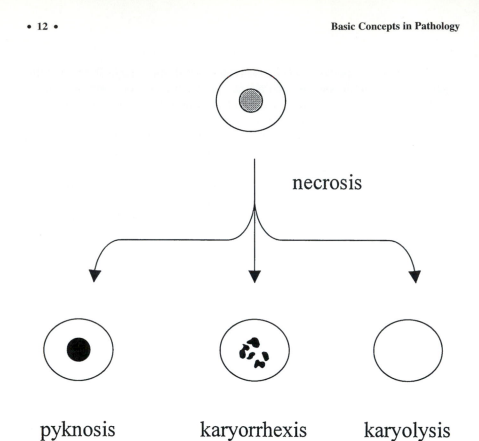

necrosis

pyknosis   karyorrhexis   karyolysis

Figure 2-2
Nuclear changes with necrosis (pyknosis)

detail in the chapter dealing with inflammation. The liquefaction results from the release of large amounts of lysosomal enzymes. Brain tissue has abundant lysosomes, and this is why infarction of the brain results in liquefactive necrosis. Additionally, inflammatory cells such as neutrophils have lots of lysosomes, which they normally use to destroy microorganisms. This is the reason why the major cause of liquefactive necrosis is bacterial infections.

There are other types of necrosis. Fat necrosis can result from either trauma or enzymes. Traumatic fat necrosis is usually found in breast tissue, while enzymatic fat necrosis is usually associated with acute pancreatitis. Caseous necrosis is an especially important cause of necrosis that is caused by *mycobacterium tuberculosis*. It is called caseous necrosis because grossly it looks like cheesy material. *Fibrinoid necrosis* is a type of necrosis associated with autoimmune diseases. This term creates a lot of confusion because its name sounds like fibrous or fibrinous. Fibrinoid necrosis is neither fibrous nor fibrinous. Fibrous refers to the deposition of collagen (a product of fibroblasts), while fibrinous refers to the deposition of fibrin (a product of blood coagulation). In contrast, fibrinoid refers only to the fact that it is pink-staining like fibrin. Fibrinoid necrosis is characterized by the deposition of immunoglobulins and necrotic material within blood vessels.

Finally, *gangrene* is a clinical term describing a type of necrosis that usually involves the extremities. Gangrene refers to black necrotic tissue that is usually the result of arterial obstruction. If the dead tissue appears dry it is called dry gangrene, but if the tissue appears moist it it called wet gangrene. The difference between these two is the presence or absence of bacteria. With little or no bacteria present, the necrosis is mainly coagulative, but if there is superimposed bacterial infection, the necrosis is liquefactive.

· C H A P T E R · 3 ·

CELL ORGANELLES

·

CELL MEMBRANES

Lipids

- Phospholipid (bilayer)
- Glycolipid
- Cholesterol

Protein

- Integral protein
- Peripheral protein

Sometimes diseases affect specific structures (organelles) within the cell. For example, we have seen how injury to cell membranes can cause cell injury. Let's briefly review the composition of cell membranes before examining several other disease processes that primarily affect cell membranes.

The cell membrane is a complex structure composed of many different substances. Its major components are lipids and proteins. The major lipids within the plasma membrane are phospholipids, glycolipids, and cholesterol. The phospholipids are amphipathic, which means they have a polar (hydrophilic) head and a nonpolar (hydrophobic) tail. These phospholipids form a bilayer by lining up so that their polar heads point to the outside and inside of the cell, and their nonpolar tails point to the middle of the cell membrane.

The proteins within the cell membrane may pass through the membrane (integral proteins), or they may be located on the inside or the outside of the membrane (peripheral proteins). The structure of the red cell membrane provides a good example of these different types of protein (Fig. 3-1). Examples of integral proteins that span the red cell membrane include protein 3 (protein C) and the glycophorins. Protein 3 forms the anion exchange channel of red cells and is responsible for the exchange of chloride and bicarbonate ions (the "chloride shift"). Glycophorins have abundant carbohydrates and give the red blood cell surface a negative charge. This charge helps the red cells repel each other, which is important in keeping them from clumping together (agglutinating) in the blood. There are several types of glycophorins in the red cell membrane. Glycophorin A, which is responsible for the MN blood types, is the binding site of plasmodium falciparum and the influenza virus. An absence of glycophorin A on red cells is associated with resistance to plasmodium falciparum. The peripheral proteins of the red cell membrane include ankyrin, protein 4.1, spectrin, and actin. Abnormalities of these proteins are associated with the development of hereditary spherocytosis.

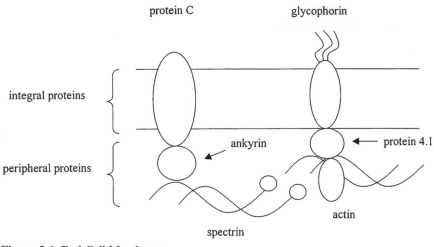

Figure 3-1 Red Cell Membrane

ABNORMALITIES OF RED CELL MEMBRANE

Hereditary spherocytosis

- Autosomal dominant inheritance
- Abnormal spectrin molecule
- Chronic hemolytic anemia
- Increased risk of pigment gallstones
- Increased osmotic fragility test

Acanthocytosis

- Red cells with irregular spikes on surface
- Abetalipoproteinemia

Hereditary spherocytosis (HS) is an autosomal dominant disorder that is characterized by an abnormality of the red cell membrane that changes their shape from normal biconcavity to spherocytic. This change in shape make the red cells prone to splenic sequestration and destruction (extravascular hemolysis). This chronic hemolytic anemia can lead to splenomegaly, jaundice, and the formation of pigmented gallstones.

The basic defect of the red cells that produces heredity spherocytosis involves the spectrin molecule. This defect causes spectrin to have less binding to protein 4.1, which decreases the amount of the red blood cell membrane, decreases the surface-to-volume ratio, and forms spherocytes. These spherocytic red cells have an increased hemoglobin concentration, which is seen clinically as an increase in the mean cell hemoglobin concentration (MCHC). Hereditary spherocytosis can be diagnosed in the laboratory by the osmotic fragility test. Because spherocytes have less surface membrane, they will explode (lyse) sooner in hypotonic solutions than normal red cells. The treatment for patients with HS is splenectomy.

Acanthocytes are red blood cells that have numerous irregularly shaped spikes on their surface. Acanthocytes can be found in the peripheral blood of patients with abetalipoproteinemia or liver disease. Abetalipoproteinemia is a disorder that results from the absence of beta lipoproteins. The formation of acanthocytes in the peripheral blood is due to increased amounts of sphingomyelin in the RBC membrane.

ABNORMALITIES OF MITOCHONDRIA

Size, shape, and numbers

- Swelling → reversible cell injury
- Giant abnormally shaped mitochondria → alcoholic liver disease or Reye's syndrome
- Cells with increased numbers of mitochondria → oncocytic cells

Inclusions

- Calcifications → irreversible cell injury
- "Parking lot" crystals → mitochondrial myopathies

Toxins

- Uncoupler of oxidative phosphorylation → dinitrophenol
- Inhibition of oxidative phosphorylation (cytochrome oxidase) → cyanide

---

We have seen how injury to cell membranes can damage mitochondria. Normally mitochondria provide energy to the cell by producing ATP through the process of oxidative phosphorylation. Injury to mitochondria decreases the energy available to the cell and results in either reversible or irreversible cell injury. Several enzyme complexes involved in the process of oxidative phosphorylation are located in the inner mitochondrial membrane. These complexes include the NADH dehydrogenase complex, the b-cl complex, and the cyto-chrome oxidase complex. Certain chemical toxins can inhibit the production of ATP by inhibiting these mitochondrial enzyme complexes. For example, cyanide inhibits oxidative phosphorylation by inhibiting the cytochrome oxidase complex.

Interestingly, not all the genes inside a cell are located on chromosomes within the nucleus. A few genes are found within mitochondrial DNA (mtDNA) and code for some of the oxidative phosphorylation enzymes, such as NADH dehydrogenase, cytochrome c oxidase, and ATP synthase. Inherited deficiencies of these enzymes produce signs and symptoms in organs that require large amounts of ATP, such as the central nervous system, muscle, liver, and kidneys. Because many of these abnormalities produce proximal muscle weakness, they are called mitochondrial myopathies. They are often associated with severe in-volvement of eye muscles (ophthalmoplegia). Histologically the abnormal mito-chondria cause the muscle to appear irregular ("ragged red fibers"). Electron microscopy reveals subsarcolemmal collections of mitochondria that are filled with "parking lot" crystallin inclusions.

These mitochondrial myopathies have non-Mendelian patterns of inheri-tance: Females transmit the disease to all their children, but only their female off-spring transmit the disease any farther. The reason for this unusual inheritance pattern is that all the mitochondrial DNA is of maternal origin and none is of paternal origin. This is because ova have large amounts of cytoplasm that contain mitochondria, but sperm have no cytoplasm with mitochondria. The mtDNA of patients with mitochondrial myopathies may be composed of either a mixture of mutant and normal DNA (*heteroplasmy*) or of mutant DNA entirely (homo-plasmy). The severity of these diseases correlates with the amount of mutant mtDNA that is present.

REYE'S SYNDROME

- Systemic mitochondrial injury
- Typical patient: young child with previous viral illness
- Questionable association with salicylates
- Encephalopathy
- Microvesicular steatosis

In some diseases, such as Reye's syndrome and alcoholic liver disease, the mitochondria can be enlarged and have abnormal shapes. Reye's syndrome is an acute postviral illness of children that is characterized by swelling of the central nervous system (encephalopathy), fatty change of the liver (microvesicular steatosis), and widespread mitochondrial injury (large budding or branching mitochondria). Mitochondrial injury results in decreased activity of the citric acid cycle and the urea cycle, and defective beta-oxidation of fats, which leads to the accumulation of serum fatty acids. The typical patient with Reye's syndrome presents with vomiting about three to five days after a viral illness. There is a questionable association of Reye's syndrome with salicylate (aspirin) ingestion. The fatality rate is quite high (up to 40%).

Finally, some epithelial cells are characterized by having increased numbers of mitochondria within their cytoplasm. The increased numbers of mitochondria cause the cytoplasm of these cells to have a "pretty pink" appearance when examined under light microscopy. These cells are sometimes called *oncocytic* cells, and a benign tumor that contains many of these cells is called an oncocytoma. Cells with the same histologic appearance line the papillary projections of a Warthin's tumor (a benign tumor found in the parotid gland) and can be found in the thyroid gland of patients with Hashimoto's thyroiditis.

LYSOSOMES

- Degrade intracellular or extracellular material
- Contain acid hydrolases

Lysosomes are cellular organelles that contain many different types of enzymes. Many of these enzymes are active in an acid environment (acid hydrolases). Lysosomal enzymes are synthesized in the rough endoplasmic reticulum (RER), packaged within the Golgi, and then transported as vesicles within the cytoplasm. At this point the vesicles are surrounded by a clathrin coat and are called *primary lysosomes* (late endosomes). Examine Figure 3-2 and note the primary lysosome that is being formed from the Golgi apparatus. The enzymes that are packaged into primary lysosomes reach these lysosomes because of mannose-6-phosphate receptors.

HETEROPHAGY AND AUTOPHAGY

- Heterophagy → ingestions and degradation of extracellular substances
- Autophagy → degradation of intracellular organelles

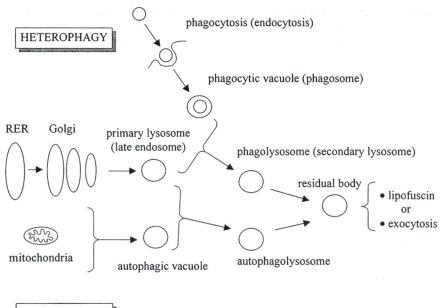

Figure 3-2 Heterophagy and Autophagy
Compare the process of heterophagy with the process of autophagy. The two processes are very similar, except that heterophagy involves the degradation of extracellular substances and autophagy involves the degradation of intracellular substances. The phagocytic vacuole is analogous to the autophagic vacuole. Each combines with the primary lysosome to form either the phagolysosome or the autophagolysosome. Both of these are broken down to form residual bodies. Note that the enzymes formed in the RER and packaged in the Golgi reach the primary lysosome because of mannose-6-phosphate receptors.

ABNORMALITIES OF LYSOSOMES
Heterophagy

- Bacterial infection
- Chédiak-Higashi syndrome
- Familial hypercholesterolemia

Autophagy

- Lysosomal storage diseases

Primary lysosomes can fuse with phagosomes to form *secondary lysosomes* (phagolysosomes). What are phagosomes and where do they come from? Phagosomes are cytoplasmic vacuoles that are formed when extracellular material is taken up by cells through their plasma membranes. The uptake of large material is called *phagocytosis*; the uptake of smaller macromolecules is called *pinocytosis*. The entire process is called *heterophagy*. Examples of heterophagy include the phagocytosis of bacteria by neutrophils and the phagocytosis of dead cells by macrophages. Within the secondary lysosomes, the hydrolytic enzymes from the lysosomes destroy the material that was within the phagosome. Defective formation of secondary lysosomes is characteristic of Chédiak-Higashi syndrome, a disorder that is associated with recurrent bacterial infections. Familial hypercholesterolemia results from defective heterophagic processes involved in the uptake of low-density lipoprotein by hepatocytes.

Autophagy is a process that is analogous to heterophagy but involves the breakdown of cellular organelles rather than extracellular material. Cellular material and organelles (mitochondria, RER, and Golgi) are first processed to form autophagic vacuoles (analogous to the phagosomes of heterophagy). The autophagic vacuoles then fuse with primary lysosomes to form autophagolysosomes (analogous to the secondary lysosomes seen during heterophagy). Within these autophagolysosomes the hydrolytic enzymes from the lysosomes destroy the cellular material within the original autophagic vacuole. Material that cannot be digested can remain within the lysosomes as residual bodies or as lipofuscin pigment. *Lipofuscin* is a fine, granular, golden-brown pigment that has been called the "wear and tear" pigment of cells. It is most commonly found in the heart of elderly individuals or patients with severe malnutrition. From a clinical standpoint, lipofuscin causes no functional abnormality.

LYSOSOMAL STORAGE DISEASES

Glycogen storage disease

- Pompe disease

Mucopolysaccharidoses

- Hurler's syndrome
- Hunter's syndrome (X-linked recessive disorder)

Sphingolipidoses

1. Phosphosphingolipid
   - Niemann-Pick disease

2. Glycosphingolipid
  a. Galactoceramide
  b. Glucoceramide
    1) Gangliosides
      • GM_1 ganglioside
      • GM_2 ganglioside (Tay-Sachs disease and Sandhoff disease)
    2) Nongangliosides
      • Gaucher disease

DISEASE	ENZYME DEFICIENCY	SUBSTANCE ACCUMULATING
• Pompe disease	α-1,4-glucosidase (acid maltase)	Glycogen
• Hurler's syndrome	α-L-iduronidase	Heparan sulfate, dermatan sulfate
• Hunter's syndrome	L-iduronosulfate sulfatase	Heparan sulfate, dermatan sulfate
• Niemann-Pick disease	Sphingomyelinase	Sphingomyelin
• Tay-Sachs disease	Hexosaminidase A	GM_2-ganglioside
• Sandhoff disease	Hexosaminidase A and B	GM_2-ganglioside and globoside
• Gaucher disease	Glucocerebrosidase	Glucocerebroside
• Fabry disease	α-galactosidase A	Ceramide trihexosidase

    Inherited deficiencies of lysosomal enzymes result in incomplete breakdown (catabolism) of substances. This leads to the accumulation of partially digested insoluble substances within lysosomes. Diseases that result from deficiencies of lysosomal enzymes are called lysosomal storage diseases. Examples of material that may accumulate in lysosomal storage diseases include glycogen, glycosaminoglycans (GAGs), and lipid (sphingolipid). There are several types of glycogen storage disease, but only one leads to accumulation of glycogen within lysosomes, and that is Pompe disease. We will discuss the glycogen storage diseases in the chapter dealing with cellular accumulations.

MUCOPOLYSACCHARIDOSES

- Autosomal recessive disorders, except for Hunter's syndrome
- Mental retardation
- Corneal clouding
- Alder-Reilly bodies (inclusions within leukocytes)
- Zebra bodies (inclusions within neurons)
- Increased glycosaminoglycans in serum and urine

Mucopolysaccharides consist of glycosaminoglycans (GAGs). The six major types of GAGs are hyaluronic acid, chondroitin sulfate, keratin sulfate, dermatan sulfate, heparan sulfate, and heparin. There are also six types of mucopolysaccharidoses (MPS), all of which are inherited as autosomal recessive traits. (The one exception is type II Hunter's syndrome, an X-linked recessive disorder.) The MPS are progressive disorders that are characterized by involvement of multiple organs, such as the liver, spleen, heart, and blood vessels. The clinical signs of patients with MPS, best illustrated by Hurler's syndrome, consist of coarse facial features, clouded cornea, joint stiffness, and mental retardation. Hunter's syndrome lacks corneal clouding and has a milder clinical course. Accumulation of GAGs within leukocytes produces inclusions called Alder-Reilly bodies; accumulation of GAGs within neurons can produce zebra bodies. The amount of GAGs (such as heparan sulfate and dermatan sulfate) are increased in the urine.

NIEMANN-PICK DISEASE

- Deficiency of sphingomyelinase
- Accumulation of sphingomyelin
- Infantile form (type A) → mental retardation, seizures, death
- Adult form (type B) → hepatosplenomegaly
- "Foam cells"
- Cherry-red macula

Abnormal accumulation of sphingolipids includes abnormal accumulation of phospholipids or glycosphingolipids. The glycosphingolipids are further divided into galactoceramide or glucoceramide. The latter is divided into the gangliosides (GM_1 ganglioside or GM_2 ganglioside) and the nongangliosides.

Niemann-Pick disease is characterized by the accumulation of sphingomyelin and cholesterol. Clinically there are four subtypes of Niemann-Pick disease: types A, B, C, and D. These types can be categorized into two major groups. One group has a deficiency of sphingomyelinase (types A and B); the other group has normal levels of sphingomyelinase, but defects in intracellular cholesterol esterification and transport (types C and D). The most common type is type A, which is the infantile type. These patients have severe neurologic symptoms (mental retardation, seizures, and ataxia) and visceral accumulation of sphingomyelin, and usually die by age 3. In contrast, type B is seen mainly in adults and is associated with enlargement of the liver and spleen, but there are no central nervous system abnormalities.

Patients with Niemann-Pick disease have an accumulation of sphingomyelin in phagocytic cells (macrophages). These cells become stuffed with droplets of lipid and have a fine vacuolated or foamy appearance histologically ("foam cells"). Lamellated myelin figures (zebra bodies) can be seen by electron microscopy. Organs affected by this disease, such as the spleen, liver, bone marrow, lymph nodes, and central nervous system, normally have a high number of phagocytic cells.

CHERRY-RED MACULA

- Niemann-Pick disease
- Tay-Sachs disease
- Sandhoff disease

In patients with Niemann-Pick disease lipid material (sphingomyelin) can accumulate in the neurons of the retina surrounding the macula. This lipid material causes this area to appear pale clinically. The macula, which normally does not have any neurons, does not accumulate any lipid and appears bright red in contrast to the surrounding lipid-filled retinal cells. Enhancement of the normal color of the macular choriod contrasts with the pallor of the swollen ganglion cells of the retina and produces a characteristic "cherry-red spot." This same clinical appearance can also be seen in patients with Tay-Sachs disease and Sandhoff disease.

TAY-SACHS DISEASE

- Decreased hexosaminidase A
- Accumulation of GM_2 ganglioside
- Ashkenazi Jews (eastern European origin)
- Cherry-red macula and blindness

Tay-Sachs disease (amaurotic familial idiocy) is one of a group of lysoso-mal storage diseases that is caused by an inability to break down GM_2-ganglio-sides (these diseases are naturally called GM_2-gangliosidoses). Breakdown of GM_2-ganglioside is accomplished by the enzyme hexosaminidase, which is formed by two subunits, an alpha subunit and a beta subunit. Hexosaminidase A is composed of both the alpha and the beta subunit, while hexosaminidase B is composed of two beta subunits. Tay-Sachs disease results from genetic mutations involving the alpha subunit, and therefore hexosaminidase A is abnormal. The disease is especially common in Jews, particularly Ashkenazi Jews (eastern Euro-pean origin). Patients with Tay-Sachs disease have an accumulation of GM_2-gan-glioside in the brain, since it is involved in ganglioside metabolism. The affected cells appear swollen and foamy and may contain cytoplasmic whorled lamellar bodies (seen with electron microscopy). The retina is usually involved and dis-closes the characteristic cherry-red spot in the macula. The retinal changes can be severe and can lead to blindness (amaurosis). There are several clinical forms of Tay-Sachs disease, but the infantile form is the most severe. Patients develop mental retardation and seizures. Death usually occurs before the age of 3.

Sandhoff disease, another GM_2-gangliosidosis, results from a mutation involving the beta subunit of hexosaminidase. Therefore, both hexosaminidase A and hexosaminidase B levels are decreased, and there is accumulation of GM_2-ganglioside and globoside. Patients are infants who present with mental retarda-tion, seizures, and blindness. These patients also have a cherry-red macula.

GAUCHER DISEASE

- Decreased beta-glucocerebrosidase
- Accumulation of glucocerebroside
- Macrophages with crinkled ("tissue paper") cytoplasm (Gaucher cells)
- Adult form (type I) → normal life span
- Infantile form (type II) → neurologic symptoms

Gaucher disease is characterized by the accumulation of glucocerebroside in the reticuloendothelial cells of the liver, spleen, and bone marrow. Glucocere-brosides are formed from the catabolism of glycolipids obtained from the cell membranes of old and dying leukocytes and erythrocytes. This accumulation leads to the formation of Gaucher cells, which microscopically have crinkled ("tissue paper") cytoplasm. Gaucher disease has been divided into three clinical subtypes. Type I, the adult chronic form, is the most common form and does not involve neurologic signs or symptoms. Glucocerebrosides accumulate most often in the spleen and skeleton (femoral head), but not the brain. The disease is found primarily in Ashkenazi Jews. Laboratory examination of the blood may find elevated levels of acid phosphatase and angiotensin-converting enzyme. In contrast to the adult form, both type II (infantile form) and type III (juvenile form) forms of Gaucher disease involve neurologic symptoms. The infantile form is the most severe type of Gaucher disease.

PEROXISOMES

Normal function

- Catabolism of very-long-chain fatty acids (VLCFA)
- Detoxify ethanol
- Contain the enzyme catalase

Abnormalities

- X-linked adrenoleukodystrophy
- Zellweger syndrome

Peroxisomes (microbodies) are small, ovoid, membrane-bound organelles. They contain three oxidative enzymes: D-amino acid oxidase, urate oxidase (uricase), and catalase. Microsomes can be identified by the cytochemical reaction to catalase, an enzyme that is important for its ability to degrade hydrogen peroxide. Abnormalities of peroxisomes include deficiencies of a single peroxisome enzyme or multiple enzymes. The latter abnormality produces an "absence" of peroxisomes and is called. Zellweger syndrome. An example of a single enzyme deficiency is adrenoleukodystrophy (ALD), an X-linked disorder that results from defective peroxisomal catabolism of very-long-chain fatty acids. Both of these diseases are quite rare.

CYTOSKELETON

- Microtubules
- Thin actin filaments
- Thick myosin filaments
- Intermediate filaments

ABNORMALITIES INVOLVING MICROTUBULES

Colchicine

- Preparation of karyotypes
- Treatment of gout

Chédiak-Higashi syndrome

- Impaired fusion of lysosomes with phagosomes
- Recurrent infections

Immotile cilia syndrome (Kartagener's syndrome)

- Abnormal dynein arms of cilia
- Bronchiectasis
- Sinusitis
- Dextrocardia

The cytoskeleton of cells consists of microtubules, thin actin filaments, thick myosin filaments, and various intermediate filaments. Microtubules are long, thin, hollow tubules that help to maintain the shape of cells. They provide for the intracytoplasmic transport of vesicles and organelles and form the mitotic spindle, which moves chromosomes during mitosis. Microtubules can be disrupted by colchicine. This chemical is used in the preparation of *karyotypes* (used to examine chromosomes), because colchicine blocks mitosis during metaphase. Colchicine is also used to treat the inflammatory response of patients with gout because it inhibits microtubules within leukocytes and stabilizes the membranes of lysosomes.

Two diseases are characterized by abnormalities involving microtubules. The Chédiak-Higashi syndrome is characterized by a defect in microtubule polymerization. This abnormality causes delayed or decreased fusion of lysosomes with phagosomes in leukocytes and impairs phagocytosis by these white blood cells. Defective organization of microtubules within cilia can result in malfunction of the cilia of the body (immotile cilia syndrome). One of the immotile cilia syndromes is Kartagener syndrome, an autosomal recessive disorder that includes the triad of bronchiectasis, sinusitis, and dextrocardia with or without situs inversus. It is caused by a structural abnormality of cilia, most commonly absent or irregular dynein arms. *Bronchiectasis* refers to abnormal dilation of the bronchi ("ectasia" means dilation). Bronchiectasis results from chronic infections of the lung, which in patients with an immotile cilia syndrome results from decreased ciliary removal of bacteria and mucus. Males with this abnormality are sterile because of the lack of sperm motility.

INTERMEDIATE FILAMENTS

- Keratin filaments
- Neurofilaments
- Glial filaments
- Vimentin
- Desmin

ABNORMALITIES INVOLVING INTERMEDIATE FILAMENTS

1. Alcoholic hyaline (alcoholic liver disease) → prekeratin intermediate filaments
2. Neurofibrillary tangles (Alzheimer's disease) → neurofilaments
3. Lewy bodies (Parkinson's disease) → neurofilaments
4. Tumors
   - Keratin → carcinoma
   - Vimentin → sarcomas, lymphomas, melanomas
   - Vimentin and desmin → muscle tumors
   - Glial filaments → glial tumors
   - Neurofilaments → neural tumors

The principal intermediate filaments are keratin filaments, neurofilaments, glial filaments (glial fibrillary acidic protein), vimentin, and desmin. Three characteristic histologic features are the result of accumulations of certain types of intermediate filaments. *Alcoholic hyaline* (Mallory body) is an eosinophilic intracytoplasmic inclusion in liver cells composed predominantly of prekeratin intermediate filaments. Neurofibrillary tangles seen in patients with Alzheimer's disease are composed of microtubule-associated proteins and neurofilaments. Neurofilaments are also found in the neuronal inclusions found in patients with Parkinson's disease (Lewy bodies). These three histologic findings are produced when intermediate filaments are combined with the protein ubiquitin, whose "housekeeping" function is to link with damaged protein.

Intermediate filaments can also be used to characterize tumors, but these findings are fairly general.

CELL DEPOSITS AND ACCUMULATIONS

·

- **Hydropic Change**
- **Fatty Change (Steatosis)**
- **Fatty Change of the Liver**
- **Protein-Energy Malnutrition**
- **Fatty Change of the Heart**
- **Accumulations in the GI Mucosal Cells**
- **Protein Deposits**
- **Amyloid**
- **Amyloidosis**
- **Alpha-1-Antritrypsin Deficiency**
- **Hyaline Change**
- **Viral Changes**
- **Hyaline Membranes of the Lungs**
- **Acute Respiratory Distress Syndrome (ARDS)**
- **Hyaline Membrane Disease**
- **Glycogen**
- **Glycogen Storage Diseases**
- **Calcium Deposits**
- **Psammoma Bodies**
- **Hypercalcemia**
- **Hyperparathyroidism**
- **Iron Deposits**
- **Abnormal Deposits of Hemosiderin**

- **Sideroblastic Anemia**
- **Hypochromic Microcytic Anemias**
- **Systemic Iron Overload**
- **Primary Hemochromatosis ("Bronze" Diabetes)**
- **Bilirubin**
- **Bilirubin Deposits**
- **Causes of Hyperbilirubinemia**
- **Hereditary Hyperbilirubinemia**
- **Hereditary Unconjugated Hyperbilirubinemia**
- **Hereditary Conjugated Hyperbilirubinemia**
- **Gallstones**
- **Copper Deposits**
- **Urate Deposits**
- **Gout**
- **Lipofuscin Deposits**
- **Black Pigments**
- **Abnormalities Involving Melanocytes**
- **Nevi**
- **Carbon Deposits**
- **Homogentisic Acid**
- **Routine Stain (H&E)**
- **Special Stains**

HYDROPIC CHANGE

- Reversibly injured cells accumulate water and swell
- Hydropic change refers to the accumulation of water within a cell

Injured cells can accumulate various types of chemicals and compounds, such as water, lipid, protein, sugar, minerals, and pigments. The accumulation of water within cells is called hydropic change and is characteristic of reversible injury.

FATTY CHANGE (STEATOSIS)

- Accumulation of triglyceride in the cytoplasm of injured cells
- Model for fatty change: the hepatocyte

FATTY CHANGE OF THE LIVER

1. Increased free fatty acids
   - Starvation
   - Corticosteroids
   - Diabetes mellitus
2. Increased formation of triglyceride
   - Alcohol
3. Decreased formation of apoprotein
   - Carbon tetrachloride
   - Protein malnutrition

The accumulation of lipid within cells is an important pathologic process. Any type of lipid can accumulate within cells, such as cholesterol, triglyceride, and phospholipid. The accumulation of cholesterol is very important in the pathogenesis of atherosclerosis. We will discuss the pathogenesis of atherosclerosis in the chapter dealing with vascular disease.

The accumulation of triglyceride is called fatty change or *steatosis*. The cell that serves as the model for fatty change is the liver cell, or hepatocyte (Fig. 4-1). Abnormalities involving any of the steps in these normal metabolic pathways can lead to fatty change of the hepatocytes. Basically fatty change results from either excess delivery of free fatty acids to the liver, increased formation of lipids within

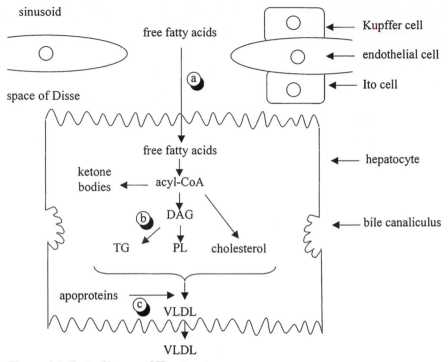

Figure 4-1 Fatty Change of Hepatocyte
In the normal scheme of the liver, free fatty acids (FFA) are taken up by hepatocytes and then are converted to cholesterol esters, triglyceride (TG), phospholipids (PL), or ketone bodies. Some of the newly formed lipids combine with specific types of proteins (apoproteins) to form a specific type of lipoprotein called VLDL (very low density lipoprotein). The lipid is then secreted into the blood as VLDL.

the liver, or decreased formation of VLDL by the liver. Excess delivery of free fatty acids to the liver occurs when there are excess levels of free fatty acids in the blood (letter "a" in Fig. 4-1). This can be the result of the increased mobilization of adipose tissue, which can occur in patients with starvation, corticosteroid use, or diabetes mellitus. Increased formation of triglycerides (letter "b") can be the result of alcohol ingestion, while decreased formation of VLDL can result from decreased production of the apoprotein needed to form VLDL (letter "c"). This decreased production of apoprotein can be due to generalized protein deficiency (protein malnutrition) or carbon tetrachloride poisoning.

Histologic examination of the liver from patients with steatosis reveals that the lipid droplets within the hepatocytes can be small or large. Small droplets (microvesicular steatosis) do not displace the nucleus, while large droplets (macrovesicular steatosis) cause the nucleus to be abnormally displaced to the side of the cell. Microvesicular steatosis is associated with acute toxic hepatocellular injury. Macrovesicular steatosis is associated with chronic hepatocellular injury, such as malnutrition or chronic alcohol abuse.

PROTEIN-ENERGY MALNUTRITION
Kwashiorkor

* Dietary protein deficiency
* Anasarca (generalized edema)
* Fatty liver
* Abnormal skin and hair
* Defective enzyme formation

Marasmus

* Dietary calorie deficiency
* General wasting

A fatty liver can be seen in patients with *kwashiorkor*, a disease of children that is characterized by a lack of protein despite adequate (although barely) caloric intake. The decreased protein leads to decreased synthesis of enzymes and proteins. Children with kwashiorkor develop generalized peripheral edema (*anasarca*), ascites, and a "moon" face, all of which are due to decreased albumin synthesis and sodium retention. These young children also develop an enlarged, fatty liver due to decreased synthesis of the lipoproteins that are necessary for the export of lipids from liver cells. Additional physical signs in these children include "flaky paint" areas of skin and abnormal pigmented streaks in their hair. These children also have mental changes (lethargy and somnolence) and anemia, the latter being due to decreased levels of iron and folate. It is important to realize that decreased synthesis of proteins and enzymes produces villous atrophy of the small intestine and decreased enzymes (disaccharidases) that are normally found on the brush border of these intestinal cells. Because of these intestinal abnormalities, even when appropriate food is given orally, children with kwashiorkor cannot digest or absorb it. This makes treatment much more difficult.

In contrast to kwashiorkor, *marasmus* is caused by lack of calories (starvation). These children develop generalized wasting, growth retardation, atrophy of muscles, and loss of subcutaneous fat ("skin and bones"). They have no edema or hepatic enlargement (they get amino acids from muscle breakdown and wasting), and they are alert and ravenous (not apathetic like children with kwashiorkor). When they are given food to eat they digest and absorb it normally.

FATTY CHANGE OF THE HEART

- Diphtheria
- Reye's syndrome

Fatty change of the myocardium can be caused by severe hypoxia or diphtheric myocarditis. *Corynebacterium diphtheria* is a gram-positive bacillus that is the causative agent of diphtheria. This disease is characterized by the formation of a pseudomembrane in the larynx that is composed of an exudate of acute inflammation and necrotic cells. *C. diphtheria* secretes an exotoxin composed of two fragments held together by disulfide bonds. The B fragment attaches to a cellular receptor, and once inside the cell, the A fragment inactivates EF-2 (elongation factor 2) by transferring ADPR to EF-2. (The mechanism of this toxin is the same as exotoxin A produced by *Pseudomonas aeruginosa*.) In addition to causing laryngeal necrosis, the diphtheria exotoxin can cause fatty myocardial change and nerve damage. The gross appearance of the fatty heart reveals alternating bands of yellow (fatty change) and red-brown (muscle). This gross change is sometimes called a "tiger skin" appearance.

ACCUMULATIONS IN THE GI MUCOSAL CELLS

Whipple's disease

- PAS-positive macrophages in mucosa of small intestines
- *Tropheryma whippelii*
- Malabsorption, fever, and arthritis

Abetalipoproteinemia

- Lipid-laden macrophages in mucosa of small intestines
- Deficiency of apolipoprotein B
- Acanthocytes in peripheral blood

Two diseases that are characterized by the accumulation of material within the mucosal cells of the small intestines are Whipple's disease and abetalipoproteinemia. Whipple's disease is a systemic disease that is associated with malabsorption, fever, and arthritis. A biopsy of the small intestine from a patient with Whipple's disease typically reveals the lamina propria to be filled with numerous macrophages that contain glycoprotein and rod-shaped bacteria (*Tropheryma whippelii*, a gram-positive actinomycete). This disorder responds well to antibiotic therapy.

Abetalipoproteinemia is a genetic defect in the synthesis of apolipoprotein B. All lipoproteins that have this apoprotein B are decreased in the blood (chylomicrons, VLDL, and LDL). A biopsy of the small intestine of a patient with abetalipoproteinemia reveals the mucosal cells to be filled with lipid (triglyceride) inclusions. The peripheral smear reveals numerous *acanthocytes* (red cells with irregular spines on the surface). The symptoms of malabsorption can be partially reversed by ingestion of medium-length triglycerides rather than long-chain-length triglycerides. The reason is that medium-length triglycerides can be absorbed directly into the portal system and do not have to be incorporated into lipoproteins.

PROTEIN DEPOSITS

- Immunoglobulin
- Neurofibrillary tangles
- Amyloid
- Alpha-1-antitrypsin
- Hyaline change

The accumulation of protein within the cytoplasm of cells is much less common than the accumulation of fat. Protein deposits may be the result of increased protein in the blood (most commonly due to increased amounts of immunoglobulin) or increased protein in the urine (due to the nephrotic syndrome). In the latter abnormality the protein can be absorbed by the renal tubular epithelial cells and can appear as hyaline deposits within the cytoplasm. The *neurofibrillary tangle* of patients with Alzheimer's disease is composed of microtubule-associated proteins and neurofilaments. Two other important diseases associated with protein deposits are amyloidosis and alpha-1-antitrypsin deficiency.

AMYLOID

- Any protein with a "beta-pleated sheet" configuration
- Special stain → Congo red
- Polarization → apple-green birefringence

AMYLOIDOSIS

Systemic

*   Multiple myeloma → deposits of amyloid light protein
*   Chronic inflammatory diseases → deposits of amyloid associated protein
*   Hemodialysis → deposits of beta2-microglobulin

Localized

*   Senile cardiac disease → deposits of amyloid transthyretin
*   Alzheimer's disease → deposits of beta2-amyloid protein
*   Medullary carcinoma of thyroid → deposits of procalcitonin
*   Type II diabetes mellitus → amyloid deposits in islets of Langerhans in pancreas

---

Amyloid is a term that describes any protein with a particular pattern. Amyloid proteins stain brown with iodine (hence the name *amyloid*, which means "starch-like"). Histologically amyloid stains pink with the routine hematoxylin and eosin stain, but dark red with the Congo red stain. When viewed under polarized light, amyloid stained with the Congo red stain displays apple-green birefringence (this is very important for diagnosis). The histologic diagnosis of amyloid is based solely on its special staining characteristics. Any fibrillar protein that has a "beta-pleated sheet" configuration will stain as amyloid.

Amyloidosis is a clinical state that refers to the deposition of amyloid material within the body. Many different proteins stain as amyloid. Conditions associated with amyloidosis can be classified by systemic or localized depositions of amyloid. Abnormalities of the immune system, such as multiple myeloma (a malignancy of plasma cells), secrete amyloid light (AL) chains, while reactive systemic diseases secrete amyloid associated protein (AA). Patients on chronic hemodialysis may develop amyloid deposits consisting of beta2-microglobulin. Patients with senile cardiac disease may develop amyloid deposits in the heart consisting of amyloid transthyretin (ATTR), while patients with senile cerebral disease, such as Alzheimer's disease, may develop amyloid deposits in the brain consisting of beta2-amyloid protein. Patients with medullary carcinoma of the thyroid, a malignancy of the calcitonin-secreting C cells of the thyroid, characteristically have amyloid deposits of procalcitonin within the tumor. Finally, patients with type II diabetes mellitus may have amyloid deposits within pancreatic islets consisting of islet amyloid polypeptide.

ALPHA-1-ANTITRYPSIN DEFICIENCY

Liver disease

- PAS-positive globules within hepatocytes
- Cirrhosis

Lung disease

- Panacinar emphysema

Alpha-1-antitrypsin is an enzyme that functions as a proteinase inhibitor. A deficiency of this enzyme, alpha-1-antitrypsin deficiency (A1ATD), is associated with severe disease of the liver and the lungs. The pathogenesis of the liver cell injury is not well understood, but microscopically there are globules of abnormal alpha-1-antitrypsin (PAS-positive) within the cytoplasm of hepatocytes. Patients with alpha-1-antitrypsin deficiency are at an increased risk for developing hepatocellular carcinoma.

There is a well-established association between A1ATD and panacinar emphysema. Emphysema is a chronic obstructive disease of the lungs that is characterized by destruction of the airways. The pathogenesis of emphysema is the result of an imbalance between proteases (elastases) and anti-proteases (anti-elastases) in the lungs (Fig. 4-2). Destruction of the lungs can result from excess func-

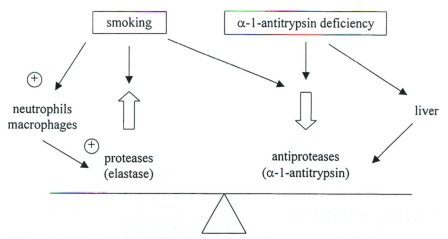

Figure 4-2 Balance Between Proteases and Anti-Proteases
Normally there is a yin-yang balance between proteases (elastase) and anti-proteases (α-1-antitrypsin) within the lung. Increasing the proteases or decreasing the anti-proteases upsets this balance and can lead to destruction of the elastic tissue in the lung. This destruction results in emphysema.

tion of elastases or decreased function of anti-elastases. Excess functioning of elastase can result from cigarette smoking; decreased functioning of anti-elastase can result from a deficiency of A1AT, since A1AT functions as an anti-elastase. Smoking causes destruction of the proximal portion of the lung acinus (centri-acinar emphysema). A1ATD causes destruction of the entire acinus (panacinar emphysema).

The enzyme A1AT is coded for by proteinase-inhibitor (*Pi*) genes on chromosome 14. There are several alleles (variants of this gene) at this site. The normal Pi allele is M, and the normal homozygote is MM. The Z allele yields the lowest level of antiprotease, and the Pi ZZ homozygote is the most deficient in alpha-1-antitrypsin. These individuals are at the greatest risk for developing severe liver disease and lung disease. Smoking increases their risk of developing emphysema even more.

HYALINE CHANGE

- Immunoglobulin deposits
- Alcoholic hyaline
- Hyaline arteriolosclerosis
- Viral inclusions
- Hyaline membranes of the lung

Hyaline is a general, nonspecific term that describes any material, inside or outside of the cell, that stains a homogenous red color with the routine hematoxylin and eosin (H&E) stain. Many different types of substances may be described as having an appearance of hyaline. Immunoglobulins may form intra-cytoplasmic (within plasma cells) or extracellular round bodies called Russell bodies. Immunoglobulin deposits within the nucleus of plasma cells are called Dutcher bodies and are seen in patients with Waldenström's macroglobulinemia. Alcoholic hyaline inclusions (Mallory bodies) are composed of prekeratin intermediate filaments. They are a nonspecific finding found in several liver diseases. Hyaline material may be found in the arterioles of kidneys in patients with benign hypertension (benign nephrosclerosis). This material is composed of basement membrane material and precipitated plasma proteins.

VIRAL CHANGES
Giant cells

- Herpes simplex virus
- Cytomegalic virus (CMV)
- Measles (Warthin-Finkeldey giant cells)
- Respiratory syncytial virus

Inclusions

- Herpes simplex virus (Cowdry A bodies)
- Smallpox virus (Guarnieri bodies)
- Rabies virus (Negri bodies)
- Molluscum contagiosum (molluscum bodies)

Ground glass change

- Nucleus = herpes simplex virus
- Cytoplasm = hepatitis B

Atypical cells

1. Atypical lymphocytes
   - Epstein-Barr virus
2. Smudge cells
   - Adenovirus (respiratory epithelial cells)
3. Koilocytosis
   - Human papillomavirus (HPV)

Viruses infect cells and typically produce inclusions within the cytoplasm or nucleus of the infected cell. These viral inclusions (cytopathic effect) often appear histologically as hyaline inclusions. This cytopathic effect produced by viruses is often a histologic clue to the diagnosis. For example, there are several types of herpes viruses, but infection with either herpes simplex virus (HSV) or varicella-zoster virus (VZV) is recognized by nuclear homogenization (ground-glass nuclei), intranuclear hyaline inclusions (Cowdry type A inclusions), and the formation of multinucleated giant cells. Epstein-Barr virus (EBV) is another herpes virus that infects B lymphocytes but has no characteristic viral inclusion. EBV instead causes CD8+ (cytotoxic) T lymphocytes to proliferate. These cells are called *atypical lymphocytes* because they have abundant cytoplasm. Cytomegalic virus (CMV), another herpes virus, enlarges infected cells (hence the name of the virus) and produces large, purple intranuclear inclusions (surrounded by a clear halo) and smaller, less prominent basophilic intracytoplasmic inclusions. Adenoviruses can produce similar inclusions, but the infected cells are not enlarged. Adenoviruses produce characteristic *smudge cells* in infected respiratory epithelial cells.

Multinucleate giant cells with up to 100 nuclei and both intracytoplasmic and intranuclear inclusions (Warthin-Finkeldey giant cells) are characteristic of rubeola (measles) infection. Human papillomavirus (HPV) infection produces a characteristic effect called *koilocytosis*—enlarged squamous epithelial cells having shrunken nuclei ("raisinoid") within large cytoplasmic vacuoles. Molluscum contagiosum is a self-limited disease of the skin caused by a poxvirus. This virus has a characteristic brick shape with a dumbbell-shaped DNA core. Clinically, multiple small, pruritic lesions are formed, typically on the trunk. Histologically, the epidermis bulges downward into the superficial dermis and numerous large intracytoplasmic inclusion bodies (molluscum bodies) are seen.

Finally, Guarnieri bodies are multiple, granular, eosinophilic intracytoplasmic inclusions that are associated with variola (smallpox) virus, and Negri bodies are round eosinophilic cytoplasmic inclusions that are associated with rabies virus.

HYALINE MEMBRANES OF THE LUNGS

* Acute respiratory distress syndrome
* Respiratory distress syndrome of the newborn

Excess proteins can be deposited as hyaline droplets in proximal renal tubular epithelial cells, or they can be part of hyaline membranes found in the alveoli of the lungs. The latter is an important histologic finding in two important diseases of the lungs—acute respiratory distress syndrome (ARDS) and respiratory distress syndrome of the newborn.

ACUTE RESPIRATORY DISTRESS SYNDROME (ARDS)

* Diffuse alveolar damage (DAD)
* Injury to endothelial cells and type I pneumocytes
* Increased capillary permeability
* Hyaline membrane formation
* Type II pneumocyte hyperplasia

The acute respiratory syndrome (ARDS) is characterized clinically by the rapid onset of severe respiratory insufficiency. (ARDS has many, many names, such as adult respiratory failure, shock lung, traumatic wet lung, pump lung, and diffuse alveolar damage.) This is a common problem that has many causes including sepsis, shock, oxygen toxicity, diffuse pulmonary infections (mostly viruses and gram-negative bacteria), burns, toxins, and drugs.

The basic lesion that produces ARDS is diffuse damage to the alveolar wall (diffuse alveolar damage is called DAD). The initial injury damages capillary endothelial cells and produces interstitial *edema* within the alveolar septa. Protein-rich edema fluid then leaks into the alveolar spaces. Accumulation of fibrinogen and cell debris produces pink membranes (hyaline membranes) that line the alveolar septa. These hyaline membranes are the histologic hallmark of ARDS. There is also damage to type I pneumocytes. As these cells are destroyed, type II pneumocytes divide and proliferate to replace them. This proliferation (hyperplasia) creates a cuboidal lining to the alveolar spaces that can be mistaken histologically for adenocarcinoma.

HYALINE MEMBRANE DISEASE
Associations

- Premature infants
- C-sections
- Maternal diabetes

Cause

- Decreased production of surfactant
- Increased endothelial permeability

A disorder in newborns that is histologically identical to ARDS is neonatal respiratory distress syndrome (hyaline membrane disease or HMD). HMD is basically a disease of premature infants. Most affected infants weight 1000 to 1500 gm. Clinical situations that are associated with the development of HMD include diabetes in the mother (maternal diabetes causes increased fetal secretion of insulin which inhibits lung maturation), and cesarean section. Infants with HMD clinically appear normal at birth, but soon afterward they develop problems breathing. Grossly their lungs are a mottled, red-purple color (they look grossly like liver). Histologically there are numerous hyaline membranes within the alveoli.

There are two basic defects in infants with HMD—a deficiency of pulmonary surfactant and increased pulmonary endothelial permeability. *Surfactant* is a lipid produced by type II pneumocytes that reduces the surface tension between air and fluid interfaces by getting between the molecules in the liquid and reducing their attraction to each other. This reduces the tendency for the alveoli to collapse with expiration. Synthesis of surfactant increases throughout fetal development, but is maximal at about 35 weeks. With a deficiency of surfactant, the lungs will collapse (*atelectasis*) with expiration. Additionally, the increased permeability of pulmonary endothelial cells produces protein-rich edema fluid in the alveoli that contributes to the formation of hyaline membranes.

In order to minimize the risk of HMD, the maturity of the lungs of a fetus must be determined. The most reliable test to determine pulmonary maturity is the lecithin-to-sphingomyelin ratio (L/S). The fetal production of lecithin (a major component of surfactant) is increased starting around 35 weeks of gestation, while levels of spingomyelin remain fairly constant. This results in an increased L/S at about 35 weeks of gestation. An L/S ratio or about 2 indicates fetal maturity, 1.2 indicates a possible risk for HMD, and below 1 a definite risk for HMD.

GLYCOGEN

1. PAS-positive, diastase-sensitive material
2. Deposits
   - Abnormal glucose metabolism → diabetes mellitus
   - Abnormal glycogen metabolism → glycogen storage diseases

---

Glycogen deposits appear histologically as clear vacuoles within the cytoplasm or the nucleus of affected cells. This clear appearance is similar to the changes produced by water (hydropic change) and fat (steatosis). The periodic acid-Schiff stain (PAS stain) is used to differentiate these substances. Glycogen is PAS positive, and this staining is sensitive to diastase.

Glycogen deposits are the result of abnormal glucose metabolism or abnormal glycogen metabolism. The most important clinical disorder of glucose metabolism is diabetes mellitus. In patients with diabetes mellitus, glycogen can be deposited in the epithelial cells of the distal convoluted tubules of the kidneys, the beta cells of the islets of the pancreas, the parenchymal cells of the liver (hepatocytes), or the muscle cells of the heart (cardiac cells).

GLYCOGEN STORAGE DISEASES

Von Gierke disease (type I)

- Deficiency of glucose-6-phosphatase
- Glycogen accumulates in liver and kidneys
- Hypoglycemia → convulsions
- Increased lipids → xanthomas
- Increased uric acid → gout

McArdle disease (type V)

- Deficiency of muscle phosphorylase
- Glycogen accumulated in muscle
- Cramps during exercise

Pompe disease (type II)

- Deficiency of alpha-1,4-glucosidase (acid maltase)
- Glycogen accumulates systemically (lysosomal storage disease)
- Main cause of death: congestive heart failure

Andersen disease (type IV)

- Deficiency of branching enzyme
- Abnormal glycogen (amylopectin) accumulates systemically
- Cirrhosis at young age

Glycogen deposits also occur in patients with one of the glycogen storage diseases. The glycogen storage diseases are characterized by abnormalities of the enzymes involved in the synthesis or catabolism of glycogen. There are eight subtypes of glycogen storage diseases, all of which are inherited as autosomal recessive traits (except for type VIII, which is an X-linked disorder). These types can be further divided into three major subgroups depending upon whether the liver is involved (hepatic forms), muscle is involved (myopathic forms), or there is systemic involvement (generalized types). The major storage sites for glycogen are the liver and muscle, but these storage areas of glycogen are used for different purposes. Liver glycogen is used to maintain blood glucose levels during times of fasting (and prevent hypoglycemia). Muscle glycogen is used to produce energy during times of exercise. Therefore, abnormalities involving liver glycogen produce hypoglycemia and convulsions, while abnormalities of muscle glycogen produce muscular symptoms with exercise.

The most important hepatic form of GSD is von Gierke disease (type I GSD). Affected individuals have a deficiency of glucose-6-phosphatase and glycogen accumulation within the cytoplasm of their hepatocytes and cortical tubular epithelial cells of their kidneys. Clinically, these patients develop enlargement of the liver and kidneys, and convulsions (due to hypoglycemia). Additionally these individuals develop *xanthomas* (from increased lipids), gout (from increased uric acid), and bleeding.

The most important myopathic form of GSD is McArdle disease (type V GSD). This disease is characterized by decreased muscle phosphorylase, which results in glycogen accumulation within the muscle. These patients have a normal expected lifespan, but with exercise they can develop cramps and myoglobinuria.

Two generalized glycogen storage diseases are Pompe disease (type II GSD) and Andersen disease (type IV GSD). Pompe disease results in a generalized (systemic) disease because there is a deficiency of the lysosomal enzyme acid maltase (alpha-1,4-glucosidase), and this lysosomal enzyme is not limited to the liver or skeletal muscle. (Pompe disease is the only glycogen storage disease that is also a lysosomal storage disease.) Patients accumulate glycogen within lysosomes especially in the heart, liver, and muscle. Cardiac involvement leads to cardiomegaly and heart failure, which can lead to death in infancy. Patients with Pompe disease are not hypoglycemic because their cytoplasmic enzymes are not affected. Finally, Andersen disease is caused by a deficiency of the branching enzyme, and this leads to the accumulation of an abnormal glycogen called amylopectin. These patients develop cirrhosis at a young age, which is lethal.

CALCIUM DEPOSITS

Dystrophic calcification

- Severe atherosclerosis
- Damaged heart valves
- Tumors

Metastatic calcification

- Hypercalcemia

Abnormal (pathologic) calcification can be the result of dystrophic calcification or metastatic calcification. It is important to understand the difference between these two processes. Dystrophic calcification occurs in abnormal (dystrophic) tissue in patients with normal serum levels of calcium. Metastatic calcification occurs in normal tissue in patients with abnormal calcium metabolism and hypercalcemia.

Dystrophic calcification occurs in damaged or necrotic tissue, such as atherosclerosis, and damaged heart valves. Calcification of an abnormal bicuspid aortic valve (AV) is one of the important causes of aortic stenosis (AS). In order to pump the blood into the aorta across a stenotic AV, the pressure in the left ventricle must be much greater than the pressure in the aorta. To produce this increased pressure, the left ventricle undergoes concentric hypertrophy. Patients with AS present clinically with chest pain (angina), because there is a mismatch between increased oxygen demand of the hypertrophied LV and decreased blood flow across the stenotic valve. Patients are also likely to develop syncopal episodes (fainting) with exertion because of the inability to increase their cardiac stroke volume when needed. AS is the most common valvular heart disease that is associated with angina and syncope. Patients eventually develop heart failure because the work necessary to contract the hypertrophied stiff heart cannot be maintained for extended periods of time.

PSAMMOMA BODIES

- Papillary tumors of the ovary
- Papillary carcinoma of the thyroid
- Meningioma
- Mesothelioma

Calcification is characteristic of some types of tumors. For example, calcifications can be seen with mammography and can be used to diagnose breast cancer while the tumors are still small. Calcifications within a brain tumor, which can be seen with an X-ray examination of the skull, are suggestive of the tumor being an oligodendroglioma. In some tumors single necrotic tumor cells may become progressively calcified (like the rings of a tree), forming laminated calcifications (*psammoma bodies*). These calcified tumors are particularly characteristic of papillary tumors, such as papillary tumors of the ovary or papillary cancer of the thyroid gland. Psammoma bodies can also be seen microscopically in meningiomas or mesotheliomas.

HYPERCALCEMIA

Increased parathyroid hormone levels

- Hyperparathyroidism

Decreased parathyroid hormone levels

- Hematologic malignancies
- Sarcoidosis
- Excess vitamin D
- Excess milk intake (milk-alkali syndrome)
- Prolonged immobilization
- Metastases to bone
- Paraneoplastic secretion of parathyroid-related protein

Metastatic calcification occurs in normal tissues in patients with hypercalcemia (Fig. 4-3). The increased blood levels of calcium can be due to excess secretion of parathyroid hormone (PTH) by the parathyroid glands (hyperparathyroidism), or to processes that do not involve the parathyroid glands. Examples of the latter include certain hematologic malignancies (multiple myeloma and adult leukemia lymphoma), sarcoidosis, excess vitamin D, excess milk consumption (milk-alkali syndrome), prolonged immobilization, and certain paraneoplastic syndromes. Note that these conditions produce hypercalcemia with decreased serum levels of PTH (box "A" in Fig. 4-3).

Tumors associated with the paraneoplastic production of calcium include lung cancer, kidney cancer, endometrial cancer, and urinary bladder cancer. These tumors produce hypercalcemia by secreting parathyoid hormone-related peptide (PTHrP), which is a normal substance produced locally by many different tissues of the body. PTHrP is distinct from parathyroid hormone (PTH), secreted by the parathyroid glands. Patients with this type of paraneoplastic syndrome have

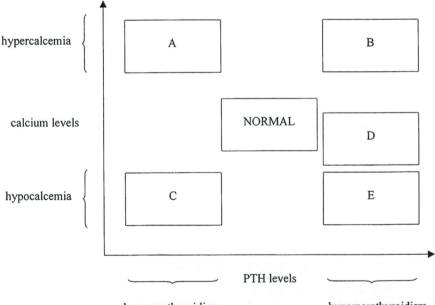

Figure 4-3 Relationship Between Calcium Levels and Parathyroid Levels
The function of parathyroid hormone (PTH) is to keep blood levels of calcium within normal limits. Increased serum levels of calcium (hypercalcemia) can be associated with increased or decreased levels of PTH, and likewise, decreased serum levels of calcium (hypocalcemia) can be associated with increased or decreased levels of PTH.

increased calcium levels but decreased PTH levels. All of the parathyroid glands in these patients are small (atrophic).

HYPERPARATHYROIDISM

Primary hyperparathyroidism

1. Increased serum calcium
2. Cause
   - Hyperplasia → all four glands enlarged
   - Adenoma → one gland enlarged, three glands small
   - Carcinoma → infiltrating tumor mass

Secondary hyperparathyroidism

- Normal or decreased serum calcium
- Most common cause: chronic renal failure

Signs and symptoms

- Bone resorption (osteitis fibrosa cystica)
- Hypercalciuria → renal stone
- Peptic ulcer disease
- Mental changes

Perhaps the most important clinical cause of hypercalcemia is hyperparathyroidism (excess production of parathyroid hormone). Hyperparathyroidism may be due to an intrinsic abnormality of the parathyroid gland itself (primary hyperparathyroidism) or it may be secondary to another disease (secondary hyperparathyroidism). The most common cause of secondary hyperparathyroidism is chronic renal failure. In these individuals, the serum calcium levels are normal or low, while the serum PTH levels are increased (box "D" in Fig. 4-3). These patients develop characteristic bone lesions because of the excess actions of PTH.

Primary hyperthyroidism is associated with hypercalcemia and increased serum levels of PTH (box "B" in Fig. 4-3). The causes of primary hyperparathyroidism include parathyroid adenomas, parathyroid hyperplasia, and parathyroid carcinoma. For the most part these diseases can be separated based on the gross appearance of the parathyroid glands. For example, a parathyroid carcinoma, which is quite rare, would enlarge a single parathyroid gland, and the malignant tumor would infiltrate into adjacent structures. A parathyroid adenoma usually affects only one gland. The excess production of PTH by the adenoma causes the remaining three normal parathyroid glands to become small (atrophy). The end result is that grossly there is one large gland and three small glands. Finally, primary hyperplasia of the parathyroids most commonly affects all four of the glands, and grossly all four glands are enlarged. (Note that this gross appearance is identical to that produced by secondary hyperparathyroidism, which is most commonly associated with hyperplasia of all four glands.)

Increased levels of parathyroid hormone (PTH) cause increased bone resorption and increased intestinal calcium absorption (due to the actions of vitamin D). PTH also increases calcium reabsorption in the distal renal tubule, but because the filtered amount of calcium exceeds the ability to reabsorb it, calcium is increased in the urine (hypercalciuria). The excess calcium in the urine increases the risk of forming kidney stones (calcium oxalate or calcium phosphate). Renal stone formation is the most common presentation of hyperparathyroidism. The hypercalcemia also causes peptic ulcer disease because of the stimulation of gastrin release and increased acid secretion by the parietal cells of the stomach. Additionally, the hypercalcemia can produce muscle weakness, fatigue, and hypomotility of the GI tract, the latter leading to constipation and nausea. Mental changes are common.

To finish explaining the boxes in Figure 4-3, notice that box "C" and box "E" are associated with decreased serum levels of calcium (hypocalcemia). Box "C" demonstrates the combination of hypocalcemia and hypoparathyroidism, which is the result of primary hypoparathyroidism. This abnormality can result from destruction of the parathyroid glands (autoimmune disease) or abnormal development of the parathyroid glands (DiGeorge's syndrome). Finally, box "E" demonstrates the combination of hypocalcemia and hyperparathyroidism. This abnormality results from abnormal functioning of parathyroid hormone, such as may occur with abnormalities of the receptors for parathyroid hormone (Albright's syndrome). Because this disorder produces hypocalcemia (a finding suggestive of hypoparathyroidism), it is sometimes referred to as pseudohypoparathyroidism.

IRON DEPOSITS

- Ferritin → small electron-dense particles of storage iron
- Hemosiderin → golden-brown particles composed of large aggregates of ferritin
- Hematin → dark brown breakdown pigment of hemoglobin

There are several forms of iron found within the body—functional forms, transport forms, and storage forms. Functional iron is found within hemoglobin, myoglobin, and certain enzymes (catalase and cytochromes). Iron is transported in the plasma bound to transferrin, which is normally about one-third saturated with iron. All storage iron is in the form of ferritin or hemosiderin. In the liver, ferritin is found within parenchymal cells, while in the spleen and bone marrow, ferritin is found within macrophages. Very small amounts of ferritin circulate in the plasma. Since ferritin is derived from the storage pool, serum ferritin levels are a good indicator of total body stores.

These different forms of iron are important when you consider the normal breakdown of old red cells. Macrophages destroy senescent erythrocytes to reuse their amino acids and the iron that is associated with hemoglobin. In this process, the globin chains separate from the heme groups, and the heme groups split into iron and protoporphyrin. The iron is processed for storage either as ferritin or hemosiderin. Iron is normally stored within the protein apoferritin to form ferritin, a protein-iron complex found in red cells, macrophages, and hepatocytes. Ferritin particles cannot be seen with routine light microscopy, but they can be seen with electron microscopy. Ferritin can be partially denatured and aggregated to form hemosiderin. Hemosiderin is packets of ferritin that is found within macrophages. These particles contain ferric iron and stain a deep blue color with Prussian blue stain.

Hematin is a black, crystalline product of the oxidation of heme (from the ferrous to the ferric state). Even though it has iron in the ferric state it is Prussian blue negative. It is associated with severe destruction of red cells (severe transfusion reactions or malaria).

ABNORMAL DEPOSITS OF HEMOSIDERIN

Reaction to hemorrhage

- Bruise
- Heart failure cells

Bone marrow

- Sideroblastic anemia
- Anemia of chronic disease

Systemic

- Hemosiderosis
- Hemochromatosis

Deposition of hemosiderin may occur locally or systemically. Local deposits of hemosiderin can be found within the bone marrow or within tissue as a result of *hemorrhage*. A bruise is a local area of hemorrhage. Consider the color reactions involved with the formation of a bruise on the skin. At first a bruise has a red-blue color due to the red-blue color of the hemoglobin that is deposited in the tissue. The color changes that follow are due to the sequential breakdown products of hemoglobin. These color changes proceed from various shades of green-blue (from the green color of biliverdin and the red color of bilirubin) to golden-yellow (from the golden-brown color of hemosiderin).

In the lungs localized hemorrhage can occur within the alveoli due to left-sided heart failure. The red cells within alveoli are eventually destroyed, and their products (hemoglobin) are ingested by alveolar macrophages to produce hemosiderin-laden macrophages ("heart failure cells").

SIDEROBLASTIC ANEMIA

1. Ring sideroblasts (iron trapped within mitochondria of red cell precursors)
2. Dimorphic red cell population in peripheral blood
3. Primary sideroblastic anemia
    • Idiopathic → a myelodysplastic syndrome
4. Secondary sideroblastic anemia
    • Drugs (INH)
    • Lead poisoning
    • Alcohol

Approximately one-third of the red cell precursors in the normal bone (normoblasts) contains ferritin granules and are called *sideroblasts*. In sideroblastic anemia a deficiency of pyridoxine and ferritin decreases the production of globin or heme, and ferritin granules accumulate within the mitochondria. Since mitochondria normally form a rim around the nucleus of red cell precursors, accumulation of iron within mitochondria produces a ring of iron (ring sideroblast). Patients with sideroblastic anemia typically have a dimorphic population of red cells in the peripheral blood, this being a combination of normal cells (normochromic normocytic) and small pale cells (hypochromic microcytic). This dimorphic population of cells can also be found in patients with treated iron deficiency anemia or patients who have received a blood transfusion. Sideroblastic anemia may be a primary disease, or it may be secondary to some other process. Primary sideroblastic anemia may be associated with a pryridoxine (vitamin B6) deficiency or some unknown (idiopathic). The latter disease is classified as being one of the *myelodysplastic* syndromes. Secondary causes of sideroblastic anemia include certain drugs (INH), lead poisoning, and alcoholism.

HYPOCHROMIC MICROCYTIC ANEMIAS

	SERUM Fe	SERUM TIBC	% SATURATION	SERUM FERRITIN	BM SIDEROBLASTS	BM Fe
• ↓ Fe	↓	↑	↓	↓	↓	↓
• Thal	normal	normal	normal	normal/↑	normal	normal/↑
• AOCD	↓	↓	↓	↑	↓	↑
• SA	↑	↓	↑	↑	↑	↑

Sideroblastic anemia (SA) is one of the four hypochromic microcytic anemias. The other three major causes of microcytic hypochromic anemias are iron deficiency (↓ Fe), anemia of chronic disease (AOCD), and thalassemia (thal). An important test to differentiate among these four causes of hypochromic microcytic anemia is to evaluate the bone marrow iron stores by using Prussian blue stain to stain ferritin and hemosiderin granules. In iron deficiency, iron stores are decreased or absent. In AOCD iron is present and increased in amount, but it is found only within macrophages. The iron is decreased in amount within marrow sideroblasts. Marrow iron is increased in patients with sideroblastic anemia, and ring sideroblasts, in which the iron is deposited in mitochondria that ring the nucleus, are present. The iron in patients with thalassemia is generally within normal limits. Serum levels of ferritin reflect the total body iron stores and are generally the same as bone marrow iron. Therefore, serum ferritin is decreased in iron deficiency anemia and increased in AOCD and sideroblastic anemia.

Additional laboratory tests can be used to differentiate among these four causes of hypochromic microcytic anemia. The serum iron and percent saturation are decreased in both iron deficiency anemia and AOCD, but they are both increased in sideroblastic anemia, and may be normal or increased in thalassemia. The total iron binding capacity (TIBC) is increased only in iron deficiency, and is normal or decreased in the others.

SYSTEMIC IRON OVERLOAD
Hemosiderosis

- Chronic hemolysis
- Multiple transfusions
- Too much iron intake (especially with alcohol ingestion)
- Too much iron absorption

Hemochromatosis

* Primary hemochromatosis
* Secondary hemochromatosis

Excess iron may be deposited systemically as hemosiderin deposits in many organs in the iron overload syndromes. Hemosiderin may be deposited within macrophages only, or it may be deposited within macrophages and parenchymal cells or organs. Systemic deposition of hemosiderin within macrophages is called *hemosiderosis* and is not associated with organ dysfunction. In contrast, systemic deposition of hemosiderin within parenchymal cells is called *hemochromatosis* and is associated with organ dysfunction. Hemochromatosis may be a primary (idiopathic) disease, or it may be secondary to some other abnormality. Secondary hemochromatosis is most common in patients with chronic hemolytic anemias (thalassemia). It may also be secondary to other abnormalities such as too many blood transfusions, too much iron in the diet, or too much absorption of dietary iron. Increased iron absorption may be seen in patients with alcoholic cirrhosis. A very strange cause of excess dietary iron is Bantu siderosis, a disease found in individuals of South Africa who use iron utensils.

PRIMARY HEMOCHROMATOSIS ("BRONZE" DIABETES)

1. Classic triad:
   * Micronodular pigment cirrhosis
   * Diabetes mellitus
   * Skin pigmentation
2. Increased risk of hepatocellular carcinoma
3. Cause of death → congestive heart failure

Primary hemochromatosis is a genetic disorder of iron metabolism that is inherited as an autosomal recessive disorder. Signs and symptoms don't appear in patients with primary hemochromatosis until middle age. They consist of the classic triad of micronodular cirrhosis, diabetes mellitus, and skin pigmentation. (The combination of diabetes and skin pigmentation is called "bronze diabetes.") These signs and symptoms are due to deposition of iron within the parenchymal cells of many organs, including the liver and pancreas. The deposition of iron within liver hepatocytes produces cirrhosis and increases the risk of developing hepatocellular carcinoma. Iron deposition in the islets of the pancreas destroys the cells of the islets of Langerhans. Destruction of the B cells leads to decreased production of insulin (diabetes mellitus). Iron deposition in joints leads to arthritis, while deposition in the testes leads to atrophy. Deposition in the adrenal cortex leads to decreased production of cortisol, which leads in turn to increased secretion of ACTH by the anterior pituitary. The precursor to ACTH has melanocyte stimulating hormone (MSH) properties. Its increase causes the skin pigmentation that is seen clinically as a bronze color. Finally, iron deposition in the heart leads to congestive heart failure, which is the main cause of death in these patients.

BILIRUBIN

Indirect bilirubin

- Unconjugated bilirubin
- Not soluble in urine
- Complexed to albumin

Direct bilirubin

- Conjugated bilirubin
- Soluble in urine
- Not complexed to albumin

Bilirubin is the end product of heme metabolism. Hemoglobin from red cells is broken down into heme and globin. The heme is converted to biliverdin by the enzyme heme oxygenase, and the biliverdin is converted to bilirubin by the enzyme biliverdin reductase. Bilirubin is transported to the liver in the blood bound to albumin. It is taken up by the liver where it is conjugated to glucuronic acid by the enzyme bilirubin UDP-glucuronosyltransferase (UGT) and secreted into the bile. Note that bilirubin bound to albumin (bound bilirubin) is not the same as bilirubin conjugated to glucuronide (conjugated or direct bilirubin). In contrast to conjugated bilirubin, unconjugated bilirubin (indirect bilirubin) is not soluble in an aqueous solution, is complexed to albumin, and cannot be excreted in the urine.

BILIRUBIN DEPOSITS

Clinical

- Icterus → yellow skin and yellow sclera
- Pruritus
- Xanthomas
- Kernicterus → in neonates

Microscopic

- Cholestasis
- Bile plugs
- Bile lakes

Increased blood levels of bilirubin produce characteristic clinical signs and symptoms. Jaundice is a descriptive clinical term for a yellow discoloration of skin and scleras produced by accumulation of bilirubin in tissues. Deposition of bile salts in the skin produces itching (*pruritus*). Impaired excretion of cholesterol leads to hyperlipidemia, and the deposition of this excess lipid in the skin produces lipid tumors called *xanthomas*. In neonates excess amounts of unconjugated bilirubin can be deposited in the brain (*kernicterus*). This deposition can severely damage the brain and produce mental retardation or death. This deposition occurs only in neonates because the blood-brain barrier is not fully developed. Additional laboratory findings in patients with jaundice include increased serum alkaline phosphatase levels and decreased levels of the fat-soluble vitamins (ADEK). The microscopic changes of the liver in patients with jaundice include the accumulation of bile pigment within hepatocytes (*cholestasis*). Depending on the cause, bile may be deposited within bile ductules (bile plugs), or extracellularly outside of bile ducts (bile lakes).

CAUSES OF HYPERBILIRUBINEMIA

Excess production of bilirubin

- Chronic hemolytic anemia

Hepatocellular disease

1. Decreased hepatic uptake of bilirubin
   - Drugs

2. Impaired conjugation of bilirubin
- Physiologic jaundice of the newborn
- Crigler-Najjar syndrome
- Gilbert's syndrome

3. Impaired canalicular transport
- Dubin-Johnson syndrome
- Rotor syndrome

Biliary obstruction

1. Gallstones
- Cholesterol stones
- Pigment (bilirubin) stones

2. Carcinoma

Increased blood levels of bilirubin (hyperbilirubinemia) results from abnormalities of bilirubin metabolism. Basically, *jaundice* can result from three types of abnormalities: hemolysis, hepatocellular disease, or obstruction to bile flow. *Hemolysis* results in excess bilirubin production and increased unconjugated bilirubin. Hepatocellular disease may cause jaundice by decreasing hepatic uptake of bilirubin, by impaired conjugation of bilirubin, or by impaired canalicular transport of bilirubin glucuronide. Obstruction to bile flow may be from intrahepatic causes or extrahepatic causes, such as gallstones or carcinoma.

Laboratory tests can be used to separate the causes of jaundice into these three general categories (hemolytic disease, hepatocellular disease, and obstructive disease). Hemolytic disease causes an unconjugated hyperbilirubinemia. Serum hemoglobin levels are characteristically decreased, and urinary urobilinogen levels are increased. (Note that unconjugated bilirubin is not found in the urine and that the serum hemoglobin levels in other causes of jaundice are normal.)

The two other general categories are hepatocellular diseases and obstructive diseases. The hepatocellular diseases may result from either abnormal conjugation of bilirubin or hepatocellular damage in general. The former produces increased unconjugated bilirubin in the blood; the latter results in increased unconjugated bilirubin and conjugated bilirubin. This conjugated bilirubin in the blood may be excreted in the urine, and urine urobilinogen levels are also increased. In addition, these hepatocellular damage diseases result in increased alkaline phosphatase and markedly increased serum aminotransferase levels (AST and ALT).

HEREDITARY HYPERBILIRUBINEMIA
Unconjugated hyperbilirubinemia

- Gilbert's syndrome
- Crigler-Najjar syndrome

Conjugated hyperbilirubinemia

- Dubin-Johnson syndrome
- Rotor syndrome

HEREDITARY UNCONJUGATED HYPERBILIRUBINEMIA
Gilbert's syndrome

- Unconjugated hyperbilirubinemia
- Mildly decreased UGT
- Asymptomatic

Crigler-Najjar syndrome

- Unconjugated hyperbilirubinemia
- Type I → no UGT
- Type II → decreased UGT

Hereditary hyperbilirubinemia may result in the increase of either unconjugated bilirubin or conjugated bilirubin. Hereditary diseases resulting in an unconjugated hyperbilirubinemia (UHBR) include Gilbert's syndrome and Crigler-Najjar syndrome (CN). Gilbert's syndrome, which affects about 7% of the population of the United States, is a mild form of UHBR. Clinically patients are asymptomatic and have a normal life span. There are two types of Crigler-Najjar syndrome. Type I is a rare autosomal recessive UHBR in which there is an absence of UGT (UDP-glucuronyl transferase) activity. The disease is almost uniformly fatal during the neonatal period because of brain disease (kernicterus). Crigler-Najjar syndrome type II is an autosomal dominant disease that is characterized by a deficiency (but not absence) of UGT activity. Patients develop a mild UHBR, but only rarely do they develop kernicterus. Treatment may be with phenobarbital, a drug that induces enzymes within the SER, one of which is UGT.

HEREDITARY CONJUGATED HYPERBILIRUBINEMIA

Dubin-Johnson syndrome

- Conjugated hyperbilirubinemia
- Defective canalicular transport of bile
- Black liver grossly
- Intracytoplasmic inclusions in hapatocytes

Rotor syndrome

- Similar to Dubin-Johnson syndrome (but no black liver)

Two hereditary diseases the produce conjugated hyperbilirubinemia (CHBR) include the Dubin-Johnson syndrome and the Rotor syndrome. Dubin-Johnson syndrome is a benign disorder characterized by chronic or intermittent CHBR. It is caused by a genetic defect in the canalicular transport of organic anions and is associated with a grossly pigmented (black) liver. Microscopically the hepatocytes have numerous pigmented inclusions in their cytoplasm. Rotor syndrome is similar to Dubin-Johnson syndrome, except there is no black pigment grossly, and the liver is unremarkable microscopically.

GALLSTONES

Cholesterol stones

- Yellow stones
- Risk factors → fat, female, fertile, forty, flatulent
- Increased incidence in Native Americans

Bilirubin (pigment) stones

- Black stones
- Risk factors → chronic hemolysis and infections of biliary tract
- Increased incidence in Asians

The obstructive liver diseases interfere with bilirubin reaching the lumen of the gut. Therefore, the pigmented products of the bacteria in the gut on bile are not produced, and the stools are pale and clay-colored. The urine also appears dark due to conjugated bilirubin increasing in the serum and spilling over into the urine. The other product of bacteria on bile, urobilinogen, is decreased, and this leads to decreased urobilinogen levels in the urine. The biliary obstruction may occur within the liver (intrahepatic) or outside the liver (extrahepatic). The latter, which may be produced by stones or cancer, is also associated with markedly elevated serum alkaline phosphatase levels.

Gallstones (cholelithiasis) are divided into two main types. Cholesterol stones are pale yellow, hard, round, radiographically translucent stones that are most often multiple. Their formation is associated with several clinical factors, such as female sex hormones (oral contraceptives), obesity, rapid weight reduction, and hyperlipidemia. They are prevalent in some Native American populations. The other main type of gallstones are the pigment stones, which are brown or black in color and are composed of bilirubin calcium salts. They are found more commonly in Asian populations and are related to chronic hemolytic states, diseases of the small intestines, and bacterial infections of the biliary tree.

COPPER DEPOSITS

Wilson's disease (hepatolenticular degeneration)

- Failure of copper to enter circulation
- Liver → fatty change and cirrhosis
- Basal ganglia (putamen) → tremor, rigidity, choreiform movements
- Cornea → Kayser-Fleischer ring

Wilson's disease (hepatolenticular degeneration) is an autosomal recessive genetic disorder of copper metabolism. Normally dietary copper is absorbed in the stomach and duodenum and is transported to the liver bound to albumin. Free copper then dissociates within hepatocytes and is incorporated into an alpha-2-globulin to form ceruloplasmin, which is then secreted into the plasma. Ceruloplasmin accounts for the majority of plasma copper.

In patients with Wilson's disease, the initial steps of copper metabolism (absorption and transport to the liver) are normal, but the copper fails to enter the circulation as ceruloplasmin and instead remains within the liver. Serum ceruloplasmin levels, therefore, are characteristically low. Early in the disease serum copper levels are decreased, but non-ceruloplasmin copper can enter the blood from the liver. Serum copper levels are therefore of no diagnostic value, since they may be low, normal, or elevated depending on the stage of the disease. Urinary excretion of copper, which normally plays a minor role in copper metabolism, is markedly increased.

Copper is deposited in the cytoplasm of hepatocytes and initially causes microvacuolar fatty change and focal liver cell necrosis. These changes are progressive and produce cirrhosis and liver failure. Copper deposition in the brain primarily involves the basal ganglia (the lenticular nucleus). This deposition produces signs of extrapyramidal dysfunction (tremor, rigidity, and choreiform or athetotic movements). Physical examination of patients with Wilson's disease reveals deposits of copper in the Descemet's membrane at the corneoscleral junction. This produces a copper-colored ring at the periphery of the corneal that is known as Kayser-Fleischer ring.

URATE DEPOSITS

- Joints → chalky white deposits
- Soft tissue → tophus formation

GOUT

1. Hyperuricemia
2. Precipitation of monosodium urate crystals
   - First MTP joint (big toe)
   - Needle-shaped negatively birefringent crystals
   - Tophus formation
3. Classification
   a. Primary gout
      - Impaired uric acid excretion
   b. Secondary gout
      - Increased production of uric acid → Lesch-Nyhan syndrome
      - Increased turnover of nucleic acid → leukemias and lymphomas
      - Decreased excretion of uric acid → chronic renal disease, ethanol intake, diabetes

---

Gout is a clinical disease that is associated with increased serum uric acid levels (although most individuals with elevated serum uric acid levels don't develop symptoms of gout). Uric acid is the main end product of purine catabolism. Abnormalities that affect the normal production or excretion of uric acid can produce gout. These abnormalities are classified clinically as being primary or secondary. Primary (idiopathic) gout usually results from impaired uric acid excretion by the kidneys. Secondary gout may be secondary to increased production of uric acid, from increased turnover of nucleic acids, or from decreased uric acid excretion. An important secondary cause of gout from a biochemical standpoint is Lesch-Nyhan syndrome, an X-linked recessive disorder caused by a deficiency of hypoxanthine-guanine phosphoribosyl transferase (HGPRT). Lesch-Nyhan syndrome clinically is characterized by gout, mental retardation, spasticity, self-mutilation, and aggressive behavior.

In patients with gout, sodium urate crystals precipitate and form chalky white deposits. The crystals are needle-shaped and negatively birefringent. (Negative birefringence means that the crystals appear yellow when aligned parallel with a compensating filter, but blue when oriented perpendicular. Hint: Think yellow, parallel, allopurinol.) The monosodium urate crystals cause an intense inflammatory response that can produce acute arthritis or renal disease. Most patients with gout present with pain and inflammation of the first metatarsophalangeal joint ("big toe"). Urate crystals may also precipitate in extracellular soft tissue, such as the helix of the ear, forming masses called tophi. Histologically these masses consist of deposits of urate crystals surrounded by fibrosis and foreign-body-type giant cells. Treatment of gout involves the drug colchicine, which stabilizes the lysosomal membranes of leukocytes and inhibits the inflammatory response. Colchicine does this by inhibiting microtubules within the cytoplasm.

One of the main abnormalities in the differential diagnosis of gout is pseudogout. Pseudogout is caused by the deposition of calcium pyrophosphate dihydrate (CPPD) in synovial membranes. These deposits form chalky white areas on cartilaginous surfaces that are similar to those seen in patients with gout. CPPD crystals are not needle-shaped like urate crystals, but are short and rhomboid shaped. They are birefringent like urate crystals, but they are weakly positively birefringent (blue when oriented parallel to the compensator). Patients typically develop an acute arthritis of the large joints of the lower extremities.

LIPOFUSCIN DEPOSITS

- Heart (brown atrophy)
- Liver
- Brain

Lipofuscin is an insoluble "wear and tear" (aging) golden-brown pigment found in residual bodies of aging cells, typically neurons, cardiac myocytes, or hepatocytes. Lipofuscin is composed of polymers of lipids and phospholipids that come from lipid peroxidation of cellular membranes by free radicals. Essentially lipofuscin is the indigestible material that is obtained by the process of autophagy. Lipofuscin is typically found in aging patients, but it can occasionally be found in patients with cachexia or severe malnutrition.

BLACK PIGMENTS

- Melanin
- Carbon
- Homogentisic acid

Tyrosine is an important amino acid that is metabolized into multiple substances including homogentisic acid, catecholamines, thyroxin, and melanin. Melanin is a dark brown-black pigment synthesized from tyrosine by melanocytes. The copper-containing enzyme tyrosinase forms dihydroxyphenylalanine (DOPA) and then dopaquinone, which is further metabolized through several steps to form melanin. (Tyrosine hydroxylase is another enzyme that forms DOPA from tyrosine. It is important to realize that tyrosine hydroxylase is not the same enzyme as tyrosinase. The pathway involving tyrosine hydroxylase subsequently forms dopamine, norepinephrine, and epinephrine.)

Blocks in the metabolic pathways involving tyrosine can lead to several different diseases. For example, a deficiency of liver phenylalanine hydroxylase leads to phenylketonuria (PKU), while a deficiency of fumarylacetoacetate hydrolase can lead to the accumulation of tyrosine (tyrosinosis). A deficiency of homogentisic oxidase (which normally breaks down homogentisic acid into carbon dioxide and water) is associated with alkaptonuria; and a deficiency of tyrosinase can lead to albinism.

ABNORMALITIES INVOLVING MELANOCYTES

Normal numbers of melanocytes

- Albinism
- Freckles
- Melasma
- Increased pituitary ACTH secretion

Decreased numbers of melanocytes

- Vitiligo

Increased numbers of melanocytes

- Lentigo
- Nevi
- Melanoma

The synthesis of melanin occurs primarily within melanocytes. Melanocytes are dendritic cells that originate in the neural crest, migrate into the basal layer of the epidermis, and contain melanosomes. Histochemical tests used to identify melanocytes include the DOPA reaction (positive in the presence of enzymes of the tyrosine-melanin pathway), S100 protein (nonspecific reaction), and HMB-45 (specific reaction).

In lower animals (but not humans) the formation of melanin by melanocytes is under the control of a hormone called melanin-stimulating hormone (MSH), produced by the pars intermedia of the pituitary gland. In humans, stimulation of melancocytes is probably related to levels of adrenocorticotropic hormone (ACTH). This is because ACTH is part of a group of hormones secreted by the anterior pituitary gland called the pro-opiomelanocortin (POMC) peptide family. The POMC protein can be cleaved into multiple products including ACTH, beta-lipotropin, and gamma-MSH. Excess secretion of ACTH by the pituitary is often associated with increased skin pigmentation due to this melanin-stimulating effect. For example, destruction of the adrenal cortex (such as by iron deposits in patients with hemochromatosis or immune destruction in patients with Addison's syndrome) leads to decreased production of cortisol and increased secretion of ACTH by the anterior pituitary. Because of this increase secretion, patients develop increased skin pigmentation. ACTH secretion may also be increased due to secretion of ACTH by a pituitary adenoma. These patients develop signs and symptoms of excess cortisol production (Cushing's syndrome), and may have increased skin pigmentation secondary to increased production of MSH or the melanogenic effect of high ACTH levels.

Abnormalities of pigmentation of the skin (hyperpigmentation or hypopigmentation) are associated with normal or abnormal numbers of melanocytes. Normal numbers of melanocytes are seen in patients with albinism, freckles, and melasma. Albinism refers to a group of disorders characterized by an abnormality in the synthesis of melanin. Two forms of oculocutaneous albinism can be differentiated by the presence or absence of tyrosinase. Because melanin normally protects individuals from the effects of the sun, patients with albinism are at a greatly increased risk for the development of squamous cell carcinomas in sun-exposed skin.

Freckles (ephelides) are characterized by increased pigmentation of the basal keratinocytes without an increase in the number of melanocytes. Freckles tend to increase with exposure to sunlight and may fade at puberty. Increased pigmentation of the basal keratinocytes without an increase in the number of melanocytes is found in the epidermal type of melasma. Melasma (chloasma) refers to a mask-like zone of hyperpigmentation on the face, which may occur secondary to pregnancy ("mask of pregnancy") or from the use of oral contraceptives. A second form of melasma (dermal type) has numerous macrophages in the superficial dermis that have phagocytized melanin.

Loss of melanocytes within the epidermis causes large areas of depigmentation of the skin (vitiligo). These irregular, sharply defined lesions are more common in dark-skinned races and tend to be symmetrical.

Increased numbers of melanocytes (melanocytic hyperplasia) cause hyperpigmentation of the skin and can be classified into several different lesions. A *lentigo* consists of melanocytic hyperplasia in the basal layers of the epidermis along with elongation and thinning of the rete ridges. Two types of lentigines are lentigo simplex (younger individuals) and lentigo senilis ("liver spots" of older individuals). These lesions do not fade from lack of sun exposure.

NEVI

Common nevi

- Junctional nevus → clusters of nevus cells at epidermal-dermal junction
- Intradermal nevus → clusters of nevus cells within the dermis
- Compound nevus → combination of junctional and intradermal nevus

Uncommon nevi

- Blue nevus → spindle nevus cells deep in dermis
- Halo nevus → peripherally depigmented nevus due to lymphocytic infiltrate
- Spitz nevus → groups of spindle-shaped nevus cells found in children
- Congenital nevus → nevus greater than 1 cm in diameter
- Dysplastic nevus → abnormal histologic appearance of nevus

Increased numbers of melanocyte precursor cells may form multiple groups or clusters of cells. These lesions are called nevocellular nevi (nevi for short) or "moles." Most nevocellular nevi are not present at birth, but begin to appear within the first two years of life. Normally these cells migrate from the neural crest of the fetus to the epidermis where they form melanocytes. Nevi are formed when the migration of these cells is stopped just before they can form the melanocytes within the epidermis. There are three basic types of nevi depending upon the location of the groups of nevus cells—junctional nevus, intradermal nevus, or compound nevus (Fig. 4-4). In addition to these three main types of nevi, there are several variant forms of nevi. Blue nevi have nevus cells that are located deep in the dermis, but do not form nests of cells. These nevus cells are spindle shaped and have long thin dendritic processes. (The blue color seen clin-

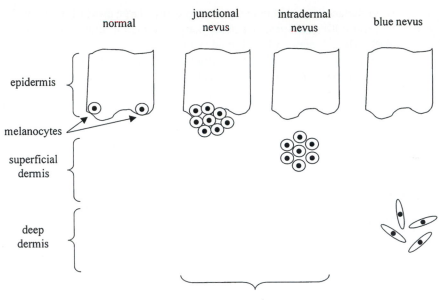

Figure 4-4 Nevi

There are three basic types of nevi depending upon the location of the groups of nevus cells. These groups of cells may be located at the epidermal-dermal junction (junctional nevus), in the superficial dermis (dermal nevus), or both the epidermal-dermal junction and the superficial dermis (compound nevus). A blue nevus has elongated dendritic nevus cells that are located deeper in the dermis.

ically is caused by the deep location of the nevus cells. Light bouncing off of these pigmented cells must travel through more collagen and this produces a blue color. This is basically the same reason why blood vessels appear blue, the sky appears blue, etc.) A halo nevus has a peripheral light color, which is due to lymphocytes infiltrating around the nests of nevus cells. The Spitz nevus (epithelioid cell nevus) is composed of groups of epithelioid and spindle melanocytes. It is found predominantly in children and young adults and may be misdiagnosed clinically as a hemangioma (because or the absence of melanin and its rich vascularity). A Spitz nevus can be misdiagnosed histologically as a malignant melanoma. These lesions, however, have no increased risk for malignant transformation.

Most melanocytic nevi eventually differentiate into delicate neuromesenchymal structures (neurotized nevus) that are histologically similar to a small skin tag (acrochordon). A few lesions persist rather than disappear. Abnormal, irregular growth patterns, without cytologic atypia, produce atypical nevi. If cytologic atypia is also present, the nevus is classified as dysplastic. Dysplastic nevi differ from ordinary moles in that they occur on both sun-exposed and non-sun-exposed areas, have a much higher incidence of malignant transformation, and may be part of a familial syndrome.

CARBON DEPOSITS

Carbon particles

* Anthracosis → carbon dust particles within macrophages

Coal dust (carbon and silica)

* Simple coal workers' pneumoconiosis → coal macules and nodules
* Complicated coal workers' pneumoconiosis → progressive massive fibrosis

---

The pneumoconiosis are non-neoplastic lung diseases caused by several types of environmental particles (dusts). Reactions to carbon particles may result in asymptomatic anthracosis, simple coal workers' pneumoconiosis, or complicated coal workers' pneumoconiosis. *Anthracosis* refers to the deposition of carbon particles within macrophages in and around the lungs. There is very little cellular reaction to these deposits. Anthracosis is commonly seen in coal miners, urban populations, and tobacco smokers, but no clinical signs or symptoms are seen. The deposition of coal dust (carbon and silica) may produce small or large deposits. Simple coal workers' pneumoconiosis is characterized by coal macules (1 to 2 mm in diameter) and slightly larger coal nodules. Patients are generally asymptomatic. In contrast, complicated coal workers' pneumoconiosis (black lung disease or progressive massive fibrosis) is associated with fibrotic nodules larger than 2 cm. These patients develop signs of severe pulmonary disease and right-sided heart failure.

HOMOGENTISIC ACID

* Normally a colorless compound
* Oxidized to a darkly pigment compound

Alkaptonuria (ochronosis) is caused by the excess formation and deposition of homogentisic acid. This disease results from a block in the metabolism of phenylalanine and tyrosine due to a deficiency of homogentisic oxidase. Excess homogentisic acid causes the urine to turn dark when it is exposed to air for a period of time. Homogentisic acid also causes some tissue (sclera, tendons, and cartilage) to turn a dark color. After years, many patients will develop a degenerative arthritis.

ROUTINE STAIN (H&E)

Hematoxylin

- Blue and basic
- Stains negatively charged structures → DNA and RNA

Eosin

- Pink and acidophilic
- Stains positively charged structures → mitochondria

SPECIAL STAINS

- Fats → oil red O
- Glycogen → PAS positive, diastase sensitive
- Iron → Prussian blue
- Hemosiderin → Prussian blue
- Amyloid → Congo red
- Alpha-1-antitrypsin → PAS positive, diastase resistant
- Calcium → von Kossa
- Copper → rhodamine stain (not worth memorizing)
- Lipofuscin → hematoxylin and eosin (H&E)
- Melanin → H&E

Now that we have finished discussing all the different types of substances that may accumulate inside or outside of cells, a brief review of the stains used to differentiate these substances is in order.

CELL ADAPTATIONS

·

- Cell Adaptation (Terms)
- Types of Dividing Cells
- Causes of Hypertrophy
- Cardiac Hypertrophy
- Hypertrophic Cardiomyopathy
- Hyperplasia
- Erythroid Hyperplasia
- Hyperplasia Involving Lymph Nodes
- Hyperplasia Involving Blood Vessels
- Hyperplasia of the Breast
- Causes of Gynecomastia
- Hyperplasia of the Endometrium
- Hyperplasia of the Prostate
- Hyperplasia of the Lung
- Hyperplasia of the Skin
- Human Papillomavirus
- Psoriasis
- Lichen Planus
- Hyperplasia of the Adrenal Glands
- 21-Hydroxylase Deficiency
- 11-Hydroxylase Deficiency
- 17-Hydroxylase Deficiency
- Metaplasia
- Myelofibrosis with Myeloid Metaplasia

· · · · · · · · · · · · ·

CELL ADAPTATION (TERMS)

- Hypertrophy → increase in the size of cells
- Hyperplasia → increase in the number of cells
- Atrophy → decrease size of an organ
- Aplasia → failure of cell production
- Hypoplasia → decrease in the number of cells
- Metaplasia → replacement of one cell type by another
- Dysplasia → abnormal cell growth

An organ or tissue can adapt to injury in many different ways (Fig. 5-1). Adaptations include changing the size of cells, changing the number of cells, or changing the type of cells. Cells can become larger (*hypertrophy*) or smaller (*atrophy*); cells can become more numerous (*hyperplasia*) or less numerous (*hypoplasia*). These cell adaptations may change the size of an organ. Typically, an organ may increase in size because of an increase in the size of cells or an increase in the number of cells. Similarly, an organ may decrease in size because of a decrease in the size of cells or a decrease in the number of cells.

Don't confuse the terms *aplasia* and *hypoplasia* with the similar sounding term *atrophy*. Atrophy refers to the decrease in size of an organ because of a decrease in the number of preexisting cells. In contrast, aplasia and hypoplasia refer to the failure of cells to proliferate and form normal structures or organs. *Aplasia* refers to the complete failure of an organ to develop. Hypoplasia refers to a reduction in the size of an organ because of a developmental abnormality that produces a decrease in the number of cells. Structurally the organ tends to be normal but small in size.

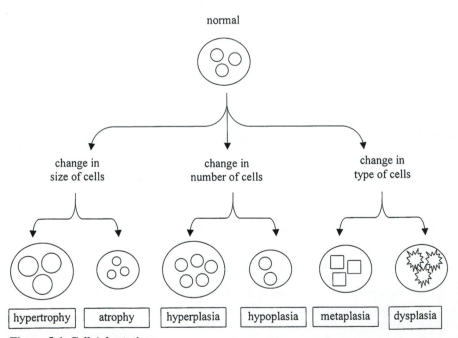

Figure 5-1 Cell Adaptations
Notice that increased cell size (hypertrophy) and increased cell numbers (hyperplasia) increase the size of an organ. In contrast, decreased cell size (atrophy) and decreased cell numbers (hypoplasia) decrease the size of an organ.

TYPES OF DIVIDING CELLS

Permanent cells

- Neurons
- Cardiac cells
- Skeletal muscle cells

Labile cells

- Bone marrow cells
- GI tract
- Epithelial cells

Stable cells

- Hepatocytes
- Smooth muscle cells
- Fibroblasts

The type of cell adaptation that results from cell injury depends to a large extent upon the type of injury that occurs, but it also depends greatly on the ability of the cell to divide and proliferate. Many, but not all, cells continue to grow and divide throughout life. There are three basic types of cells with regard to their ability to divide. Cells that cannot divide are permanent cells; cells that are continuously dividing are labile cells; and cells that are not dividing but are capable of dividing when necessary are stable cells. Both labile cells and stable cells can proliferate and increase in number (hyperplasia). In contrast, permanent cells cannot divide and adapt by increasing their size (hypertrophy).

CAUSES OF HYPERTROPHY

Skeletal muscle

- Exercise
- Steroid use

Smooth muscle

- Congenital pyloric stenosis

Cardiac muscle

- Aortic stenosis and regurgitation
- Hypertension (systemic and pulmonic)
- Hypertrophic cardiomyopathy

Hypertrophy usually occurs in tissue composed of permanent (nondividing) cells, such as skeletal muscle, cardiac muscle, and smooth muscle. The increase in the size of the cells is the result of an increase in the number and size of cell organelles along with increased protein synthesis. Before examining the process of hypertrophy in depth, one specialized type of hypertrophy found in the liver needs to be mentioned. It is caused by certain drugs (xenobiotics) that cause proliferation of the smooth endoplasmic reticulum (SER). These drugs, such as phenobarbital, cause proliferation of the SER by inducing microsomal mixed-function oxidases, such as cytochrome P-450. This reaction is used beneficially for the treatment of one type of inherited deficiency of the hepatic enzyme bilirubin UDP-glucuronosyltransferase (UGT), which conjugates bilirubin with glucuronic acid. In this particular disease, type II Crigler-Najjar syndrome, phenobarbital is used to induce the proliferation of the SER. UGT is found within the SER and is increased in amount.

For the most part, hypertrophy of muscle results from increased work (functional demand), such as skeletal muscle hypertrophy from increased exercise or smooth muscle hypertrophy of the pylorus of the stomach because of obstruction. The latter is seen in infants with congenital hypertrophic pyloric stenosis, who present in the second or third week of life with symptoms of regurgitation and persistent severe vomiting. The vomiting is of nonbilious material, because the obstruction is proximal to the sphincter of Oddi. (Duodenal atresia, in contrast, produces bilious vomiting, because the obstruction is distal to the sphincter.) Physical examination reveals a firm palpable mass ("olive") in the region of the pylorus. Surgical splitting of the hypertrophic muscle in the stenotic region cures this condition.

CARDIAC HYPERTROPHY
Concentric hypertrophy

- Response to pressure overload
- Sarcomeres proliferate in parallel
- Increased ventricular thickness
- No change in size of ventricular cavity

Eccentric hypertrophy

- Response to volume overload
- Sarcomeres proliferate in series
- No increase in ventricle thickness
- Increase in size of ventricular cavity

The cardiac muscle cells of the ventricles of the heart respond to increased pressure or increased volume of blood by adapting via the process of hypertrophy (Fig. 5-2). There are two basic types of cardiac hypertrophy. Pressure overloads cause concentric hypertrophy of the heart, while volume overloads cause eccentric hypertrophy. Concentric hypertrophy is characterized by a parallel duplica-

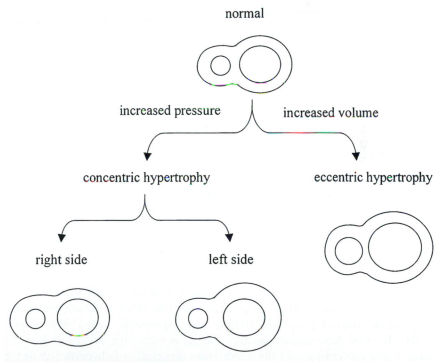

Figure 5-2 Cardiac Hypertrophy
Compare the different types of hypertrophy. Increased pressure causes concentric hypertrophy, which is characterized by an increase in the thickness of the wall of the ventricle, but no increase in the size of the lumen. In contrast, increased volume of blood causes eccentric hypertrophy, which is characterized by an increase in the size of the lumen, but no increase in the thickness of the wall of the ventricle.

tion of sarcomeres, which increases the ventricular wall thickness, but not the size of the ventricular cavity (hypertrophy without dilation). The wall becomes thicker and stiffer. In contrast, eccentric hypertrophy is characterized by proliferation of sarcomeres in series in response to the dilation of the ventricular cavity. The result is increase in the size of the ventricular cavity, but not in the thickness of the ventricular wall. The wall is less stiff (increased ventricular compliance). In hypertrophied cardiac muscle, the capillaries of the interstitium of the heart do not increase in number and eventually will not be able to supply the blood that is needed by the hypertrophied muscle fibers. The fibers will fail and congestive heart failure will develop.

Examples of increased pressure (afterload) include hypertension (systemic or pulmonic) and aortic stenosis; an example of increased volume (preload) is aortic regurgitation. Hypertensive heart disease (HHD) can be divided into systemic HHD and pulmonary HHD. Systemic hypertensive heart disease is the result of systemic hypertension, which produces left ventricular (LV) hypertrophy. By definition no other cardiac disease present could cause LV hypertrophy. In systemic HHD the LV is stiff because there is decreased LV compliance. Pulmonary HHD is characterized by right ventricular hypertrophy that is the result of pulmonary disease (the heart disease in this instance is called *cor pulmonale*). Pulmonary diseases that can cause cor pulmonale include diseases of the lung parenchyma (COPD and interstitial fibrosis) and diseases of the pulmonary vessels (multiple pulmonary emboli or pulmonary vascular sclerosis).

HYPERTROPHIC CARDIOMYOPATHY

- Autosomal dominant inheritance
- Mutation in gene for beta-myosin heavy chain
- Asymmetrical hypertrophy of interventricular septum
- Characteristic histologic finding: myofiber disarray
- Risk of sudden death in young adult

Another important heart disease associated with myocardial hypertrophy is hypertrophic cardiomyopathy. Other names for this disease include idiopathic hypertrophic subaortic stenosis (IHSS) and asymmetric septal hypertrophy (ASH). Both of these names describe the gross pathology of this disease. In hypertrophic cardiomyopathy the major gross abnormality is hypertrophy of the interventricular septum, which is thicker than the wall of the left ventricle (causing an appearance of asymmetric hypertrophy). Histologically, the myofibers are disorganized, hypertrophied, and have hyperchromatic nuclei. The disease is thought to result from a mutation in the cardiac beta-myosin heavy chain gene. Hypertrophic cardiomyopathy is characterized by hypercontractility that predisposes patients to the risk of sudden death. (Up to one-third of these patients may die from sudden cardiac death, usually related to physical exertion.) Therefore, treatment for patients is with drugs that decrease contractility.

HYPERPLASIA

Physiologic hyperplasia

- Breast enlargement
- Uterine enlargement

Compensatory hyperplasia

- Liver
- Kidney

Pathologic hyperplasia

- Erythroid hyperplasia
- Hyperplasia of lymph nodes
- Hyperplasia of smooth muscle cells of arteries
- Hyperplasia of the breast (gynecomastia and fibrocystic change)
- Endometrial hyperplasia
- Prostatic hyperplasia
- Hyperplasia of the lung
- Congenital adrenal hyperplasia

In contrast to hypertrophy, hyperplasia usually occurs in tissue with labile cells and stable cells. It may be the result of physiologic processes, compensatory processes, or pathologic processes. (Sometimes physiologic hyperplasia and compensatory hyperplasia also involve hypertrophy of cells. In fact, these combinations could be classified as being mixed hyperplasia-hypertrophy reactions.) Many times hyperplasia is the result of stimulation by hormones, for example, physiologic hyperplasia of the breast at puberty or during pregnancy (hyperplasia of the glands) or hyperplasia of the uterus during pregnancy (hyperplasia of the smooth muscle).

Loss of one kidney results in compensatory enlargement of the other kidney. This enlargement is due to an increase in the number of cells and size of the cells. Perhaps the best example of compensatory hyperplasia is the liver. A majority of the liver can be removed surgically, and the remaining tissue will regenerate and restore the normal function of the liver.

ERYTHROID HYPERPLASIA

Relative polycythemia

- Prolonged vomiting
- Diarrhea
- Excessive use of diuretics

Absolute polycythemia

1. Primary polycythemia
   - Polycythemia rubra vera
2. Secondary polycythemia
   a. Appropriate polycythemia
   - Lung disease
   - Cyanotic heart disease
   - High altitude
   - Abnormal hemoglobins with increased oxygen affinity
   b. Inappropriate polycythemia
   - Kidney cancer
   - Liver cancer

There are many examples of pathologic hyperplasia, and most are the result of stimulation by hormones. For example, erythropoietin, produced by the peritubular cells in the kidney, is essential for the differentiation of erythroid precursors. Increased levels of erythropoietin produces increased numbers of red blood cells (*polycythemia*). But increased numbers of red cells are not always the result of stimulation by erythropoietin. In fact, polycythemia may be a relative polycythemia due to a decrease in the plasma volume (hemoconcentration), or it may be an absolute polycythemia due to a real increase in the total red cell mass.

Absolute polycythemia may be a primary disorder, or it may be secondary to an increase in the production of erythropoietin. Primary polycythemia is due to a defect in myeloid stem cells and is called polycythemia rubra vera. In patients with polycythemia rubra vera, a myeloproliferative disorder, the red cell mass is increased, but the levels of erythropoietin are normal or decreased. The erythropoietin levels are low because the total oxygen content of the blood is actually increased, and there is no stimulus for increasing the secretion of erythropoietin.

In contrast to primary polycythemia, secondary polycythemias are the result of increased levels of erythropoietin. This increased erythropoietin may be appropriate (in response to tissue hypoxia) or inappropriate (due to paraneoplastic secretion of erythropoietin).

HYPERPLASIA INVOLVING LYMPH NODES

Follicular hyperplasia

- Chronic inflammation
- Rheumatoid arthritis
- AIDS (early)
- Toxoplasmosis

Paracortical hyperplasia

- Viral infections
- Vaccines
- Drugs
- SLE

Sinus histiocytosis

- Nonspecific reactions

Reactive processes involving lymph nodes typically involve different and specific portions of the lymph nodes depending upon the type of cell that is proliferating. For example, reactive B lymphocytes produce hyperplasia of the lymphoid follicles and germinal centers (follicular hyperplasia). Examples of disease that are associated with follicular hyperplasia include chronic inflammation caused by organisms, rheumatoid arthritis, and AIDS. Lymph nodes from patients with AIDS have characteristic changes that initially reveal follicular hyperplasia with loss of mantle zones, intrafollicular hemorrhage ("follicle lysis"), and monocytoid B cell proliferation. Next there is depletion of lymphocytes (CD4+ lymphocytes) in both the follicles and the interfollicular areas. Toxoplasmosis lymphadenitis is a mixed pattern of lymph node hyperplasia characterized by prominent follicular hyperplasia, *monocytoid B cell* hyperplasia, and small collections of epithelioid histiocytes infiltrating into the follicles.

In contrast to B cell hyperplasia, reactive T lymphocyte proliferations produce hyperplasia involving the T cell areas of the lymph node—the interfollicular regions and the paracortex. Examples of clinical situations producing a T lymphocyte response include viral infections (infectious mononucleosis), vaccinations (smallpox vaccinations), some drugs (Dilantin), and systemic lupus erythematosus.

Finally, the sinusoidal pattern of reaction involves expansion of the sinuses by increased numbers of macrophages as seen in reactive proliferations of the mononuclear-phagocytic system. The reaction (sinus histiocytosis) is non-specific.

HYPERPLASIA INVOLVING BLOOD VESSELS

- Malignant hypertension
- Atherosclerosis

The smooth muscle cells in the wall of arteries may proliferate in response to stretching of the wall (hypertension) or injury to the blood vessel (atherosclerosis). These two diseases will be discussed in detail in the chapter dealing with hemostasis and infarction.

HYPERPLASIA OF THE BREAST

Fibrocystic change

1. Nonproliferative changes
   - Fibrosis
   - Cysts
2. Proliferative changes
   - Epithelial hyperplasia
   - Papillomatosis
   - Sclerosing adenosis
   - Radial scar
   - Atypical hyperplasia

Gynecomastia

- Epithelial hyperplasia
- Periductal edema
- Hyalinized stroma

Two conditions of the breast associated with hyperplasia of the epithelial cells of the ducts are fibrocystic change (female breast) and gynecomastia (male breast). Fibrocystic change of the breast is one of the most common features seen in the female breast. It is most likely associated with an endocrine imbalance that produces an abnormality of the normal monthly cyclic changes of the breast. These fibrocystic changes are subdivided into nonproliferative and proliferative changes. Nonproliferative changes include fibrosis of the stroma and cystic dilatation of the terminal ducts (which when large may form blue-domed cysts). A common feature of the ducts in nonproliferative changes is *apocrine metaplasia*, which consists of epithelial cells with abundant eosinophilic cytoplasm and apical cytoplasmic "snouts." Proliferative changes include hyperplasia of the epithelial cells lining the ducts. These hyperplastic cells may form papillary structures (papillomatosis), or they may be cytologically abnormal (atypical hyperplasia).

Two benign, but clinically important, forms of proliferative fibrocystic change include sclerosing adenosis and radial scar. Both of these may be mistaken histologically for infiltrating ductal carcinoma, but the histologic finding of myoepithelial cells is a helpful sign that indicates the benign nature of the proliferation. Sclerosing adenosis is a disease of the terminal lobules that is seen in middle-aged female patients. It produces a firm mass, typically in the upper outer quadrant. Microscopically there is florid proliferation of small ductal structures in a fibrous stroma. Low power examination reveals the lesion is stellate in appearance, but it maintains the normal lobular architecture of the breast.

Fibrocystic change of the breast is not a premalignant change, but several features are associated with a greater than average risk for the subsequent development of breast carcinoma. Generally, this association is proportional to the degree of epithelial hyperplasia and atypia. Changes that do not have an increased risk of breast carcinoma include fibrosis, cystic change, apocrine metaplasia, and mild degrees of epithelial hyperplasia. Changes associated with a slightly increased risk include moderate to marked epithelial hyperplasia, marked ductal papillomatosis, and sclerosing adenosis. Changes associated with a significantly increased risk include atypical hyperplasia, which is characterized histologically by cellular and architectural atypia.

CAUSES OF GYNECOMASTIA

- Puberty
- Testicular tumors
- Alcoholic cirrhosis
- Klinefelter's syndrome
- Testicular feminization
- Increased prolactin
- Drugs

Gynecomastia, enlargement of the male breast, histologically reveals epithelial hyperplasia within ducts that are surrounded by hyalinized fibrous tissue and periductal edema. It is caused by an increase in the estrogen to androgen ratio. This abnormality may be found in males at the time of puberty. Other causes of gynecomastia include testicular tumors, alcohol-induced cirrhosis of the liver, Klinefelter's syndrome (decreased secretion of testosterone), testicular feminization (androgen insensitivity), increased prolactin levels, and certain drugs (digoxin). Testicular neoplasms that are associated with gynecomastia are tumors that secrete human chorionic gonadotropin (hCG). This hormone increases the synthesis of estradiol. Testicular tumors associated with the production of hCG include germ cell tumors (choriocarcinoma and seminoma), Leydig cell tumors, and Sertoli cell tumors.

HYPERPLASIA OF THE ENDOMETRIUM

- Simple hyperplasia → histologically similar to proliferative endometrium
- Cystic hyperplasia → simple hyperplasia with some dilated glands
- Complex hyperplasia → crowded endometrial glands without atypia
- Atypical hyperplasia → complex hyperplasia with atypia

Hyperplasia of the endometrium is the result of estrogen stimulation that is unopposed by progesterone. (Estrogen causes the normal proliferation of the endometrium during the first part of the menstrual cycle, the proliferative phase.) Sources for abnormal unopposed estrogen include polycystic ovarian disease (Stein-Leventhal syndrome), functional ovarian tumors, excess function of adrenal cortex, and prolonged administration of estrogen without progesterone.

There are several histologic types of endometrial hyperplasia including simple hyperplasia, complex hyperplasia, and atypical hyperplasia. Simple hyperplasia was previously classified as mild hyperplasia, but now is sometimes called cystic hyperplasia if some of the glands are dilated ("Swiss cheese" hyperplasia). Endometrial hyperplasia is important because of its relation to the development of cancer of the endometrium. The histologic feature that is most associated with cancer is the presence of cytologic atypia. Therefore, the type of hyperplasia that is most associated with cancer is atypical hyperplasia (which used to be called adenomatous hyperplasia with atypia).

HYPERPLASIA OF THE PROSTATE

- Increased levels of dihydrotestosterone (DHT)
- Hyperplastic glands (large, well developed, and separated from each other by intervening stroma)
- Hyperplastic stromal cells (smooth muscle cells and fibroblasts)
- Originates in transition zone around urethra
- Urinary obstruction

Hyperplasia of the prostate (benign prostatic hyperplasia or BPH) is an extremely common disorder and is associated with increased levels of dihydrotestosterone (DHT). The most significant metabolic product of testosterone is dihydrotestosterone (DHT), which is formed by the action of the enzyme 5alpha-reductase. DHT is responsible for the development of the prostate during fetal growth and at the time of puberty. With aging, DHT levels are increased in the prostate, where it binds to nuclear DNA and causes prostatic hyperplasia. This hyperplastic effect by DHT is augmented by both estrogen and testosterone.

The hyperplastic nodules of BPH characteristically originate around the urethra in the transitional zone of the prostate (median lobe and more central portions of the lateral lobes). This is in striking contrast to the distribution of prostatic carcinoma, which usually involves the posterior lobe. The location of these hyperplastic nodules is important clinically because the enlargement of the prostate impinges on the urethra and causes symptoms of urinary obstruction. These signs include urinary frequency, nocturia (increased urination at night), difficulty in starting and stopping urination, dribbling, and *dysuria*.

HYPERPLASIA OF THE LUNG
Type II pneumocyte hyperplasia
- Acute respiratory distress syndrome
- Usual interstitial pneumonitis

Two important lung diseases are associated with hyperplasia of type II pneumocytes—acute respiratory distress syndrome (ARDS) and usual interstitial pneumonitis (UIP). The alveoli of the lungs are lined by two main cell types, flattened type I pneumocytes (membranous pneumocytes) and rounded type II pneumocytes (granular pneumocytes). Type I pneumocytes are much more numerous (they cover about 95% of the alveolar surface), but type II pneumocytes are important because they are the source of pulmonary surfactant. They are also the main cells of repair of alveolar epithelium after destruction of type I pneumocytes. That is, destruction of type I pneumocytes results in proliferation of type II pneumocytes.

The basic lesion in ARDS is diffuse damage to the alveolar wall (DAD). There is damage to type I pneumocytes, and type II pneumocytes divide to replace them. This creates a cuboidal lining to the alveolar spaces that can be easily mistaken histologically for adenocarcinoma.

Interstitial pulmonary fibrosis (IF) is a slowly progressive pulmonary disease with no known etiology. The pathogenesis of UIP is similar to the initial damage-producing ARDS—damage to type I pneumocytes with subsequent hyperplasia of type II pneumocytes. Additionally, secretion of growth factors by macrophages produces interstitial fibrosis, which accounts for the major pathology of this disease.

HYPERPLASIA OF THE SKIN

- Acanthosis → hyperplasia of the epidermis
- Hyperkeratosis → increased keratin layer
- Hypergranulosis → hyperplasia of the granular layer
- Papillomatosis → epidermis forms papillary folds

HUMAN PAPILLOMAVIRUS

Verruca vulgaris

- HPV types 1, 2, and 4

Condyloma acuminata

- HPV types 6, 10, and 40 through 45

Cervical neoplasia

- Low risk → types 6 and 11
- Intermediate risk → 31, 33, 35, and 51
- High risk → 16 and 18

Hyperplasia of the cells of the epidermis causes the epidermis to become thick (*acanthosis*); hyperplasia of the keratin layer of the skin is called hyperkeratosis. Both of these changes can be seen in many different skin diseases, such as infection with human papillomavirus (HPV). There are many different subtypes of HPV, and each of these subtypes is associated with certain diseases, such as warts, laryngeal *papillomas*, and *dysplasia* of the cervix. Skin warts (verruca vulgaris) are caused by HPV types 1, 2, and 4. Histologic sections reveal increased keratin (hyperkeratosis) and an increase in the granular cell layer (hypergranulosis) with the formation of prominent keratohyaline granules. Often the hyperplastic epidermis forms papillary folds (papillomatosis). Anogenital warts (condyloma acuminata) are caused by HPV types 6, 10, 11, and 40 through 45. Finally, dysplasia of the cervix (precursor lesions of squamous cell carcinoma) is related to HPV types 16, 18, 31, 33, and 35. A characteristic histologic feature of

HPV infection of the cervix is *koilocytosis* (dark, shrunken, shriveled nuclei surrounded by clear spaces).

PSORIASIS

1. Red plaques covered by silver scales (extensor surfaces)
2. Increased turnover of epidermal cells
3. Microscopic features
   - *Parakeratosis*
   - Decreased granular cell layer
   - Regular elongation of rete ridges
4. Positive Auspitz sign and Koebner phenomenon

Two important diseases that are associated with hyperkeratosis of the skin are psoriasis and lichen planus. It is important to understand the clinical and pathologic differences between these two diseases. Psoriasis is a chronic skin disease that clinically is characterized by the formation of large, sharply defined, silver-white scaly plaques. These skin lesions are usually found on the extensor surfaces of the elbows and knees, the scalp, and the lumbosacral areas. If the scale of psoriasis is lifted, multiple, minute areas of bleeding will form. This is referred to as an Auspitz sign and is due to increased, dilated vessels within the papillary dermis. The formation of new lesions at sites of trauma is referred to as the Koebner phenomenon. This sign is also present in patients with psoriasis.

In patients with psoriasis, trauma may cause thickening of the epidermis (acanthosis), downward regular elongation of the rete ridges, hyperkeratosis, and parakeratosis. These changes may be related to faulty beta-adrenergic receptors and decreased activity of adenylyl cyclase in the lower epidermis. The pathogenesis of psoriasis is not well understood, but involves a faster turnover time of the epidermal kerotinocytes (about 3 days rather than the normal 28 days). Since the keratinocyte turnover time is faster, there is no granular cell layer.

LICHEN PLANUS

1. Pruritic purple papules and plaques (flexor surfaces)
2. Decreased turnover of epidermal cells
3. Microscopic features
   - Hyperkeratosis
   - Increased granular cell layer
   - Acanthosis with bandlike lymphocytic infiltrate at epidermal-dermal junction

---

Lichen planus is characterized by the formation of "pruritic, purple, polygonal papules" usually on flexor surfaces of the extremities (wrists and elbows). These lesions may also have white dots or lines within them (Wickham's striae). The basic defect in lichen planus is a decreased rate of keratinocyte proliferation (the exact opposite of the increased rate of keratinocyte proliferation in psoriasis).

Histologically the skin reveals a characteristic bandlike lymphocytic infiltrate in the superficial dermis. This infiltrate destroys the basal cell layer of the epidermis and causes a "saw-toothing" of the rete ridges. Additionally, anucleate, necrotic basal epidermal cells may be found in the inflamed papillary dermis. These cells are called colloid bodies or Civatte bodies. Because of the decreased rate of keratinocyte proliferation, there is an increase in the size of the granular cell layer (again, the opposite of psoriasis).

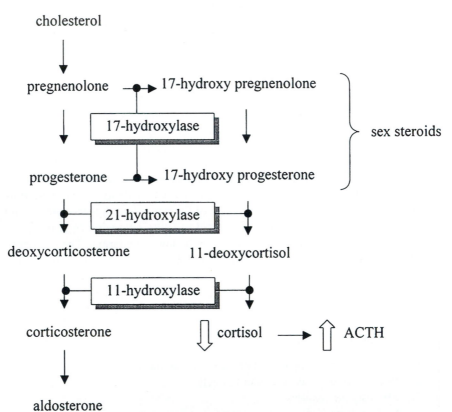

Figure 5-3 Congenital Adrenal Hyperplasia
Congenital adrenal hyperplasia is associated with deficiencies of either 17-hydroxylase, 21-hydroxylase, or 11-hydroxylase. All of these enzyme deficiencies produce a deficiency of cortisol, and a deficiency of cortisol produces an increase in ACTH. This in turn causes hyperplasia of the adrenal cortex.

HYPERPLASIA OF THE ADRENAL GLANDS

Congenital adrenal hyperplasia

1. Enzyme deficiency
   - 21-hydroxylase deficiency
   - 11-hydroxylase deficiency
   - 17-hydroxylase deficiency
2. Decreased cortisol
3. Increased ACTH

Congenital adrenal hyperplasia (CAH) is a syndrome characterized by decreased synthesis of cortisol and hyperplasia of the cortex of the adrenal glands. Decreased levels of cortisol lead to excess secretion of ACTH by the anterior pituitary, and this produces the adrenal hyperplasia. The defect in the synthesis of cortisol is the result of a deficiency in one of the enzymes in the normal pathway of cortisol synthesis, such as 21-hydroxylase of 11-hydroxylase (Fig. 5-3).

21-HYDROXYLASE DEFICIENCY

Salt-wasting syndrome

- Complete loss of 21-hydroxylase
- Decreased cortisol → increased ACTH
- Decreased aldosterone
- Sodium loss in the urine
- Hyperkalemic acidosis
- Virilism in females

Simple virilizing adrenogenitalism

- Partial loss of 21-hydroxylase
- Decreased cortisol → increased ACTH
- Aldosterone not decreased
- No sodium loss in the urine (not salt wasting)
- Virilism in females

Most cases of CAH result from deficiency of 21-hydroxylase. There are two forms of 21-hydroxylase deficiency: salt-wasting adrenogenitalism and simple virilizing adrenogenitalism. The salt-wasting syndrome results from a complete lack of the hydroxylase. This deficiency causes no synthesis of both mineralo-corticoids and glucocorticoids. A deficiency of mineralocorticoids (aldosterone) produces marked sodium loss in the urine, hence the name "salt-wasting" syndrome. Aldosterone normally causes increased potassium and hydrogen ion excretion in the urine. The serum results of decreased aldosterone are decreased sodium levels (hyponatremia), increased potassium levels (hyperkalemia), and increased hydrogen ion levels (acidosis). A deficiency of glucocorticoids (cortisol) produces increased levels of ACTH, which stimulates the cells of the adrenal cortex. Because of the enzyme block, increased amounts of 17-hydroxyprogesterone are shunted into the production of testosterone. In female infants this increased testosterone production can cause virilism (pseudohermaphroditism). Genetic XX females with CAH develop ovaries, female ductal structures, and external male genitalia. The Müllerian ducts develop into the fallopian tubes and uterus, while the Wolffian ducts regress.

More commonly, however, there is only a partial deficiency of 21-hydroxylase (simple virilizing adrenogenitalism). This leads to decreased production of both aldosterone and cortisol. The decreased cortisol levels causes increased production of ACTH by the pituitary and adrenal hyperplasia. Because there is only a partial deficiency of 21-hydroxylase, the hyperplasia of the cells of the adrenal cortex is enough to maintain adequate serum levels of aldosterone and cortisol. Therefore, there is no sodium loss or salt wasting. The excess stimulation by ACTH, however, again leads to increased production of androgens, which may cause virilism (pseudohermaphroditism) in female infants.

11-HYDROXYLASE DEFICIENCY

- Loss of 11-hydroxylase
- Decreased cortisol → increased ACTH
- Decreased aldosterone
- Increased DOC and 11-deoxycortisol → increased mineralocorticoid effects
- Sodium retention → hypertensive form of CAH
- Hypokalemic alkalosis
- Virilism in females

A deficiency of 11-hydroxylase, which is rare, also leads to decreased cortisol production and increased ACTH secretion. This again causes hyperplasia of the adrenal cortical cells, but because the levels of 21-hydroxylase are normal there is increased synthesis of deoxycorticosterone (DOC) and 11-deoxycortisol. Both of these substances are strong mineralocorticoids (like aldosterone). Therefore instead of developing signs of aldosterone deficiency (as with 21-hydroxylase deficiency), patients with a deficiency of 11-hydroxylase develop signs of aldosterone excess—increased sodium retention by the kidneys with loss of potassium and hydrogen ions. Retention of salt and water produces hypertension (hence the name being the hypertensive form of CAH). Serum levels of potassium are decreased (hypokalemia) and hydrogen ions are decreased (alkalosis). Patients also develop virilization due to androgen excess.

17-HYDROXYLASE DEFICIENCY

- Loss of 17-hydroxylase
- Decreased cortisol → increased ACTH
- No decreased aldosterone
- Decreased sex hormones
- Females → primary amenorrhea
- Males → pseudohermaphrodites

Patients with a deficiency of 17-hydroxylase also have impaired cortisol production, increased ACTH, and secondary increased DOC. In contrast to 21-hydroxylase and 11-hydroxylase deficiencies, however, patients with a deficiency of 17-hydroxylase cannot synthesize normal amounts of androgens and estrogens. This is because the gene that codes for 17 α hydroxylase is the same in the adrenal cortex and the gonads, and the deficiency is the same in both organs. Because of decreased sex hormones, genotypic females develop primary *amenorrhea* and fail to develop secondary sex characteristics. Genotypic males present as pseudohermaphrodites. Additionally, plasma LH levels are increased because of decreased feedback inhibition.

METAPLASIA

Squamous metaplasia

- Cervix
- Respiratory tract

Gastric metaplasia

- Barrett's esophagus

Intestinal metaplasia

- Atrophic gastritis

Myeloid metaplasia

• Myelofibrosis

Osseous metaplasia

• Myositis ossificans

Metaplasia is the replacement of one cell type by another. For example, squamous metaplasia is the formation of stratified squamous epithelium in a site that normally does not have stratified squamous epithelium. Common locations for squamous metaplasia are the respiratory tract and the cervix. Squamous metaplasia of the respiratory tract is commonly the result of smoking.

Squamous metaplasia of the cervix of the uterus involves the "transformation zone." It is important to realize that this transformation zone is not the same as the transition zone of the cervix. The latter refers to the squamocolumnar junction of the cervix that is the demarcation between the squamous epithelium of the ectocervix and the columnar epithelium of the endocervix. This junction initially is located at the internal os of the cervix. In most women, the columnar epithelium will extend beyond the os onto the ectocervix, this change being called an endocervical ectropion. The area from this squamocolumnar junction to the internal cervical os, which appears clinically as reddish discolorations (and clinically is referred to incorrectly as "erosions"), will then undergo squamous metaplasia. This area of squamous metaplasia is called the transformation zone. The importance of knowing about this area is that the transformation zone is the area where almost all cervical intraepithelial neoplasia (CIN) begin.

Another example of metaplasia is Barrett's esophagus. In patients with persistent gastroesophageal reflux, the distal esophagus may become lined with columnar secretory epithelium (gastric or intestinal type epithelium) instead of the usual stratified squamous epithelium. This is an example of a metaplastic change. (Intestinal metaplasia may be seen in Barrett's esophagus and atrophic gastritis.) Barrett's esophagus appears grossly as a red, velvety plaque in the distal esophagus. In patients with Barrett's esophagus, the columnar epithelium may become dysplastic and may lead to the development of invasive adenocarcinoma. Adenocarcinoma represents the most serious complication of Barrett's esophagus. This is in contrast to the most common carcinoma of the esophagus, which is squamous cell carcinoma (infiltrating groups of squamous epithelial cells).

MYELOFIBROSIS WITH MYELOID METAPLASIA

- Bone marrow → fibrosis
- Spleen → myeloid metaplasia
- Peripheral blood → leukoerythroblastosis plus teardrop red cells

---

Myelofibrosis is a *myeloproliferative syndrome* which is characterized by a hypocellular, fibrotic bone marrow (myelofibrosis) and a proliferation of myeloid stem cells in the spleen (myeloid metaplasia). The cause of the myelofibrosis is not known, and the disease is sometimes called agnogenic (idiopathic) myeloid metaplasia. The fibroblasts that replace the marrow do not belong to the neoplastic hematopoietic clone of myeloid stem cells. These marrow fibroblasts may be stimulated by an inappropriate release from megakaryocytes of PDGF (platelet-derived growth factor) and transforming growth factor beta (also found within the platelets).

The peripheral smear of patients with myelofibrosis is markedly abnormal. Immature red cells (nucleated red cells) and immature white cells are seen. Platelets are decreased in number and are abnormal in size, shape, and function. The combination of teardrop red blood cells, immature red cells and white cells (*leukoerythroblastosis*), and abnormal platelets in the peripheral smear is highly suggestive of myeloid metaplasia with myelofibrosis.

CELL SIGNALING

·

- Cell signaling
- Receptors
- Normal Processes Involving Intracellular Receptors
- Examples of Second Messengers
- Protein Kinases
- G Proteins
- Forms of G Proteins
- Second Messengers of G Proteins
- Infections Associated with G Proteins
- Cytoplasmic Calcium Regulation
- Calcium-Binding Proteins
- Substances that Use Gs Protein Receptors
- Substances that Use Gi Protein Receptors
- Substances that Use Gq Protein Receptors
- Substances that Use Gt Protein Receptors
- Processes Involving Second Messengers
- Adrenergic Receptors
- Adrenergic Effects
- Abnormal Processes Involving Gs Protein Receptors
- Abnormal Processes Involving Gi Protein Receptors
- Abnormal Processes Using Gq Protein Receptors
- Asthma
- Arachidonic Acid
- Normal Processes Involving Arachidonic Acid Products
- Leukotrienes
- Prostaglandins
- Tyrosine Kinases
- Ion Channels
- Cystic Fibrosis

CELL SIGNALING

Signaling without involving the extracellular fluid

* Gap Junctions

Signaling involving the extracellular fluid

* Neural signaling → release of a neurotransmitter from a nerve cell at a synaptic junction
* Autocrine effect → actions on the cell that produced the chemical signal
* Paracrine effect → actions on cells in the vicinity of the cell that produced the chemical signal
* Endocrine effect → actions on many cells systemically
* Juxtacrine effect → action on a nearby cell by a chemical signal attached to a cell surface

---

A tremendous number of diseases involve abnormal communication between cells. Before we can examine these abnormal processes, we first need to discuss the normal process through which cells communicate with other cells. Cells communicate with other cells by means of chemical messengers (signaling molecules). These messengers include proteins, peptides, amino acids, steroids, and fatty acid derivatives. Basically these chemical transmitters can travel from cell to cell directly (through gap junctions) or indirectly through the extracellular fluid (ECF). In the latter process the signaling cell secretes a signaling molecule that binds to a receptor on the target cell. These receptors may be located on the surface of the cell membrane, or they may be located in the cytoplasm of the target cell.

Chemical signaling molecules have their effects in one of several ways. Neural signaling basically involves the release of a neurotransmitter from a nerve cell at a synaptic junction. This neurotransmitter crosses a synaptic cleft to reach a postsynaptic cell. *Autocrine effects* refer to actions on the cell that produced the chemical signaling molecules. *Paracrine effects* refer to actions on cells in the vicinity of the cell that produced the chemical signal, while *endocrine effects* refer to actions on many cells systemically. Hormones generally act via an endocrine effect. Finally, sometimes a transmitter is attached to the surface of a cell and interacts with a receptor on a nearby cell. This is called juxtacrine communication, an example of which is transforming growth factor α.

RECEPTORS

Cell membrane receptors

- Ion-channel-linked
- G-protein-linked
- Enzyme-linked (protein kinases and arachidonic acid metabolism)

Non–cell membrane receptors

- Intracellular receptors

NORMAL PROCESSES INVOLVING INTRACELLULAR RECEPTORS

- Thyroid hormones
- Steroid hormones
- Vitamin A
- Vitamin D

Indirect cell communication involving the extracellular fluid (including the blood) results in chemical messengers binding to cell receptors. These receptors can be attached to the cell membrane, or they can be located within the cytoplasm. Substances that use intracellular receptors are lipid-soluble molecules (lipophilic) that can pass right through the lipid plasma membrane. (Since these substances are hydrophobic, they must be transported in blood attached to carrier proteins.) Examples of substances that use this mechanism are some hormones (thyroid hormones and steroid hormones) and fat-soluble vitamins (mainly A and D). Once inside the cell, these substances generally go to the nucleus and bind to the hormone response element (HRE) of DNA. HRE is part of the regulatory DNA region that is found 5′ to the gene to be regulated.

EXAMPLES OF SECOND MESSENGERS

- cAMP
- cGMP
- Inositol triphosphate (IP3)
- Diacylglycerol (DAG)
- Calcium
- Arachidonic acid

PROTEIN KINASES

Phosphorylation of serine or threonine residues

1. Calmodulin-dependent
2. Calcium-phospholipid-dependent
   - Protein kinase C
3. Cyclin nucleotide–dependent
   - cAMP
   - cGMP

Phosphorylation of tyrosine residues (tyrosine kinase activity)

- Insulin receptor
- Epidermal growth factor receptor
- Platelet-derived growth factor receptor
- M-CSF receptor

The chemical messengers that do not bind to intracellular receptors instead bind to receptors located on the cell membrane and cause the release of different intracellular chemical messengers. The extracellular chemical messenger (ligand) that binds to the cell membrane receptor is called the "first messenger"; the intracellular chemical messenger is called the "second messenger." Second messengers generally function by activating protein kinases, which are enzymes that can phosphorylate amino acid residues. The main types of amino acids that are phosphorylated by these protein kinases include serine, threonine, and tyrosine.

G PROTEINS

- Inactive → bound to GDP
- Active → bound to GTP

The two most important second messengers are cyclic AMP (cAMP) and calcium. The intracellular concentrations of these two substances are under the control of cell membrane receptors linked to substances that interact with GTP. Substances that bind to GTP (the guanosine analogue of ATP) are called *G proteins*. Basically G proteins may be bound to either GDP or GTP. When these proteins are bound to GDP they are inactive, but when they are bound to GTP they are active. When a chemical messenger binds to the inactive G protein, GTP is exchanged for the bound GDP, causing the G protein to become active. These active GTP-bound G proteins have inherent GTPase activity that converts the

GTP back to GDP. This reaction inactivates the G proteins (they turn themselves off).

GTP-binding proteins generally need two additional components that can catalyze each of these two steps—the activating step where GDP is exchanged for GTP, and the inactivating step where GTP is converted to GDP. Guanine-nucleotide-releasing proteins (GNRP) catalyze the exchange of GDP for GTP, while GTPase-activating proteins (*GAP*) catalyze the hydrolysis of GTP.

FORMS OF G PROTEINS

Monomeric G proteins

- *Rab* proteins → regulate intracellular transport vesicles
- *Ras* proteins

Trimeric G proteins

1. Adenyl cyclase
   - Gs
   - Gi
2. Guanyl cyclase
   - Gt
3. Phospholipase C
   - Gq

SECOND MESSENGERS OF G PROTEINS

Cyclic AMP

- Gs
- Gi

Calcium

- Gp

Cyclic GMP

- Gt

G proteins basically exist in one of two forms: small monomeric forms and larger trimeric forms. The smaller monomeric forms of G proteins are involved in three basic functions: interactions between the cytoskeleton and the cell membrane, regulation of the transport of intracellular vesicles, or control of cell growth. Of these three main functions, the most important is the *ras* protein, which is involved in the control of cell growth.

The trimeric G proteins are a part of a larger membrane receptor complex that consists of the receptor, the catalytic enzyme (such as adenyl cyclase), and a coupling unit between the receptor and the enzyme. The coupling unit consists of the trimeric G proteins. The three fragments of the trimeric G proteins consist of the α unit, the β unit, and the γ unit. The α units are active only when bound to GTP and are inactive when bound to GDP.

The G proteins are subclassified according to the type of α subunit that is present. Basically there are four groups of trimeric G proteins: Gs, Gi, Gt, and Gq. These four groups involve only three membrane enzymes. Gs and Gi are involved with membrane adenyl cyclase, Gt with guanylate cyclase, and Gq with phospholipase C. The two most important enzymes of this group are adenyl cyclase and phospholipase C. Adenyl cyclase basically modulates the intracytoplasmic levels of cAMP, while phospholipase C (PLC) modulates the intracytoplasmic levels of calcium.

The two G proteins associated with adenyl cyclase may be either stimulatory (Gs) or inhibitory (Gi). Basically they either increase or decrease the intracytoplasmic levels of cAMP (Fig. 6-1). How does this occur? Adenyl cyclase, located on the inner surface of the plasma membrane, catalyzes the formation of cAMP from ATP. Binding of a substance to the Gs receptor causes stimulation of adenyl cyclase and increases the cytoplasmic levels of cAMP. Think of the Gs receptor as being the "on" switch. This "on" switch is in the "on" position when Gαs is bound to GTP and is stimulating adenyl cyclase. When Gαs is bound to GDP there is no stimulation of adenyl cyclase and the "on" switch is in the "off" position.

Once formed cAMP generally converts inactive protein kinases into active protein kinases. Therefore stimulation of Gs receptors increases the production of active protein kinases, while stimulation of Gi receptors decreases their production. Importantly, cAMP is inactivated by being converted to $5'$ AMP by the enzyme phosphodiesterase. This enzyme is inhibited by methylxanthines, such as caffeine and theophylline (letter "c" in Fig. 6-1). These methylxanthines, therefore, prolong the effects of cAMP and prolong the effects of Gs-stimulatory substances.

In contrast to Gs receptors, binding of a substance to the Gi receptor inhibits adenyl cyclase and decreases the cytoplasmic levels of cAMP. Think of this as being the "off" switch. This "off" switch is in the "on" (functioning) position when Gαi is bound to GTP and is inhibiting adenyl cyclase. When Gαi is bound to GDP there is no inhibition of adenyl cyclase and the "off" switch is in the "off" (nonfunctioning) position. One more important effect of Gi proteins is to activate potassium ion channels in atrial myocardial cells. This receptor complex, which can be stimulated by muscarinic cholinergic agonists, hyperpolarizes the myocardial cell.

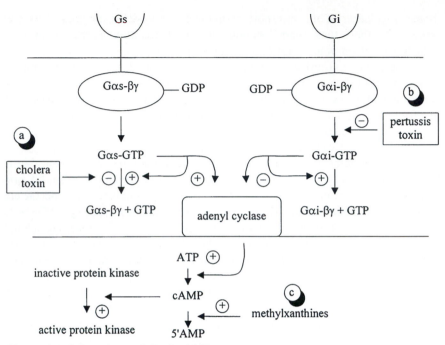

Figure 6-1 G Proteins and Cyclic AMP
G proteins are inactive when bound to GDP, but are active when bound to GTP. Gs proteins when bound to GTP (active) activate adenyl cyclase; Gi proteins when bound to GTP (active) inhibit adenyl cyclase. G proteins bound to GTP have GTPase activity, which can convert the bound GTP to GDP. This intrinsic activity enables active G proteins to inactivate themselves.

INFECTIONS ASSOCIATED WITH G PROTEINS

Gs protein receptors

- *Vibrio cholera* toxin
- *Escherichia coli* toxin

Gi protein receptors

- *Bordetella pertussis*

Cholera toxin and pertussis toxin both act by altering the adenyl cyclase pathway (Fig. 6-1). Cholera enterotoxin inhibits the conversion of Gαs-GTP to Gαs-βγ and GDP. (*Enterotoxins* are exotoxins that act upon intestinal mucosal cells.) The mechanism of the enterotoxins produced by *Escherichia coli* is similar to the vibrio toxin. These toxins are ADP-ribosyl transferases that transfer

NAD to membrane Gαs-proteins and inhibit them. Think of these toxins as keeping the "on" switch in the "on" position (letter "a" in Fig. 6-1). In the colonic crypts chloride flows through chloride channels from inside the cell into the colonic lumen. These chloride channels are controlled by cAMP, and increased intracellular cAMP levels cause these channels to open wider. Both of the enterotoxins produce a secretory type of diarrhea. *Vibrio cholera* produces "rice water" stools, while enterotoxigenic *E. coli* is a major cause of "traveler's diarrhea."

In contrast, pertussis toxin (produced by *Bordetella pertussis*, the causative agent for whooping cough) is an ADP-ribosyl transferase that inhibits the activation of Gαi-βγ to Gαi-GTP. Think of pertussis toxin as keeping the "off" switch in the "off" position (letter "b" in Fig. 6-1). *Bordetella pertussis* is a small, gram-negative coccobacillus that kills ciliated respiratory epithelial cells and produces prolonged coughing paroxysms (whooping cough). The pertussis toxin also causes a characteristic, pronounced peripheral lymphocytosis. (Both cholera toxin and pertussis toxin prolong the functioning of adenyl cyclase and increase intracellular cAMP, but the mechanisms are different. Cholera toxin keeps the "on" switch in the "on" position, while pertussis toxin keeps the "off" switch in the "off" position.)

Another important G protein uses Gq membrane receptors (Fig. 6-2). These receptors activate membrane phospholipase C (PLC) and eventually function by increasing intracellular calcium levels. This is a very important and very common second messenger system. Attachment of a substance to a cell surface receptor that is coupled to a Gq protein activates phospholipase C. This enzyme converts phosphatidylinositol 4,5-diphosphate (PIP2) to diacylglycerol (DAG) and inositol triphosphate (IP3). DAG is glycerol plus 2 fatty acids (in contrast triglycerides are glycerol plus 3 fatty acids). Increased DAG stimulates protein kinase C, which produces a response by phosphorylating proteins. Increased IP3 causes the release of calcium from intracellular storage sites such as the sarcoplasmic reticulum and mitochondria. Increased intracytoplasmic calcium may bind to calmodulin, which in turn may activate many different enzymes, such as adenylate cyclase, glycogen synthase, and pyruvate kinase.

CYTOPLASMIC CALCIUM REGULATION

Increased entry of calcium into cells

- Voltage-gated calcium channels
- Ligand-gated calcium channels

Increased release from intracellular stores

- Endoplasmic reticulum
- Mitochondria

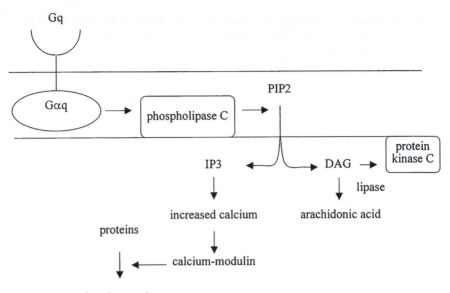

Figure 6-2 G Proteins and Intracellular Calcium
Binding of a chemical messenger to a Gq receptor stimulates membrane phospholipase C and increases intracellular levels of IP3 and DAG. IP3 increases intracytoplasmic calcium levels. DAG forms arachidonic acid and stimulates protein kinase C. (Don't confuse phospholipase C with protein kinase C.)

CALCIUM-BINDING PROTEINS

- Skeletal muscle → troponin
- Smooth muscle → calmodulin

Calcium is a very important intracellular second messenger, and the intracellular calcium concentration is an important regulator of many processes. Cytoplasmic calcium levels can be increased by increasing the entry of calcium into the cell or by releasing calcium from intracellular stores. Calcium can enter cells via two types of membrane channels: voltage-gated channels and ligand-gated channels. Voltage-gated channels are opened by depolarization of the membrane; ligand-gated channels are opened by the binding of different types of neurotransmitters and hormones. The main process by which second messengers increase intracytoplasmic calcium, however, is by stimulating the release of stored calcium (the main intracellular storage site of calcium is the endoplasmic reticulum). IP3 is the major second messenger that causes this increased release of calcium stores.

Increased intracytoplasmic calcium functions by binding to intracytoplasmic substances, such as troponin and calmodulin. Troponin is the calcium-binding protein that is involved in the contraction of skeletal muscle. Calmodulin is a calcium-binding protein that is capable of activating several types of kinases, such as phosphorylase kinase (which activates glycogen breakdown) and myosin light-chain kinase (which activates smooth muscle contraction).

In contrast to Gs and Gi, Gt receptors activate guanylate cyclase, an enzyme that converts GTP to cGMP (Fig. 6-3). The membrane receptor is bound to Gαt which when activated stimulates guanylate cyclase. Increased intracellular cGMP converts inactive protein kinases to active protein kinases. This mechanism is analogous to the functioning of Gs and adenyl cyclase, but in contrast to Gs receptors (which are very common), very few substances use cGMP as a second messenger. Examples of substances that use this mechanism include rhodopsin, atrial natriuretic factor, and nitrous oxide.

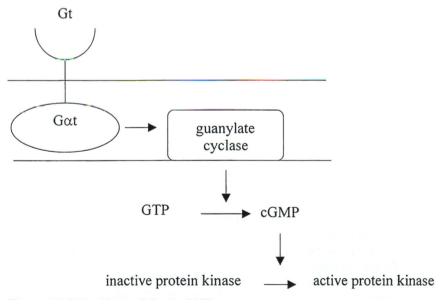

Figure 6-3 G Proteins and Cyclic GMP
Binding of a chemical messenger to a Gt receptor stimulates membrane guanylate cyclase and increases intracellular cGMP. This mechanism is very similar to Gs receptors and intracellular cAMP.

SUBSTANCES THAT USE Gs PROTEIN RECEPTORS

1. Peptide hormones
   - Thyroid stimulating hormone (TSH)
   - Luteinizing hormone (LH)
   - Follicle stimulating hormone (FSH)
   - Adrenocorticotrophic hormone (ACTH)
   - Parathyroid hormone (PTH)
   - Vasopressin (antidiuretic hormone, ADH), via V2 receptor
   - Calcitonin
   - Glucagon
   - Human chorionic gonadotropin (HCG)
2. Catecholamines
3. Prostaglandins

SUBSTANCES THAT USE Gi PROTEIN RECEPTORS

- Catecholamines
- Prostaglandins

SUBSTANCES THAT USE Gq PROTEIN RECEPTORS

1. Peptide hormones
   - Vasopressin (ADH), via V1 receptors
   - Angiotensin II
   - Thrombin
   - Gonadotropin releasing hormone (GnRH)
   - Thyrotropin releasing hormone (TRH)
   - Gonadotropin releasing hormone (GHRH)
2. Catecholamines
   - Acetylcholine
3. Prostaglandins
   - Thromboxane
4. Leukotrienes

SUBSTANCES THAT USE Gt PROTEIN RECEPTORS

- Rhodopsin
- Atrial natriuretic factor (ANF)
- Nitrous oxide

There are many different substances that function via G protein receptors. Lists like these are hard to memorize, and are exceptionally difficult to remember for any length of time. It is better to look instead at the individual processes involving these chemical messengers.

PROCESSES INVOLVING SECOND MESSENGERS

Growth factors

- Cell growth
- Neoplasia

Hormones

- Metabolic processes
- Secretion and absorption

Blood-associated processes

- Inflammation
- Hemostasis

Catecholamines

- Cardiovascular
- Metabolic processes
- Fluids and electrolytes

Many processes, both normal and abnormal, involve cell communication via second messengers. These processes can be grouped into four general categories: growth factors, hormonal processes, blood-associated processes, and processes associated with catecholamines. Growth factors obviously are concerned with cell growth, but they are quite important in abnormal processes, such as the formation of cancer.

Hormonal functions associated with second messengers involve metabolism (regulating fat cells, liver cells, and muscle) or secretion and absorption (an example being the intestinal cell). Blood-associated factors include inflammation (which involves white blood cells) and hemostasis (which involves platelets and endothelial cells).

ADRENERGIC RECEPTORS

Gs receptors

- β1 and β2 adrenergic
- Dopaminergic type 1

Gi receptors

- α2 adrenergic
- Dopaminergic type 2

Gq receptors

- α1 adrenergic

ADRENERGIC EFFECTS

Alpha Receptors

1. α1
   - Vasoconstriction of peripheral blood vessels
   - Increased blood pressure
   - Constipation
2. α2
   - Decreased CNS sympathetics
   - Decreased blood pressure
   - Increased blood glucose

Beta Receptors

1. β1
   - Increased cardiac output (increased heart rate and stroke volume)

> **2. β2**
>   - Vasodilation of blood vessels in heart and skeletal muscle
>   - Decreased blood pressure
>   - Smooth muscle relaxation in lungs (bronchodilation)

Many hormones and catecholamines function by binding to cell membrane G protein receptors. Importantly, the effects of the autonomic system are mediated by second messengers through the actions of G proteins. To review briefly, the autonomic system influences both the heart and peripheral blood vessels. The actions of the sympathetic system are through the release of norepinephrine by nerves and epinephrine from the adrenal medulla.

There are two major types of adrenergic receptors, namely α and β. Norepinephrine stimulates α1 receptors and β1 receptors of the heart. Epinephrine stimulates α1 receptors and β1 receptors, but also β2 receptors. In contrast, the parasympathetic system decreases the heart rate by the release of acetylcholine from the vagus nerve, which stimulates M2 receptors.

How do these different receptors relate to the different types of G protein receptors? β1 (found mainly on the heart), β2 (found in the lungs), and β3 receptors (found in lipocytes) activate Gs receptors and increased intracellular cAMP levels. In contrast, α2 receptors and M2 receptors (found in the heart) act via Gi receptors to decrease intracellular cAMP levels. Alpha1 receptors contract vascular smooth muscle cells in the skin and GI tract and act via Gq receptors to activate membrane phospholipase C.

ABNORMAL PROCESSES INVOLVING Gs PROTEIN RECEPTORS

- Defective formation of the α subunit of Gs
- Infections
- Asthma

ABNORMAL PROCESSES INVOLVING Gi PROTEIN RECEPTORS

- Infections

We are very interested in how abnormalities of these normal processes can result in disease. For example, several diseases result from defects involving the gene that codes for the α subunit of Gs. One defect inhibits the functioning of parathyroid hormone (PTH), one of the many hormones that bind to Gs membrane proteins. This defect produces an end-organ insensitivity to the actions of PTH and manifests clinically as decreased serum calcium levels (hypocalcemia). Usually hypocalcemia is the result of decreased production of PTH (hypoparathyroidism), but in patients with a defective Gs, the serum levels of PTH are increased. The combination of decreased calcium levels and increased PTH levels is called pseudohypoparathyroidism.

Another defect involving the α subunit of Gs produces hyperpigmented skin lesions and increased serum cortisol levels. These patients (Albright's hereditary osteodystrophy) have other characteristic signs and symptoms including short stature, subcutaneous calcifications, reduced intelligence, and abnormally short metacarpal and metatarsal bones.

A third mutation in the α subunit of Gs decreases the intrinsic GTPase activity in G proteins. This defect is associated with increased cyclic ATP levels in the cells of the pituitary and is associated with an increased incidence of neoplasms (pituitary adenomas).

ABNORMAL PROCESSES USING Gq PROTEIN RECEPTORS

Blood-associated processes

1. Inflammation
   - Leukocyte activation
   - Leukocyte chemotaxis
   - Mast cell activation
2. Hemostasis
   - Platelet activation

Growth factors

- Neoplasia

Other

- Asthma

Examples of functions that utilize the phospholipase C pathway include leukocyte chemotaxis and activation, platelet activation, and neoplasia. We will discuss leukocyte chemotaxis and activation in the chapter on inflammation, platelet activation in the chapter dealing with hemostasis, and neoplasia in a separate chapter by itself.

For now we will look at one important disease that involves the contraction of the smooth muscle cells that line the airways. Asthma is an obstructive disease of the lungs that is characterized by excessive contraction of the smooth muscle cells of the airways. This excess bronchoconstriction results in obstruction of expiratory airflow, marked *dyspnea*, and wheezing. To understand the pathogenesis of asthma we need to first review briefly the normal functioning of the airway smooth muscle cell (Fig. 6-4). Basically contraction of the airway smooth muscle cell (ASM) is the result of increased intracytoplasmic levels of calcium. The calcium binds to calmodulin and activates myosin light-chain kinase to phosphorylate myosin. This causes contraction of the ASM cell. (This is different from contraction in heart muscle and skeletal muscle, where calcium binds to troponin C.)

Normally the parasympathetic system stimulates ASM contraction (via the vagus and acetylcholine release), while the sympathetic system inhibits ASM

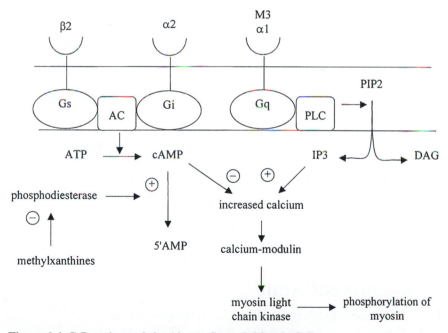

Figure 6-4 G Proteins and the Airway Smooth Muscle Cell
Asthma results from excess contraction of the airway smooth muscle cell. Contraction results from increased intracytoplasmic calcium. Gq receptors increase intracellular IP3 and calcium. In contrast, Gs receptors increase intracellular cAMP and decrease intracellular calcium.

contraction (via epinephrine release from the adrenal medulla). M3 cholinergic and α1 adrenergic receptors are attached to Gq receptors that stimulate membrane phospholipase C and increase intracytoplasmic calcium. This causes contraction of the ASM cell. This system is balanced by β2 receptors, which are bound to Gs. Stimulation of these receptors activates adenyl cyclase and increases intracytoplasmic levels of cAMP. This counteracts the increased cytoplasmic levels of calcium.

ASTHMA

1. Obstructive lung disease
2. Expiratory obstruction
3. Wheezing and coughing
4. Excess contraction of airway smooth muscle cells
5. Types
   • Immunologic extrinsic
   • Nonimmunologic intrinsic

There are two types of asthma: immunologic extrinsic asthma and nonimmunologic intrinsic asthma. Immunologic asthma is the most common type of asthma and occurs primarily in children. Exposure to certain antigens (dust, pollens, foods, and drugs) results in an IgE-mediated type I hypersensitivity reaction in which mast cells release multiple mediators, such as histamine, leukotrienes, and prostaglandins. These substances cause bronchoconstriction and increased mucus secretion.

The nonimmunologic form of asthma is thought to result from an abnormality of the parasympathetic control of airway function. As stated above and seen in Figure 6-4, cholinergic and alpha-adrenergic stimulation causes bronchoconstriction and mucosal secretion, whereas beta-adrenergic stimulation does the reverse. It is thought that cold temperature, exercise, and air pollution can stimulate excess cholinergic and alpha-adrenergic vagal effects and lead to excess bronchoconstriction and the characteristic changes of asthma.

ARACHIDONIC ACID

• Polyunsaturated fatty acid found in membranes of cells
• Formed by the actions of phospholipase A2 or DAG
• Steroids inhibit phospholipase A2
• Metabolism by lipoxygenase produces leukotrienes
• Metabolism by cyclooxygenase produces prostaglandins

Another important second messenger system involves receptor activation of phospholipase A2 and formation of arachidonic acid. Take a look at Figure 6-5. It briefly describes the pathways involved in the metabolism of arachidonic acid. Although this is a complicated pathway, it is quite important and well worth the time spent in understanding it.

Arachidonic acid (AA) is a polyunsaturated fatty acid that is normally found within the phospholipids of the membranes of cells. (Fatty acids have long alkyl chains and the side chain of arachidonic acid is 20 carbons in length.) How is arachidonic acid formed? It is released from membrane phospholipid by the activation of certain phospholipases, such as phospholipase A2. (One way to remember this is to associate "A2" with the two first letters of arachidonic acid.) Very important is the fact that steroids can inhibit this step and thus can inhibit the formation of arachidonic acid. This is the basis for one of the reasons why steroids can be used to treat some of the signs of acute inflammation. It is impor-

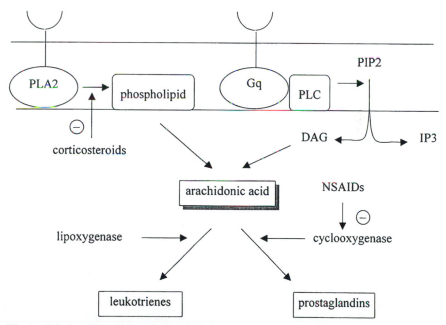

Figure 6-5 Arachidonic Acid Formation
Arachidonic acid can be formed from membrane phospholipid by the action of phospholipase A2 (PLA2) or from DAG by the action of lipase. Corticosteroids inhibit the formation of arachidonic acid by inhibiting the enzyme PLA2. Arachidonic acid is then converted into leukotrienes or prostaglandins. Nonsteroidal anti-inflammatory drugs (NSAIDs), such as aspirin and indomethacin, inhibit the formation of prostaglandins by inhibiting the enzyme cyclooxygenase.

tant to realize that arachidonic acid can also be formed from DAG by the enzyme lipase. This pathway is part of the second messenger system using the G protein Gq.

Arachidonic acid can then be metabolized by one of two pathways. The enzyme cyclooxygenase converts arachidonic acid into prostaglandins, while lipoxygenase converts arachidonic acid into leukotrienes. All of these products of arachidonic acid metabolism are called eicosanoids. (One of the ways to remember which enzyme goes with which product is to associated the "l" in lipoxygenase with the "l" in leukotrienes.)

NORMAL PROCESSES INVOLVING ARACHIDONIC ACID PRODUCTS

Vascular effects

1. Vasodilation
   - PGE2 and PGI2
2. Vasoconstriction
   - PGF2, thromboxane, LTC4, D4, and E4

Platelet aggregation

- Stimulation → TxA2 (thromboxane)
- Inhibition → PGI2 (prostacyclin)

Lipolysis

- Stimulation → PGI2
- Inhibition → PGE2

Sodium and water balance

1. Increased renin secretion
   - PGE2 and PGI2

Gastrointestinal effects

1. Inhibition of gastric acid production
   - PGE2 and PGI2
2. Inhibition of insulin secretion
   - PGE2

LEUKOTRIENES

Leukotriene B4

- Chemotaxis
- Leukocyte aggregation and adhesion

Leukotrienes C4, D4, and E4

- Increased vascular permeability
- Vasoconstriction

Let's discuss the leukotriene pathway first. Through a series of intermediates, lipoxygenase converts arachidonic acid into the leukotrienes (Lt's). The leukotrienes have many actions that are similar to histamine, such as causing increased vascular permeability and bronchospasm. Leukotriene B4 is a potent chemotactic agent that also causes aggregation and adhesion of leukocytes. Leukotrienes C4, D4, and E4 can cause increased vascular permeability and vasoconstriction. (See Fig. 6-6.)

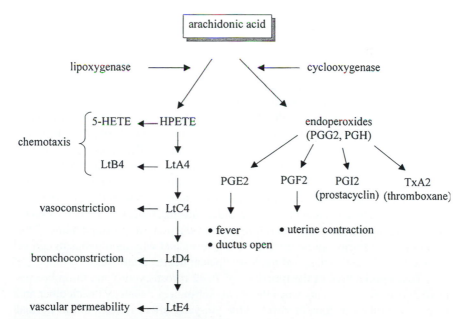

Figure 6-6 Arachidonic Acid Metabolism
Arachidonic acid is converted into leukotrienes or prostaglandins. Leukotrienes cause bronchospasm and increased vascular permeability. Leukotrienes C4, D4, and E4 are collectively known as slow-reacting substance of anaphylaxis.

PROSTAGLANDINS

Prostaglandin E2

- Fever
- Keeps the ductus arteriosus open

Prostaglandin F2

- Uterine contraction
- Bronchoconstriction

Prostaglandin I2 (prostacyclin)

- Inhibits platelet aggregation
- Vasodilation
- Bronchodilation

Thromboxane

- Stimulates platelet aggregation
- Vasoconstriction
- Bronchodilation

Next, let's discuss the prostaglandin pathway. Through a series of intermediates, arachidonic acid is converted into several important products: thromboxane A2 (TxA2), prostacyclin (PGI2), and the more stable prostaglandins, PGE2 and PGF2. PGE2 produced in the anterior hypothalamus (in response to interleukin-1 released from leukocytes) produces fever. PGE2 also keeps open a patent ductus arteriosus and can produce pain in patients with a rare type of bone tumor (osteoid osteoma). PGF2 causes uterine contractions, and excess production of PGF2 can cause pain during menstruation (dysmenorrhea). Note that aspirin, indomethacin, and other nonsteroidal anti-inflammatory drugs (NSAIDs) inhibit cyclooxygenase and therefore the production of prostaglandins. This explains why aspirin can be used to treat a fever and why indomethacin can be used to treat dysmenorrhea and to close a patent ductus arteriosus.

Take special note of the functions of PGI2 (prostacyclin) and thromboxane (TxA2) (Fig. 6-7). In many ways these two substances counteract each other and help to keep their actions in check. This yin-yang effect is common in normal human physiology, and abnormalities of these delicate balances between substances is a recurrent theme for the pathogenesis of disease. Thromboxane is produced by platelets, while prostacyclin is produced by the endothelial cells of blood vessels. (It's helpful to remember which is which by noting that platelets

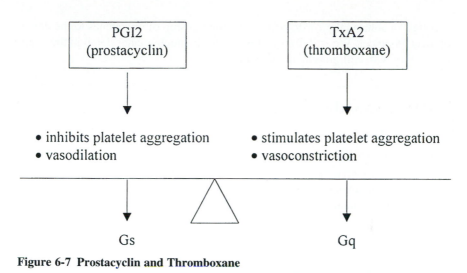

Figure 6-7 Prostacyclin and Thromboxane

are also called thrombocytes, hence the name thromboxane.) Platelets want to stop blood flow by contracting blood vessels and producing blood clots. There-fore, thromboxane causes vasoconstriction and stimulates platelet aggregation. In contrast, endothelial cells want to keep blood vessels open and the blood flowing. Therefore prostacyclin causes vasodilation and inhibits platelet aggregation. Also note that PGI2 functions via Gs receptors, while TxA2 functions via Gq recep-tors. Gs receptors activate membrane adenyl cyclase, while Gq receptors activate membrane phospholipase C. (Interestingly omega-3 fatty acids found in fish oils can decrease platelet aggregation by decreasing the production of thromboxane synthesis by platelets.)

TYROSINE KINASES

- Insulin receptor
- Epidermal growth factor receptor
- Platelet-derived growth factor
- M-CSF receptor

Some normal growth factors bind to surface receptors that are connected to a protein kinase located on the inner surface of the plasma membrane. The pro-tein kinase is usually a tyrosine kinase that can stimulate the transcription of growth regulatory genes. These genes naturally code for growth factors, such as insulin, platelet-derived growth factor (PDGF), epidermal growth factor (EGF), and multi-colony stimulating factor (M-CSF). Since this second messenger sys-tem involves normal growth factors, it is not unexpected that this same system is involved in abnormal growth, such as the relationship of oncogenes to the development of cancer. We will discuss this system in much greater detail in the chapter dealing with cell growth and neoplasia.

ION CHANNELS
Electrolytes

- Sodium channels
- Potassium channels
- Chloride channels
- Calcium channels

Neurotransmitters

- Acetylcholine channels
- Glutamate channels
- GABA channels

Finally, some substances, rather than binding to membrane receptors or crossing the membrane directly, cross the plasma membrane by way of ion channels. These channels are formed by proteins within the cell membrane (integral proteins). When the channels are open they permit the passage of certain substances and ions. Substances that utilize ion channels include electrolytes and neurotransmitters, such as acetylcholine and glutamate (stimulatory) and glycine and GABA (inhibitory). Ion channels can be voltage-gated channels or ligand-gated channels. Voltage-gated channels are opened by depolarization of the cell membrane; ligand-gated channels are opened by the binding of different types of neurotransmitters and hormones.

CYSTIC FIBROSIS
Genetics

- Autosomal recessive disorder
- Defect in CFTR gene on chromosome 7

Pancreas

- Dilation of ducts
- Atrophy of acini
- Fibrosis of interstitium

Lungs

- Fibrosis and dilated bronchi (bronchiectasis)
- Recurrent infections (*Pseudomonas*)

Gastrointestinal

- Meconium ileus (newborn)
- Malabsorption and steatorrhea

Skin

- Increased sodium chloride (salt) in sweat

The primary abnormality in patients with cystic fibrosis (CF) involves the epithelial transport of chloride. Normally, binding of a ligand to a membrane surface receptor activates adenyl cyclase and leads to increased intracellular cAMP. This is turn activates protein kinase A, which phosphorylates the cystic fibrosis transmembrane conductance regulator (CFTR), causing it to open and release chloride ions. Sodium ions and water follow to maintain the normal viscosity of mucus. Several abnormalities of the CFTR can be present in patients with CF, but the most common abnormality involves decreased glycosylation of the CFTR so that it is never incorporated into the cell membrane. A lack of chloride channels results in decreased chloride, sodium, and water secretion. This produces a very thick mucus (hence the other name of CF, which is mucoviscidosis). These thick mucus plugs may block pancreatic ducts, causing fibrosis and cystic dilatation of the ducts (hence the name cystic fibrosis). Decreased excretion of pancreatic lipase leads to malabsorption of fat and *steatorrhea*. This may lead to deficiency of fat-soluble vitamins.

Thick mucus may also cause intestinal obstruction in neonates (meconium ileus). Abnormal mucus secretion in the lungs leads to atelectasis, fibrosis, bronchiectasis, and recurrent pulmonary infections, especially with *staphylococcus aureus* and *Pseudomonas* species. Obstruction of the vas deferens and seminal vesicles in males leads to sterility, while obstruction of the bile duct produces jaundice. The skin of a child with cystic fibrosis may taste salty because of increased sweat electrolytes (the result of decreased reabsorption of electrolytes from the lumens of sweat ducts).

CELL GROWTH

·

- **Cell Growth**
- **Growth Factors**
- **Abnormalities Involving Growth Factors**
- **Second Messenger Systems of Growth Factors**
- **Control of Cell Growth**
- **Normal Oncogene Expression**
- **Abnormal Oncogene Expression**
- **Cancer Suppressor Genes**
- **Abnormal Functioning of Cancer Suppressor Genes**
- **Neurofibromatosis**

· · · · · · · · · · · ·

CELL GROWTH

- Stimulation by growth factors
- Growth factors act via second messenger systems
- Controlled by growth-inhibiting system

Cell injury can stimulate the proliferation of cells. This is one way that cells can respond to injury. To understand abnormal proliferation of cells, you must understand the normal process of cell growth. Throughout life some cells need to be able to proliferate at certain times in response to different needs. Examples include cells of the epidermis, bone marrow, and gastrointestinal tract. These proliferating cells need to be able to stop proliferating at appropriate times also. Control of cell growth is accomplished by two contrasting systems acting in a yin-yang fashion: a growth-stimulating system and a growth-inhibiting system.

The growth-stimulating system (Fig. 7-1) activates cell growth via classic cell communication pathways that involve second messenger systems. These systems involve an extracellular ligand (growth factor) that binds to a receptor on cell membranes (growth factor receptor). This binding causes the activation of a second intracellular transducing signal (second messenger) that results finally in the activation of DNA polymerase and duplication of DNA.

GROWTH FACTORS

Growth of various cell types

- Platelet-derived growth factor (PDGF)
- Epidermal growth factor (EGF)
- Fibroblast growth factors (FGF)
- Tumor growth factors (TGF)
- Insulinlike growth factor I (IGF-1)

Cytokines

- T-cell growth factor (interleukin-2)

Colony-stimulating factors

- Erythropoietin
- M-CSF

Growth factors are chemicals that are associated (obviously) with cell growth. There are three basic types of growth factors. One type can stimulate the growth of many different types of cells; a second type stimulates the growth of cells of the immune system (*cytokines*); and a third type stimulates the growth of red blood cells and white blood cells (colony-stimulating factors).

Platelet-derived growth factor (PDGF) is found in platelets, activated macrophages, endothelial cells, and smooth muscle cells and can cause migration and proliferation of fibroblasts, smooth muscle cells, and monocytes. Epidermal growth factor can cause proliferation of many types of epithelial cells and also fibroblasts and hepatocytes. There are two types of fibroblast growth factor (FGF): acidic FGF and basic FGF. The former is found in neural tissue; the latter is produced by activated macrophages. Obviously FGF can induce the proliferation of fibroblasts. Additionally, basic FGF is capable of inducing all of the stages of blood vessel proliferation (angiogenesis).

There are also two types of tumor growth factors (TGF): alpha TGF and beta TGF. The former is similar to EGF and can bind to the EGF receptor. (In fact,

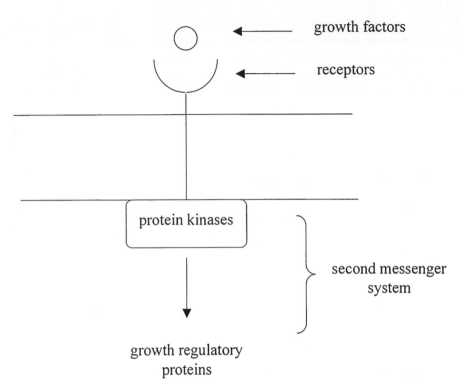

Figure 7-1 Growth-Stimulating System

these two together form the epidermal growth factor family.) Beta TGF, produced by platelets, endothelial cells, T cells, and macrophages, is associated with fibrosis. In low concentrations it causes the synthesis and secretion of PDGF, but in high concentrations it is growth inhibitory due to inhibition of the expression of PDGF receptors.

ABNORMALITIES INVOLVING GROWTH FACTORS
Smooth muscle proliferation → atherosclerosis

1. Growth promoters
   - PDGF
   - Basic fibroblast growth factor
   - IL-1
2. Growth inhibitors
   - Heparan sulfate
   - Nitric oxide

- Gamma-IFN
- Beta-TGF

Fibroblast proliferation → myelofibrosis

1. Growth promoters
   - PDGF
   - TGF-beta

Obviously abnormal growth is associated with the production of tumors. This process is so important that we will deal with it later in this chapter and also in a separate chapter. For now we will examine two non-neoplastic abnormalities associated with excess production of growth factors: atherosclerosis and myelofibrosis.

One of the important basic concepts involving atherosclerosis is that there is abnormal growth of smooth muscle cells within these atherosclerotic plaques. Normally there is a balance between factors that stimulate the growth of smooth muscle cells and factors that inhibit this growth. Growth promoters of smooth muscle cells include PDGF, basic fibroblast growth factor, and IL-1. In contrast, growth inhibitors include heparan sulfate, nitric oxide, gamma-IFN, and beta-TGF. Vascular injury stimulates smooth muscle cell growth and intimal hyperplasia by disrupting the normal balance between these growth factors and growth inhibition. The proliferating smooth muscle cells undergo changes that promote the development of atherosclerosis. These changes include increased synthesis of extracellular matrix substances, loss of thick myosin filaments, and increased organelles associated with protein synthesis. The result is a shift from contractile functioning smooth muscle cells to proliferative-type smooth muscle cells.

Myelofibrosis is a myeloproliferative syndrome that is characterized by a hypocellular and fibrotic bone marrow (myelofibrosis). The marrow fibrosis is due to a non-neoplastic proliferation of fibroblasts that secrete collagen. These marrow fibroblasts are stimulated to proliferate by an inappropriate release PDGF and transforming growth factor beta from proliferating megakaryocytes.

SECOND MESSENGER SYSTEMS OF GROWTH FACTORS

Membrane-bound protein kinases

- Epidermal growth factor
- Platelet-derived growth factor

Phosphatidyl-inositol-diphosphate (PIP2) system

- Insulinlike growth factors
- Cytokines

p21 system

- Many

The cell membrane receptors of growth factors are coupled to second messenger systems. This provides a way of converting the binding of a growth factor to the stimulation of DNA polymerase. This conversion usually involves a protein kinase, which may or may not be attached to the growth factor receptor (Fig. 7-2). In fact, most growth factor receptors have intrinsic protein kinase activity. They consist of an extracellular region (the receptor), a hydrophobic transmembrane region, and a intracellular region that has protein kinase activity (usually tyrosine kinase activity).

There are a few other growth factor receptors (cytokines and colony-stimulating factors) that do not have intrinsic tyrosine kinase activity. These receptors,

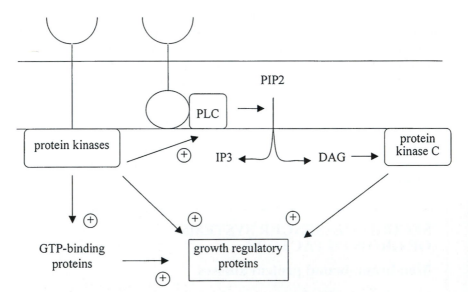

Figure 7-2 Growth Factor Receptors and Second Messenger Systems
Growth factor receptors may or may not be directly attached to protein kinases. Those receptors that are not directly bound to protein kinase still activate similar enzymes (protein kinase C) through second messenger systems (phospholipase C).

however, stimulate tyrosine kinase activity within the cytoplasm by other means, such as the PIP2 system. For example, the PIP2 pathway increases intracellular calcium and produces diacylglycerol (DAG). DAG activates protein kinase C, a serine threonine kinase attached to the cell membrane whose function is analogous to membrane-bound tyrosine kinase.

It is important to realize that the crucial link in most of the growth-activating systems are *ras* proteins (Fig. 7-3). The normal protein product of *ras* is p21, which is a monomeric form of a G protein. As with all G proteins, p21 flips back

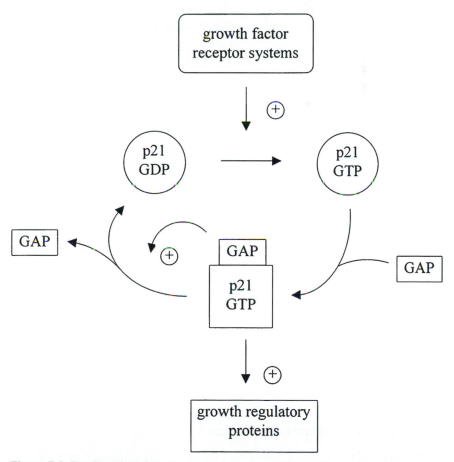

Figure 7-3 *Ras* Protein (p21)
The most important GTP-binding protein that functions as a second messenger for membrane receptor-bound protein kinases is p21, the product of the *ras* gene. Like all other G proteins, p21 is inactive when bound to GDP and active when bound to GTP. The activity of p21-GTP can be greatly increased by binding to GTPase activating protein (GAP). GAP essentially increases the GTPase activity of p21-GTP. This GTPase activity converts the bound GTP back to GDP and inactivates p21.

and forth between an activated form and an inactive form. In the inactive state, p21 binds GDP, but when cells are stimulated (by growth factors, for example) p21 becomes activated by exchanging GDP for GTP. Once active, p21 initiates a cascade of phosphorylations of serine or threonine residues that converge on mitogen-activated protein kinases (MAP kinases), which then relay the growth signal to the nucleus. For example, *ras* protein can activate *raf-1*, a serine threonine kinase that can activate the MAP kinase cascade.

In normal cells, the active stage of p21 is transient because its intrinsic GTPase activity can hydrolyze its own GTP to GDP. This returns active p21 to its inactive state. The GTPase activity of the normal *ras* protein is accelerated by GTPase-activating proteins (GAPs), which function to prevent uncontrolled *ras* activity by accelerating its own inactivation.

CONTROL OF CELL GROWTH

- Stimulation of cell growth → oncogenes
- Inhibition of cell growth → anti-oncogenes

NORMAL ONCOGENE EXPRESSION

Code for growth factors

- *c-sis* → beta chain of platelet-derived growth factor

Code for growth factor receptors

- *c-erb B1* → receptor for epidermal growth factor
- *c-neu* → receptor for epidermal growth factor
- *c-fms* → receptor for colony-stimulating factor

Code for membrane protein kinase not associated with a membrane receptor

- *c-abl* → membrane tyrosine kinase

Code for GTP-binding proteins

- *ras* → p21

Code for nuclear regulatory proteins

- *c-myc*
- *c-jun*
- *c-fos*

What genes are involved in these growth-controlling systems? The growth-stimulating system is controlled by oncogenes, while the growth-inhibiting system is controlled by anti-oncogenes. *Proto-oncogenes* (p-oncs) are the cellular genes that promote normal growth and differentiation. The protein products of proto-oncogenes have many different functions, but basically they code for growth factors, receptors for growth factors, or enzymes involved in the second messenger system of these growth factors.

The products of oncogenes (oncoproteins) can be classified into five main categories: growth factors, growth factor receptors, membrane-bound protein kinases not associated with a membrane receptor, GTP-binding proteins, and nuclear regulatory proteins. An example of an oncogene that acts similarly to growth factors is *c-sis*, which encodes for the beta chain of PDGF. Examples of growth factor receptors that are coded for by oncogenes include the receptor for epidermal growth factor (EGF) (coded for by *c-erb* and *c-neu*) and the receptor for colony-stimulating factor-1 (CSF-1) (coded for by *c-fms*). The product of the *ras* oncogene (p21) is a monomeric G protein that is important in relaying growth signals to the nucleus. Finally, some oncoproteins are associated with proteins that regulate the nucleus directly. These nuclear regulatory proteins include *myc*, *jun*, and *fos*.

ABNORMAL ONCOGENE EXPRESSION

Code for growth factors

- *c-sis* → astrocytomas and osteogenic sarcomas

Code for growth factor receptors

- *c-erb B1* → breast cancer and squamous cell carcinoma of the lung
- *c-neu* → breast cancer
- *c-fms* → leukemia

Code for membrane protein kinase not associated with a membrane receptor

- *c-abl* → chronic myelocytic leukemia

Code for GTP-binding proteins

- *ras* → adenocarcinomas

Code for nuclear regulatory proteins

- *c-myc* → Burkitt's lymphoma
- *N-myc* → neuroblastoma

To reiterate, proto-oncogenes (p-oncs) are cellular genes that promote normal growth and differentiation. An important basic concept of cancer is that abnormal functioning of oncogenes can cause cancer. A normal cellular proto-oncogene can function as an abnormal cancer oncogene if it produces more of its product than it should. Certain tumors are associated with characteristic uncontrolled expression of specific oncogenes.

For example, overexpression of the product of *c-sis* (the beta chain of PDGF) is seen in certain tumors of the central nervous system (astrocytomas) and malignant tumors of the bone (osteosarcomas). Overexpression of growth factor receptors can also result in excess growth. *c-erb B1*, the EGF receptor gene, is overexpressed in many squamous cell carcinomas of the lung, while *c-erb B2* is overexpressed in adenocarcinomas of the breast, ovary, lung, and stomach. *c-fms* codes for the receptor for CSF-1 and is associated with leukemias. Dysregulation of *c-myc* expression occurs in Burkitt's lymphoma and small cell carcinoma of the lung, while mutations involving the *ras* gene are the single most common oncogene abnormality in human tumors.

Finally, sometimes a chromosomal abnormality involves a normal oncogene and produces a new abnormal protein. The best example of this is chronic myeloid leukemia. In patients with chronic myeloid leukemia (CML), *c-abl* on chromosome 9 fuses with part of the break-point cluster region (bcr) on chromosome 22 and forms a hybrid gene with potent tyrosine kinase activity.

CANCER SUPPRESSOR GENES

Regulation of signal transduction

* *NF-1* gene

Regulation of the cell cycle

* *Rb* gene
* *p53* gene

Cancer suppressor genes represent another class of genes that are important in the formation of neoplasms. These genes, also called *anti-oncogenes*, normally function to regulate and prevent growth. They balance the stimulation of growth provided by oncogenes.

Examples of cancer suppressor genes include *NF-1*, *Rb*, and *p53*. These genes code for proteins that regulate signal transduction and nuclear transcription. *NF-1* is associated with regulating signal transduction. GAP, which binds to *p21* to increase its GTPase activity, is coded for by *NF-1*. Loss of normal functioning of *NF-1* causes *ras* to be trapped in its active state and leads to uncontrolled growth.

Genes that regulate the cell cycle include *Rb* and *p53*. In order to understand the functioning of these anti-oncogenes you need to understand the normal mechanics of the cell cycle (Fig. 7-4). Stable (nondividing) cells at G0 can enter the cell cycle at G1 (gap 1) when stimulated by an appropriate signal. From there the cells enter the S phase ("S" for synthesis) where they actively synthesize DNA and form double chromatids. Next follows the second gap (G2) phase and then the M phase ("M" for mitosis) where mitosis occurs. This is followed by G1, where no DNA synthesis occurs, and the cycle is completed. The product of the *Rb* gene is a nuclear phosphoprotein that regulates the cell cycle at several points. It exists as an active unphosphorylated form (*pRb*) and an inactive phosphorylated form (*pRb-P*). The active unphosphorylated form (*pRb*) stops the cell cycle from going from G0 to S. It does this by binding to transcription factors such as the product of *c-myc* (recall that the product of *c-myc* functions as a nuclear regulatory protein). When *pRb* is phosphorylated (inactive) the cell can enter S and complete the cell cycle. Inactivation of the *pRb* stop signal causes the cell to continuously cycle and undergo repeated mitosis. Some DNA viruses, such as SV40 and human papillomavirus, function by inactivating *pRb*.

The product of the *p53* gene is also a protein that regulates DNA replication. *p53* normally prevents the replication of cells with damaged DNA. It does this by stopping cells during G1 and giving them time to repair damaged DNA. Loss of function of *p53* (which can be due to several types of DNA viruses) allows damaged DNA to replicate.

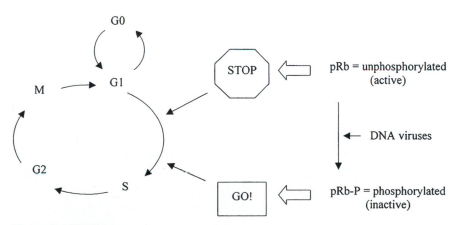

Figure 7-4 *Rb* Gene
The product of the *Rb* gene (retinoblastoma gene) is called *pRb*. When this protein is unphosphorylated it actively stops the cell cycle from proceeding to the S phase. When this protein is phosphorylated (*pRb-P*) it is inactive and the cell cycle can proceed. Do not get confused with the similar terms "*pRb*" and "*pRb-P*." The former is active, the latter is inactive.

ABNORMAL FUNCTIONING OF CANCER SUPPRESSOR GENES

- *Rb* → retinoblastoma and osteogenic sarcoma
- *p53* → many tumors and the Li-Fraumeni syndrome
- *WT-1* → Wilms' tumor and aniridia
- *NF-1* → neurofibromatosis type 1

Abnormal functioning of tumor suppressor genes is basically the result of deletions of these anti-oncogenes. Since there are two copies of each of these genes (one on each chromosome pair) it takes the deletion of both genes to lead to the development of neoplasms. This fact was first described by Knudson, who developed a "two-hit" hypothesis of anti-oncogene function. He explained that the two clinical forms of retinoblastoma (a sporadic form and a familial form) were the result of the fact that it took "two hits" (two deletions) to produce the malignant tumor. In the familial form, the first hit was an inherited deletion and the second hit was an acquired deletion. In contrast, the sporadic form results from two acquired deletions. The *Rb* gene (retinoblastoma gene), located on chromosome 13, is the cancer suppressor gene whose deletion is associated with the development of retinoblastomas. It is important to note that patients with an inherited deficiency of one of the *Rb* genes also have an increased risk for the subsequent development of osteosarcomas.

Other examples of tumor suppressor genes include *p53*, *WT-1*, and *NF* type 1. *p53*, located on chromosome 17, is the most common chromosomal location that is associated with human cancer. Abnormalities of this gene are associated with numerous cancers, including carcinomas of the breast, colon, and adrenal. Inheritance of a mutant *p53* is seen in patients with the Li-Fraumeni syndrome.

WT-1 (Wilms' tumor gene) is found on chromosome 11 and is associated with the formation of Wilms' tumor, a malignant renal tumor found in children. This tumor also occurs in a sporadic and familial form. Patients with the loss of WT-1 develop Wilms' tumor and may have an absence of the irises of their eyes (aniridia). Histologically these tumors (nephroblastomas) reveal a combination of undifferentiated mesenchymal cells and immature kidney tissue (immature tubule or glomerular formation).

NEUROFIBROMATOSIS

Neurofibromatosis type 1

- Defect in *NF1* gene
- Multiple neural tumors (neurofibromas and schwannomas)
- Plexiform neurofibroma is diagnostic
- Café-au-lait spots on the skin
- Pigmented nodules of iris (Lisch nodules)

Neurofibromatosis type 2

- Bilateral acoustic neuromas

NF (neurofibromatosis) type 1 gene (*NF-1*) is found on chromosome 17 and is associated with the development of tumors originating from Schwann cells (schwannomas). These tumors histologically are composed of spindle cells and have cellular (Antoni A) areas and less cellular (Antoni B) areas. In the Antoni A areas the cells may line up in a row and form Verocay bodies. Patients with abnormalities of the *NF1* gene can develop many of these neural tumors. Clinically this syndrome is called neurofibromatosis type 1. Characteristic of this disorder is the development of a distinctive type of neurofibroma called the plexiform neurofibroma. Other inherited defects are seen in patients with neurofibromatosis type 1, such as pigmented nodules of the iris (Lisch nodules) and cutaneous hyperpigmented macules (café-au-lait spots) of the skin.

· C H A P T E R · 8 ·

CELL DEGENERATIONS

·

- Atrophy
- Abnormalities of Regression of Tissue
- Examples of Pathologic Atrophy
- Renal Artery Stenosis
- Atrophy of the Stomach
- Atrophy of the Small Intestines
- Atrophy Involving the Nervous System
- Alzheimer's Disease
- Atrophy Involving the Striatum
- Huntington's Disease
- Parkinson's Disease
- Degeneration of Myelin
- Atrophy of Muscle
- Muscle Fiber Types
- Denervation Atrophy
- Amyotrophic Lateral Sclerosis
- Degeneration of Muscle
- Degeneration of Bone

ATROPHY

1. Reversible decrease in size of an organ or tissue
2. Decrease in the size of cells
3. Causes of physiologic atrophy
   • Decreased workload or use
   • Decreased endocrine stimulation
   • Aging
4. Causes of pathologic atrophy
   • Decreased blood supply
   • Decreased nutrition
   • Loss of innervation

Don't confuse atrophy with similar-sounding terms that describe abnormal organ development, namely aplasia and hypoplasia. Atrophy is a reversible decrease in the size of an organ or tissue that is due to a decrease in the size of the cells. Technically speaking there is no decrease in the number of cells. (A decrease in the number of cells is hypoplasia.)

Atrophy can be a physiologic or a pathologic process. Classic examples of physiologic atrophy involve atrophy of heart muscle or skeletal muscle with decreased work or disuse, or atrophy of sex characteristics associated with aging or decreased hormone stimulation. In contrast, pathologic atrophy results from decreased blood flow, nutrition, or innervation to tissue.

ABNORMALITIES OF REGRESSION OF TISSUE

• Thyroglossal duct cyst
• Gartner duct cyst
• Patent ductus arteriosus

Physiologic atrophy can also be an important process in fetal development (in which case it can be called regression). Regression can involve ducts (thyroglossal duct and mesonephric duct) or blood vessels (ductus arteriosus). Lack of the appropriate regression of these structures can produce pathologic abnormalities such as cysts. For example, remnants of the thyroglossal duct may form a cyst (thyroglossal duct cyst) in the anterior part of the neck. Another cyst found in the neck is a branchial cleft cyst, but this cyst is located in the anterolateral part of the neck. Each of these cysts may histologically reveal a lining that is composed of squamous epithelium or pseudostratified columnar epithelium. Branchial cleft cysts may have lymphoid tissue. Thyroglossal duct cysts may move up and down as the patient swallows.

Another cyst that forms from a lack of regression is the Gartner duct cyst, which is formed by the lack of regression of the Wolffian (mesonephric) duct rests or remnants. This type of cyst is located in the lateral walls of the vagina. Cysts derived from the same Wolffian duct may also be found on the lateral aspect of the vulva and are called mesonephric cysts.

An example of regression involving a blood vessel is the ductus arteriosus. The ductus is a normal vascular channel of the fetus that connects the pulmonary artery to the aorta. Closure of the ductus usually occurs a few hours to a few days after delivery when the pulmonary vascular resistance falls and the blood flow changes from right-to-left to left-to-right. The oxygenated blood flowing from the aorta into the ductus inhibits prostaglandin production, and this closes the ductus arteriosus. Failure of regression of the ductus can be found in premature infants and in infants with respiratory distress syndrome at birth. Sometimes treatment with oxygen or prostaglandins will induce closure. Indomethacin inhibits the enzyme cyclooxygenase and suppresses production of the vasodilator PGE2. This drug can help to induce closure. Note that in some diseases, such as transposition of the great vessels, it can be lifesaving to keep the ductus arteriosus patent. In these patients PGE2 may be given therapeutically to keep the ductus open. If the PDA does not close, there will be shunting of blood from the aorta (high pressure) to the pulmonary circulation (low pressure). This left-to-right shunting of blood can produce a "machinery"-type murmur. With time, a large PDA will produce pulmonary hypertension and reversal of the blood flow (Eisenmenger's syndrome).

EXAMPLES OF PATHOLOGIC ATROPHY

- Renal artery stenosis
- Chronic atrophic gastritis
- Celiac disease
- Alzheimer's disease
- Denervation atrophy

RENAL ARTERY STENOSIS

- Atheromatous plaque → older men
- Fibromuscular dysplasia → younger women
- Stenotic kidney is small (ischemic atrophy)
- Nonstenotic kidney is normal size
- Increased renin → increased aldosterone
- Hypertension
- Hypernatremia and hypokalemic alkalosis

Pathologic atrophy results in a decrease in the size of a tissue or an organ. Most commonly pathologic atrophy is the result of decreased blood flow (ischemia). For example, ischemia to a kidney causes that kidney to become small and atrophic. This is best illustrated by examining the clinical situation of decreased blood flow to one kidney, which can occur with obstruction of the renal artery (renal artery stenosis). This obstruction may occur secondary to an atheromatous plaque at the orifice of the renal artery or fibromuscular dysplasia of the renal artery. The former is more common in elderly men, while the latter is more common in young women. The kidney with the stenotic vessel will grossly become small (atrophic) due to the chronic ischemia. The decrease in blood flow to the kidney with the renal artery obstruction (the Goldblatt kidney) causes hyperplasia of the juxtaglomerular apparatus and increased renin production. This produces increased aldosterone secretion by the adrenal cortex, which causes the kidneys to retain sodium and water (and lose potassium and hydrogen ions). The end result is that patients develop hypertension, hypernatremia, and a hypokalemia alkalosis.

ATROPHY OF THE STOMACH

Type A → autoimmune gastritis

- Autoantibodies to parietal cells and intrinsic factor
- Decreased vitamin B12 → megaloblastic anemia
- Increased serum gastrin levels
- Histologic changes found in fundus of stomach

Type B → environmental

- No autoantibodies present
- Associated with *Helicobacter pylori*
- Decreased serum gastrin levels
- Histologic changes found in antrum of stomach

Atrophy of the stomach (atrophic gastritis) is characterized histologically by a decrease in the number of parietal cells. There are two types of atrophic gastritis, type A and type B. Autoimmune gastritis, also known as diffuse corporal atrophic gastritis or type A atrophic gastritis, is characterized by the presence of antibodies to parietal cells or intrinsic factor. This type of gastritis is associated with pernicious anemia and decreased production of acid (achlorhydria or hypochlorhydria). Pernicious anemia is a type of anemia caused by a deficiency of vitamin B12. A lack of vitamin B12 affects the normal maturation of cells. Abnormally maturing red blood cell precursors are called megaloblasts, and this type of anemia is called *megaloblastic anemia*. Patients with a deficiency of vitamin B12 are likely to develop a demyelinating disease of the spinal cord called subacute combined disease of the spinal cord. Histologic examination of the stomach in patients with type A atrophic gastritis reveals diffuse atrophy (decreased mucosal thickness), decreased numbers of glands, widespread intestinal metaplasia, and variable numbers of acute and chronic inflammatory cells. These changes are found predominantly in the body and fundus mucosa and are usually absent in the antrum. Patients with autoimmune atrophic gastritis have an increased risk for gastric cancer, but they do not develop peptic ulcers because of the lack of acid production.

Type B (environmental) atrophic gastritis is also associated with gastric atrophy and intestinal metaplasia of the antrum of the stomach. In contrast, this type of gastritis is not associated with autoimmune antibodies, but instead there is an association with *Helicobacter pylori* infection.

ATROPHY OF THE SMALL INTESTINES

Tropical sprue

- Acquired disease
- Found in Caribbean, Asia, and India
- Associated with chronic bacterial infection
- Treatment: antibiotic therapy

Nontropical sprue

- Inherited disease
- Associated with sensitivity to gluten
- Treatment: dietary restriction of gluten

Atrophy of the small intestines is characteristic of two diseases called sprue—tropical sprue and nontropical sprue. Histologically each of these diseases reveals atrophy of the small intestines with blunted or absent villi, lengthened crypts, and an increased mononuclear cell infiltrate in lamina propria. Tropical sprue is an acquired disease found in tropical areas, such as the Caribbean, Asia, and India. It is the result of a chronic bacterial infection, and treatment is with antibiotics. In contrast, nontropical sprue (celiac sprue) is a disease of malabsorption that is related to a sensitivity to gluten (a substance found in wheat, oats, barley, and rye). Patients may develop antibodies against gliadin, a glycoprotein component of gluten. Treatment for this disease is to remove gluten from the diet.

ATROPHY INVOLVING THE NERVOUS SYSTEM

- Diffuse atrophy of cerebral cortex → Alzheimer's disease
- Unilateral frontal or temporal lobe atrophy → Pick's disease
- Caudate and putamen → Huntington's disease
- Substantia nigra → Parkinson's disease

ALZHEIMER'S DISEASE

Clinical

- Slowly progressive dementia
- Memory loss
- Decreased cognitive function

Gross changes

- Diffuse cortical atrophy

Microscopic changes

- Neurofibrillary tangles (abnormally phosphorylated tau protein)
- Senile plaques (beta amyloid core)
- Granulovacuolar degeneration
- Hirano bodies

Possible etiology

- Decreased choline acetyltransferase
- Abnormal amyloid gene expression
- Presence of apoprotein E4
- Abnormalities involving nucleus basalis of Meynert

Diffuse atrophy of the cerebral cortex is seen in patients with Alzheimer's disease. Gross examination of the brain will reveal variable cortical atrophy with widening of the cerebral sulci that is most pronounced in the frontal, temporal and parietal lobes. The progressive loss of neurons in the entire cortex leads to slowly progressive mental deterioration. Clinical symptoms include the loss of recent memory (the most common early sign) and the loss of long-term memory. The disease is progressive and leads to immobility in about ten years.

The two major microscopic findings in the brains of patients with Alzheimer's disease are neurofibrillary tangles and neuritic (senile) plaques. Neurofibrillary tangles are bundles of filaments in the cytoplasm of neurons that contain an abnormal form of a microtubule-associated protein (tau protein). In contrast, neuritic plaques are focal collections of neuritic processes surrounding a central amyloid core (composed of amyloid beta-protein). Two other common abnormalities that can be found within the pyramidal cells of the hippocampus include granulovacuolar degeneration (small, clear, cytoplasmic vacuoles with an argyrophilic granule) and Hirano bodies (elongated, glassy, eosinophilic paracrystalline arrays of filaments, mainly actin).

The etiology of Alzheimer's disease is unknown, but several possible mechanisms have been suggested. For example, acetylcholine normally plays a role in learning and short-term memory. Perhaps an abnormality involving acetylcholine could be involved in the pathogenesis of the memory problems seen in patients with Alzheimer's disease. Possible mechanisms for the production of the neurofibrillary tangles and senile plaque have also been suggested. For example, neurofibrillary tangles are composed of intracytoplasmic bundles of filaments and microtubules. Perhaps the presence of an abnormal protein (apoprotein E4) could lead to the formation of neurofibrillary tangles. This apoprotein E4 is less effective at stabilizing microtubules than the normal apoprotein E2. In contrast, *senile plaques* have a central amyloid core. The gene for this amyloid protein is found on chromosome 21. Perhaps an abnormal expression of this gene could lead to the formation of senile plaques. (It is interesting to note that most patients with trisomy 21, Down's syndrome, will develop signs and symptoms of Alzheimer's disease during their adult life.)

Pick's disease is clinically very similar to Alzheimer's disease except that it occurs much less frequently. The cortical atrophy in patients with Pick's disease is unilateral and localized to a frontal or temporal lobe. This is in contrast to the diffuse, symmetrical atrophy seen in patients with Alzheimer's disease. Microscopically severe neuronal loss is present in the outer layers of the cortex, and the remaining neurons may be swollen (Pick cells) or contain Pick bodies (round to oval, filamentous inclusions that stain strongly with silver stains).

ATROPHY INVOLVING THE STRIATUM

- Atrophy of caudate and putamen → Huntington's disease
- Atrophy of substantia nigra → Parkinson's disease

The basal ganglia of the brain include the caudate nucleus, putamen, globus pallidus, amygdala, and claustrum. The caudate nucleus and putamen are sometimes referred to together as the striatum, while the putamen and the globus pallidus together are called the lenticular (lentiform) nucleus. Several neuronal circuits of the brain involve the basal ganglia. To briefly summarize the more important connections involving these circuits (Fig. 8-1): The striatum (caudate and putamen) receives input from the cortex, the thalamus (centromedian nucleus), and the substantia nigra. The fibers from the substantia nigra release dopamine and are inhibitory. The striatum in turn sends GABA fibers (inhibitory) to the substantia nigra and globus pallidus. The globus pallidus receives input from the striatum and the subthalamic nuclei and sends fibers back to the subthalamic nuclei and the thalamus.

These basal ganglia circuits regulate the initiation, degree, and speed of movement. Diseases of the basal ganglia produce unexpected, unplanned movements. Examples include *chorea* (sudden jerky and purposeless movements), *athetosis* (slow, writhing, snakelike movements), and *hemiballismus* (sudden wild flailing of one arm).

HUNTINGTON'S DISEASE

1. Etiology
    * Expansion of trinucleotide repeat on chromosome 4
    * Autosomal dominant inheritance
2. Location of atrophy → caudate and putamen
3. Decreased GABA and acetylcholine → decreased inhibition → increased movement
4. Signs
    * Depression
    * Progressive dementia
    * Choreiform movements
5. Treatment → dopamine antagonists

Huntington's disease is an autosomal dominant disorder characterized by atrophy of the caudate nuclei and putamen. Patients develop choreiform movements and progressive dementia after the age of 30. Huntington's disease is one of four diseases that are characterized by long repeating sequences of three nucleotides (the other diseases being fragile X syndrome, myotonic dystrophy, and spinal and bulbar muscular atrophy). The mutant gene is found on chromosome 4.

The pathophysiology of Huntington's disease relates to degeneration of GABA neurons in the striatum. GABA neurons are typically inhibitory neurons. Decreased functioning of inhibitory neurons leads to increased movement. Therapy for excessive movement (hyperkinetic) disorders can be attempted with dopamine antagonists. Examine Figure 8-1. Decreased dopamine in the striatum should theoretically cause a relative increase in acetylcholine (stimulatory) and an increase in excitation of GABA neurons in the striatum. Increased GABA will cause increased inhibition of movement. Note that the same result could theoret-

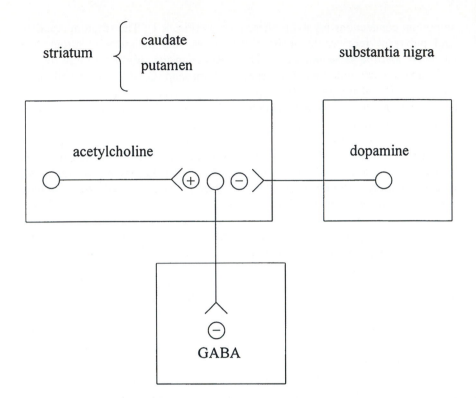

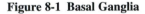

Figure 8-1 Basal Ganglia

ically be achieved with inhibition of acetylcholine breakdown (cholinesterase inhibitors).

PARKINSON'S DISEASE

1. Etiology (multiple)
   - Idiopathic (most common)
   - Postencephalitis
   - Autoimmune dysfunction
   - Trauma
   - Drugs (illicit drug MPTP)
2. Location → substantia nigra
3. Decreased dopamine in corpus striatum

4. Signs
    • Cogwheel rigidity
    • Akinesia
    • Tremor
5. Treatment → dopamine agonists

It is important to compare Huntington's disease (excessive movement) to Parkinson's disease (decreased movement). Parkinson's syndrome is characterized clinically by an expressionless (masklike) face, resting ("pill-rolling") tremors, slowness of voluntary movements (*bradykinesia*), and muscular rigidity. As patients walk they stoop forward and have a typical shuffling gait.

In patients with Parkinson's disease there is degeneration and loss of pigmented cells in the substantia nigra, which results in decreased synthesis of dopamine. Lewy bodies, eosinophilic intracytoplasmic inclusions, are found in the remaining neurons of the substantia nigra. The decreased synthesis of dopamine by neurons originating in the substantia nigra leads to decreased dopamine in the striatum (Fig. 8-1). This results in decreased dopamine inhibition and a relative increase in acetylcholine function (excitatory) in the striatum. This excitation, however, is to increase the functioning of GABA neurons, which are inhibitory. The final effect, therefore, is increased inhibition or decreased movement.

Most cases of Parkinson's disease have no known cause (idiopathic). Signs and symptoms of Parkinson's disease can be seen with many other disorders. Von Economo's encephalitis was a transient infectious disorder that occurred from 1915 to 1918 (concurrent with influenza pandemic) and was associated with postencephalitic parkinsonism. Other causes of Parkinson's disease include trauma (boxers), certain drugs and toxins (MPTP, a meperidine analog found in illicit drugs), and copper (Wilson's disease).

DEGENERATION OF MYELIN
Multiple sclerosis

- Demyelination of CNS (periventricular plaques)
- Young adults and northern latitudes
- Oligoclonal bands in CSF
- Triad → scanning speech, intention tremor, nystagmus

Guillain-Barré syndrome

- Demyelination of peripheral nerves
- Ascending paralysis

Multiple sclerosis (MS) is associated with the formation of focal plaques of demyelination anywhere in the CNS. Most often the plaques are located in the white matter near the angles of the lateral ventricles (periventricular). MS primarily affects young adults between 20 and 40 years of age and is more common in northern latitudes. Early clinical findings include weakness of the lower extremities and visual abnormalities with retrobulbar pain. The classic (Charcot) triad of patients with MS is scanning speech, intention tremor, and *nystagmus*. Also pathognomonic for MS is internuclear ophthalmoplegia (INO), which results from demyelination of the medial longitudinal fasciculus (MLF syndrome). It produces medial rectus palsy on attempted lateral gaze and monocular nystagmus in the abducting eye with convergence. Examination of the CSF in patients with MS reveals increased T lymphocytes, increased protein, and normal glucose. Protein electrophoresis of the CSF reveals oligoclonal bands (individual *monoclonal* spikes), although this latter finding is not specific for MS.

ATROPHY OF MUSCLE

Examples of muscle atrophy

- Denervation atrophy
- Disuse atrophy
- Amyotrophic lateral sclerosis
- Werdnig-Hoffmann disease

Examples of muscular dystrophy

- Duchenne muscular dystrophy
- Becker muscular dystrophy

MUSCLE FIBER TYPES

	TYPE 1 FIBERS	TYPE 2 FIBERS
• color	red	white
• speed of contraction	slow	fast
• number of mitochondria	abundant	few
• lipid	abundant	little
• glycogen	little	abundant
• myosin ATP-ase pH 9.4	light	dark
• myosin ATP-ase pH 4.3	dark	light

DENERVATION ATROPHY

* Atrophic muscle fibers (small and angulated)
* Group atrophy
* Target fibers
* Reinnervation produces fiber type grouping

Denervation of skeletal muscle causes atrophy of the skeletal muscle fibers. Histologically the cross sections of these atrophic muscle fibers appear small and angulated. Since a single motor neuron normally supplies many myofibers, denervation initially results in randomly scattered atrophic fibers. With further denervation, however, small groups of fibers become atrophic (group atrophy). The atrophic fibers are a mixture of type 1 (red) and type II (white) fibers. Another histologic change seen in denervated muscle is the presence of distinctive three-zoned fibers called target fibers. The denervated muscle fibers may become reinnervated by collateral sprouting of nearby axons. Since the muscle fiber type is determined by the motor neuron, all of the reinnervated fibers will be converted to a single fiber type. This phenomenon is described as fiber type grouping. This is in contrast to the mixed "checkerboard" pattern of type I (red) and type II (white) fibers of normal skeletal muscle. In contrast, atrophy of primarily type II fibers is characteristic of disuse atrophy.

AMYOTROPHIC LATERAL SCLEROSIS

1. Degeneration of motor neurons
   * Anterior horn cells of spinal cord
   * Motor nuclei of brain stem
   * Upper motor neurons of cerebral cortex
2. Lower motor neuron disease
   * Weakness
   * Fasciculations
3. Upper neuron disease
   * Spasticity
   * Hyperreflexia
   * Positive Babinski reflex
4. Theory of pathogenesis
   * Decreased SOD activity produces apoptosis of motor neurons

---

There are a large number of abnormalities of lower motor neurons and peripheral nerves that produce denervation muscle atrophy. These abnormalities include traumatic injuries and degenerative diseases of the central nervous system (amyotrophic lateral sclerosis and Werdnig-Hoffmann disease). Amyotrophic lateral sclerosis (ALS), Lou Gehrig disease, is a degenerative disorder of motor neurons, principally the anterior horn cells of the spinal cord, the motor nuclei of the brain stem, and the upper motor neurons of the cerebral cortex. Clinical signs and symptoms of Lou Gehrig disease include a combination of *lower motor neuron (LMN)* disease (weakness and fasciculations) and *upper motor neuron (UMN)* disease (spasticity and hyperreflexia). Early symptoms include weakness and cramping, followed by muscle atrophy and fasciculations. Reflexes are hyperactive in upper and lower extremities, and a positive extensor plantar (Babinski) reflex is found (loss of upper motor neurons). The clinical course is progressive, and death can result from respiratory complications.

Theories about the etiology of ALS include many different possible causes, such as viruses, immunologic injury, or oxidative stress. The latter is related to a defect in the zinc-copper binding superoxide dismutase (SOD) on chromosome 21. Decreased SOD activity leads to apoptosis of spinal motor neurons.

Werdnig-Hoffmann disease is a rare autosomal recessive disorder that results in degeneration of brain stem and spinal cord motor neurons. The disorder may be discovered prenatally due to decreased fetal movement or during the first few years of life with profound weakness and hypotonia ("floppy infant"). Affected children generally die from respiratory complications soon after the onset of the disease.

DEGENERATION OF MUSCLE
Duchenne muscular dystrophy

- X-linked recessive disorder
- Deficiency of dystrophin
- Rounded atrophic muscle fibers mixed with hypertrophied fibers
- Pseudohypertrophy of calf muscles
- Gowers maneuver is characteristic

Becker muscular dystrophy

- X-linked recessive disorder
- Abnormal form of dystrophin
- Less severe disease

Variation in size and shape along with degenerative changes and intrafascicular fibrosis are features of muscular dystrophy. The muscular dystrophies are a heterogeneous group of degenerative disorders that are characterized by degeneration and atrophy of skeletal muscle. Many classifications have been proposed to separate these disorders based on mode of inheritance, age of onset and pattern of involvement. Duchenne muscular dystrophy is a noninflammatory inherited myopathy that causes severe and progressive weakness and degeneration of muscles, particularly the proximal muscles (pelvic and shoulder girdles). Weakness usually becomes evident when the child first starts to walk. The weakness produces clumsiness, and difficulty climbing steps. Involvement of the pelvic girdle muscle results in the clinical finding that the child uses the stronger arm and shoulder muscles to rise up from the floor (*Gowers maneuver*). The disease is progressive, and patients develop problems walking, followed eventually by involvement of respiratory muscles. Death from respiratory failure may occur before the age of 20.

Duchenne muscular dystrophy is the most severe of the muscular dystrophies and is transmitted as an X-linked recessive disorder. The basic defect has been localized to a gene on the X chromosome that codes for *dystrophin*, a protein found on the inner surface on the sarcolemma. Sporadic cases are common because of the high rate of spontaneous mutations. (The gene for dystrophin is quite large, and this large size increases the probability of spontaneous mutation.)

Histologically the muscle fibers show variations in size and shape (rounded, atrophic fibers mixed with hypertrophied fibers), degenerative and regenerative changes in adjacent myocytes, and necrotic fibers invaded by histiocytes. Necrosis of muscle fibers causes the serum creatine kinase levels to become elevated. The weak muscles are replaced by fibrofatty tissue, and this causes the muscles to appear grossly enlarged (pseudohypertrophy).

Patients with Becker muscular dystrophy have dystrophin, but the molecular weight of the protein is abnormal. Like Duchenne dystrophy, this form of muscular dystrophy is transmitted as an X-linked recessive trait, or it may result from spontaneous mutations. The pathologic changes are similar to Duchenne muscular dystrophy, but they are less severe. Weakness appears during the first to third decades and progresses slowly. Most patients are able to walk for many years after the onset of the disease. Contractures of muscle are not found, cardiac involvement is minimal, and patients often have a nearly normal life span.

DEGENERATION OF BONE

Osteoarthritis

1. Degenerative joint disease
2. Loss of articular cartilage → smooth subchondral bone (eburnation)
3. Osteophyte formation
   - DIP → Heberden's nodes
   - PIP → Bouchard's nodes
4. Joint pain worse in evening

Osteoarthritis, degenerative joint disease, is a very common type of joint disease. Essentially it is a "wear and tear" disorder in which destruction of the articular cartilage results in smooth subchondral bone formation (eburnated, "ivorylike"). This loss of cartilage results in new bone formation at the edges of the bone (*osteophytes*). Osteophytes located over the distal interphalangeal (DIP) joints are called Heberden's nodes; osteophytes located at the proximal interphalangeal (PIP) joints are called Bouchard's nodes. Fragments of cartilage may also break free into affected joint spaces producing loose bodies called "joint mice." Patients develop pain, stiffness, and swelling of the affected joints without acute inflammation. A characteristic clinical appearance is the presence of crepitus, a grating sound produced by friction between adjacent areas of exposed subchondral bone.

DEVELOPMENTAL ABNORMALITIES

- Abnormal Organ Development
- Renal Agenesis
- Aplasia of the Bone Marrow
- Aplastic Anemia
- Pure Red Cell Aplasia
- DiGeorge's Syndrome
- Hypoplasia of Ganglia
- Neural Tube Developmental Defects
- Spina Bifida
- Hypoplasia Involving the Posterior Fossa
- Arnold-Chiari Malformation
- Dandy-Walker Malformation
- Syringomyelia
- Hypoplasia of the Gonads
- Atresia
- Coarctation of the Aorta
- Atresia of the Gastrointestinal Tract
- Developmental Abnormalities of the Heart
- Ventricular Septal Defects (VSD)
- Atrial Septal Defects (ASD)
- Patent Ductus Arteriosus (PDA)
- Tetralogy of Fallot
- Transposition of the Great Vessels

ABNORMAL ORGAN DEVELOPMENT
Terms

- Anlage → primitive mass of cells
- Aplasia → complete failure of an organ to develop (anlage present)
- Agenesis → complete failure of an organ to develop (no anlage present)
- Hypoplasia → reduction in size of an organ due to a decrease in number of cells
- Atrophy → decrease in size of an organ due to a decrease in number of preexisting cells

Examples of aplasia and hypoplasia

- Renal agenesis
- Aplastic anemia
- Pure red cell aplasia
- DiGeorge's syndrome

Don't confuse the terms *aplasia, agenesis*, and *hypoplasia* with the similar-sounding term *atrophy*. Atrophy refers to the decrease in size of an organ due to a decrease in the number of preexisting cells. In contrast, aplasia, agenesis, and hypoplasia refer to the failure of cells to proliferate and form normal structures or organs (Fig. 9-1). This usually, but not always, refers to processes that are associated with normal fetal development. Aplasia refers to the complete failure of an organ to develop. *Agenesis* is a similar term which also refers to the complete failure of an organ to develop. With aplasia, however, an undeveloped *anlage* (primitive mass of cells) or vascular pedicle can be found; these structures are absent with agenesis. Hypoplasia refers to a reduction in the size of an organ due to a developmental abnormality that produces a decrease in the number of cells. Structurally the organ tends to be normal but small in size.

RENAL AGENESIS
- Failure of metanephric diverticulum to develop
- Potter's sequence
- Oligohydramnios
- Characteristic facial features

Failure of the metanephric diverticulum to develop leads to agenesis of both kidneys (bilateral renal agenesis). This developmental abnormality leads to a

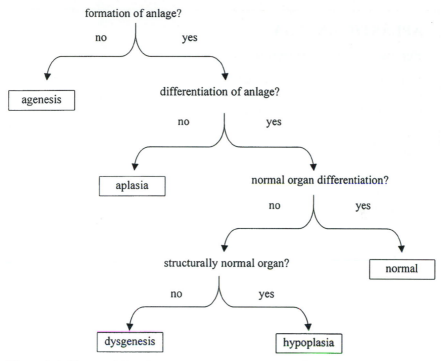

Figure 9-1 Abnormal Development

combination of signs called Potter's sequence. Normally the kidneys are important for the circulation of amniotic fluid. The fetus swallows amniotic fluid and absorbs it within the respiratory and digestive tracts. Waste products cross the placental membrane and enter the maternal blood through the intervillous space. Excess water is excreted by the fetal kidneys into the amniotic fluid. Developmental abnormalities that impair fetal swallowing of amniotic fluid (esophageal atresia or severe anomalies of the CNS) lead to *polyhydramnios* (too much amniotic fluid), while agenesis of the kidneys or urinary obstruction leads to *oligohydramnios* (too little amniotic fluid). Normally one of the functions of amniotic fluid is to cushion and protect the fetus. With a lack of amniotic fluid the fetus is pressed up against the uterus, and this produces the characteristic facial features of Potter's sequence, which include wide-set eyes, low-set floppy ears, and a broad-flat (parrot-beak) nose.

APLASIA OF THE BONE MARROW

- Aplasia of all cell lines → aplastic anemia
- Aplasia of red cell precursors → pure red cell aplasia

APLASTIC ANEMIA

Peripheral pancytopenia

- Decreased red cells → anemia
- Decreased white cells → infections
- Decreased platelets → bleeding

Causes

1. Inherited
   - Fanconi's anemia
2. Acquired
   - Drugs and chemicals
   - Radiation
   - Infections
   - Paroxysmal nocturnal hemoglobinuria

Aplasia can affect all of the proliferating cells in the marrow, or only specific proliferating cells. Normally the bone marrow consists of three types of proliferating cells: erythroid cells, myeloid cells, and megakaryocytes. Erythroid cells give rise to red blood cells, myeloid cells give rise to leukocytes, and megakaryocytes give rise to platelets. All of these cells arise from a common precursor stem cell. Aplastic anemia results from a defect involving the precursor stem cell and causes decreased production of all of the cells in the marrow. Patients with aplastic anemia present with symptoms related to the decrease of all cell lines in the peripheral blood (*pancytopenia*). Decreased red cells produce anemia, decreased white cells lead to infections, and decreased platelets (thrombocytopenia) lead to bleeding.

Aplastic anemia may be inherited or acquired. Fanconi's anemia, one of the chromosome instability syndromes (along with xeroderma pigmentosa, ataxia-telangiectasia, and Bloom syndrome), is an inherited cause of aplastic anemia. Patients develop other congenital abnormalities including hypoplastic kidneys, hypoplastic thumbs, and the absence of radii. The most common cause of aplastic anemia, however, is marrow suppression by drugs. Other causes include chemicals (benzene and "glue sniffers"), radiation, and certain types of infections (hepatitis C). Certain predisposing conditions, such as paroxysmal nocturnal hemoglobinuria, are associated with an increased risk of developing aplastic anemia.

PURE RED CELL APLASIA

1. Acute
   - Parvovirus (B19) infection
   - Patient with chronic hemolytic anemia
2. Chronic
   - Young patient → primary (congenital)
   - Older patient → secondary to thymoma

Decreased numbers of red cell precursors without any decrease in the number of white cell precursors or megakaryocytes is called pure red cell aplasia (PRCA). This decreased production of red cells leads to decreased numbers of red cells in the peripheral blood. Pure red cell aplasia can occur suddenly (acute), or it may develop over a longer period of time (chronic). Acute PRCA is usually the result of a parvovirus infection (B19) in a patient with chronic hemolytic anemia. Chronic PRCA may present in the young or in older individuals. In the young, chronic PRCA is usually primary (congenital), while in older individuals, chronic PRCA is usually secondary to another disease, most commonly a thymoma. These unusual tumors are associated with many abnormalities including pure red cell aplasia and myasthenia gravis.

DiGEORGE'S SYNDROME

1. Hypoplasia of pharyngeal pouches 3 and 4
2. Hypoplasia of thymus → defective cell-mediated immunity
3. Hypoplasia of parathyroid glands → hypocalcemia
   - Numbness and tingling
   - Tetany
   - Positive Chvostek's sign and Trousseau's sign

DiGeorge's syndrome results from abnormal development of the third and fourth pharyngeal pouches. Patients with DiGeorge's syndrome have hypoplasia or aplasia of the thymus and the parathyroid glands. Hypoplasia of the thymus leads to defective production of T lymphocytes and defective cell-mediated immunity. Hypoplasia of the parathyroid glands leads to decreased production of parathyroid hormone (primary hypoparathyroidism). Lack of parathyroid hormone leads to decreased blood levels of calcium (hypocalcemia) and increased blood levels of phosphorous (hyperphosphatemia). The signs of hypoparathyroidism are mainly due to the effects of hypocalcemia, which may produce numbness and tingling of the hands, feet, and lips, or *tetany* (spontaneous tonic muscular contractions). Two clinical tests to demonstrate tetany are Chvostek's sign (tapping on the facial nerve produces twitching of the ipsilateral facial muscles) and Trousseau's sign (inflating a blood pressure cuff for several minutes produces painful carpal muscle contractions).

HYPOPLASIA OF GANGLIA

Hirschsprung's disease

- Congenital megacolon
- Absence of the myenteric plexus and the submucosal plexus in the distal colon
- Constipation early in life

Congenital aganglionic megacolon (Hirschsprung's disease) is caused by failure of the neural crest cells to migrate all the way to the anus. The result is that a portion of distal colon lacks ganglion cells and both Meissner's submucosal and Auerbach's myenteric plexuses. The aganglionosis starts at the anorectal junction and extends proximally. In the anatomically abnormal areas, the absence of the myenteric plexus produces a lack of peristalsis. This abnormal portion of the colon may become obstructed due to spastic contraction of the muscles. The anatomically normal portion of the colon proximal to this constricted area will become dilated (*megacolon*). Symptoms of Hirschsprung's disease include the failure to pass meconium soon after birth followed by constipation. The treatment for this disease is surgery. The constricted (anatomically abnormal) portion is resected, but the anatomically normal (but dilated) portion is not resected.

NEURAL TUBE DEVELOPMENTAL DEFECTS

- Cranial abnormalities → anencephaly
- Caudal abnormalities → spina bifida

Neural tube developmental defects are caused by defective closure of the neural tube during fetal development. These defects, which may occur anywhere along the entire extent of the neural tube, are associated with maternal obesity and decreased folate during pregnancy. Neural tube defects are classified as being either caudal or cranial defects. Failure of development of the cranial end of the neural tube results in anencephaly. This abnormality, which is not compatible with life, is characterized by the absence (aplasia) of the forebrain. Instead, there is a mass of vascularized neural tissue in this area that is called the cerebrovasculosa.

SPINA BIFIDA

1. Failure of cerebral vertebra to close
2. Associated with decreased folate during pregnancy
3. Forms:
   a. Spina bifida occulta
      • Mildest form
   b. Spina bifida cystica
      • Meningocele
      • Myelomeningocele
      • Myeloschisis

Spina bifida is a general term that refers to abnormal fusion of the lowest vertebral arches (usually the sacrolumbar region). There are several disorders in this group of developmental abnormalities that have varying degrees of severity (Fig. 9-2). Spina bifida occulta is the mildest form and is characterized by failure of the vertebral arches to form (hypoplasia). In spina bifida occulta the spinal cord and meninges are normal. The remaining types of spina bifida are associated with the formation of a cyst and are classified as spina bifida cystica. Spina bifida with a meningocele is characterized by protrusion of a meningeal sac that is filled with cerebrospinal fluid (CSF). Because the spinal cord is in its normal location there are minimal neurologic deficits. Next in severity is spina bifida with a myelomeningocele characterized by herniation of the cord and a meningeal sac through the vertebral defect. This abnormality is often associated with severe neurologic defects in the lower extremities, bladder, and rectum. The most severe form of spina bifida, spina bifida aperta (myeloschisis), results from a complete failure of the fusion of the caudal end of the neural plate that instead lies open on the skin surface. This also results in severe neurologic defects in the legs, bladder, and rectum.

HYPOPLASIA INVOLVING THE POSTERIOR FOSSA

• Hypoplasia of posterior fossa → Arnold-Chiari malformation
• Hypoplasia of cerebellar vermis → Dandy-Walker malformation

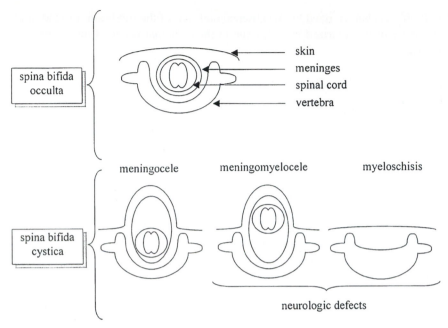

Figure 9-2 Spina Bifida
Spina bifida results from defective formation of the vertebra. Notice that the vertebra are incompletely formed because there is no bone between the spinal cord and the skin. If no cyst forms, the defect is called spina bifida occulta. If a cyst forms it is called spina bifida cystica. If the cyst contains only the meninges it is a meningocele; if the cyst contains both the meninges and the spinal cord it is a meningomyelocele.

ARNOLD-CHIARI MALFORMATION

- Hypoplasia of posterior fossa
- Elongation of medulla and cerebellum through foramen magnum
- Hydrocephalus
- Spina bifida with meningomyelocele
- Syringomyelia

Developmental abnormalities of the brain include the Arnold-Chiari malformation and the Dandy-Walker malformation, both of which involve hypoplasia involving the posterior fossa. The Arnold-Chiari malformation is characterized by a small posterior fossa. This results in elongation of the cerebellum and medulla into the foramen magnum (the medulla being S-shaped). This defect also blocks CSF from flowing naturally within the subarachnoid space (*hydrocephalus*). The Arnold-Chiari malformation is also associated with flattening of the base of the skull (platybasia), spina bifida with meningomyelocele, and syringomyelia (see below).

DANDY-WALKER MALFORMATION

- Hypoplasia of cerebellar vermis
- Enlarged posterior fossa
- Hydrocephalus
- Occipital meningocele
- Agenesis of corpus callosum

In contrast to the Arnold-Chiari malformation, the Dandy-Walker malformation is associated with an increase in the size of the posterior fossa that is due to the presence of a large cyst within the posterior fossa. This large cyst can block the foramina of Luschka and Magendie and produce an obstructive hydrocephalus. Additionally there may be severe hypoplasia or absence (aplasia) of the cerebellar vermis. The Dandy-Walker malformation is also associated with an occipital meningocele and agenesis of the corpus callosum.

SYRINGOMYELIA

- Cavity in central portion of cervical spinal cord
- Damage to crossing fibers of spinothalamic tract
- Bilateral loss of pain and temperature sensation in arms
- Preservation of touch

Syringomyelia refers to a cleftlike cavity (syrinx) being formed in the inner portion of the spinal cord. At first the syrinx involves and destroys the crossing fibers of the ventral white commissure, namely, the fibers that are involved with pain and temperature sensation (at the level of the lesion). Since a syringomyelia is usually found in the cervical area (C5–T5), this loss of pain and temperature sensation affects the upper trunk and both arms (Fig. 9-3). Touch sensation is not involved by a syringomyelia because some fibers involved with touch do not cross.

HYPOPLASIA OF THE GONADS

- Female hypogonadism → Turner syndrome
- Male hypogonadism → Klinefelter's syndrome

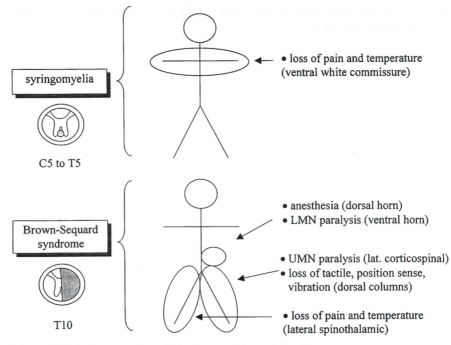

Figure 9-3 Syringomyelia and the Brown-Séquard Syndrome
It is important to compare the signs and symptoms produced by syringomyelia (due to a cystic cavity at the level of C5 to T5) with those associated with the Brown-Séquard syndrome (due to hemitransection of the spinal cord at level T10). The structures within the parentheses indicate the structure or tract that is producing the sign or symptom.

Hypoplasia of the gonads (hypogonadism) may result from abnormalities of the sex chromosomes. Lack of one X chromosome produces Turner syndrome, an important cause of hypogonadism in phenotypic females. In contrast, two or more X chromosomes and one or more Y chromosomes produce Klinefelter's syndrome, an important cause of male hypogonadism. We will discuss these two disorders in depth in the chapter dealing with genetics.

ATRESIA

- Hypoplasia or aplasia of a segment of a tubular structure
- Atresia of the aorta → coarctation of the aorta (preductal and postductal types)
- Atresia of the bile ducts → biliary atresia

COARCTATION OF THE AORTA

Preductal coarctation

- Stenosis proximal to ductus arteriosus

Postductal coarctation

- Stenosis distal to ductus arteriosus
- Hypertension in upper extremities → dizziness and headaches
- Hypotension in lower extremities → claudication
- Rib notching

Hypoplasia or aplasia of a segment of a tubular structure (blood vessels, bile ducts, esophagus, or intestines) is called *atresia*. An example of atresia of a vascular structure is coarctation of the aorta. This condition refers to narrowing (atresia) of the distal portion of the aortic arch and is divided into a preductal (infantile) type and a postductal (adult) type. The coarctation produces a discrepancy between the blood pressure in the upper and lower extremities. The blood pressure is increased in the upper extremities, but it is decreased in the lower extremities. Hypertension proximal to the obstruction produces dizziness and headaches, while hypotension distal to the obstruction produces weakness, *claudication*, and *pallor*. Increased collateral circulation in the internal mammary arteries results in notching of the inner surface of the ribs.

Another example of atresia is atresia of the bile ducts (biliary atresia). This disease is found in neonates and can produce obstruction and signs of jaundice. Histologic examination of the liver may reveal bile stasis in the interlobular bile ducts and bile duct proliferation in the portal areas. Characteristic large areas of bile (bile lakes) may be seen.

ATRESIA OF THE GASTROINTESTINAL TRACT

- Esophogeal atresia → associated with tracheo-esophagela fistula
- Intestinal atresia → imperforate anus associated with fistulas to the bladder or vagina

---

Most cases of atresia of the esophagus are associated with tracheo-esophageal fistula (TEF; the most common congenital anomaly of the esophagus). Congenital anomalies of the esophagus are classified into 5 types, but only 4 types are associated with esophageal atresia (Fig. 9-4). Type A abnormality

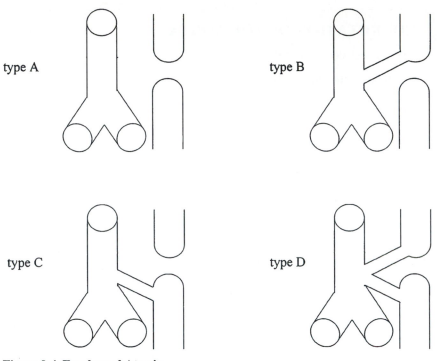

Figure 9-4 Esophageal Atresia
In each of these diagrams, the trachea is on the left and the esophagus is on the right. Each segment of esophagus has severe atresia that separates the esophagus into an upper and a lower segment. Sometimes one of these segments is attached to the trachea and forms a fistula. Type A congenital esophageal abnormality has no fistula. The trachea is connected to the upper esophageal segment in type B, to the lower segment in type C, and to both the upper and lower segments in type D.

consists of atresia of the esophagus without a connection to the trachea (no fistula). Type B consists of atresia of the esophagus with a fistula between the trachea and the blind upper segment, while type C (the most common type) is characterized by atresia of the esophagus with a fistula between the trachea and the distal esophageal segment. Type D has esophageal atresia with a fistula between both segments and the trachea. Finally, type E is characterized by a fistula between a normal esophagus and the trachea. This abnormality has no atresia and is not seen in Figure 9-4. (To summarize, type A has no fistula, type B connects to the upper segment, type C to the lower segment, and type D to both segments.)

These defects are dangerous because material that is swallowed may pass into the trachea (aspiration) either directly (types B, D, and E) or indirectly through reflux if there is a blind upper pouch present (types A and C). Additionally gastric dilatation can occur due to "swallowed" air in those anomalies in which the trachea communicates with the lower esophagus (types C, D, and E). Also important is the fact that any defect that interferes with fetal swallowing in utero will produce polyhydramnios.

Intestinal atresia is very rare, and patients present with abdominal symptoms. Patients with imperforate anus obviously present with the failure to pass any stools. These patients commonly have fistulas that connect to either the bladder or the vagina.

DEVELOPMENTAL ABNORMALITIES OF THE HEART

Left-to-right shunts

- Ventricular septal defects
- Atrial septal defects
- Patent ductus arteriosus

Right-to-left shunts

- Tetralogy of Fallot

No shunts

- Coarctation of the aorta
- Transposition of the great vessels

Developmental abnormalities of the heart may or may not cause shunting of blood between the systemic and pulmonary circulations. This provides a basic way to separate the congenital heart defects. Many congenital disorders are associated with shunting of blood, but examples of defects with no shunting include coarctation of the aorta (see above) and transposition of the great vessels (see below). The disorders that produce shunting of blood can be further divided into those that produce a left-to-right shunt (from the higher pressure left side to the lower pressure right side) and those that produce a right-to-left shunt. In the latter disorders, the blood is shunted away from the lungs and produces cyanosis.

Examples of defects that initially involve a left-to-right shunt include ventricular septal defects, atrial septal defects, and patent ductus arteriosus. These defects initially are not cyanotic (because the blood does not bypass the lungs), but cyanosis may develop later (cyanosis tardive) if the shunt shifts right-to-left due to increased pulmonary vascular resistance (Eisenmenger complex). A defect that initially is a right-to-left shunt is the tetralogy of Fallot, which is the most common cyanotic congenital heart disease in older children and adults.

VENTRICULAR SEPTAL DEFECTS (VSD)

- Initial left-to-right shunt
- Muscular septal defects usually close spontaneously
- Membranous defects associated with endocardial cushion defect

Ventricular septal defects (VSD) are the most common congenital cardiac abnormality and can occur anywhere in the intraventricular septum. They may be classified according to their location (membranous, infundibular, muscular) or their size (large, medium, small). Small VSDs are common and are usually located in the muscular septum. This type of defect is called Roger disease and can produce loud pansystolic murmurs, but they usually cause little functional abnormalities. These muscular holes tend to close as the heart becomes larger. Some VSDs occur in the membranous septum (membranous VSD) and are close to the bundle of His. High defects in the membranous septum are not uncommonly associated with an endocardial cushion defect.

ATRIAL SEPTAL DEFECTS (ASD)

1. Patent foramen ovale
   - Most common heart anomaly (not defect)
2. Ostium secundum ASD
   - Most common ASD
   - Located at level of fossa ovalis
3. Sinus venous ASD
   - Located near superior vena cava
   - Incomplete incorporation of sinus venosus into right atrium

Atrial septal defects (ASD) are located in the atrial wall at different locations that are related to the embryologic development of the interatrial septum. The initial connection between the left and right atria (ostium primum) is closed by the septum primum, which extends down from the roof of the atrium to join with the interior endocardial cushions. Before these form a complete septum, a second connection between the atria (ostium secundum) develops in the septum primum. A second septum (septum secundum) develops to the right of the septum primum and grows downward toward the endocardial cushions to close this ostium secundum. A patent foramen is left, however, at the midportion of the septum and is called the foramen ovale. This foramen is sealed off after birth and is called the fossa ovalis. The most common ASD is the ostium secundum type, which is located in the middle portion of the septum at the level of the fossa ovalis. Other types of ASDs may be located high in the atrial septum near the superior vena cava (sinus venous defect), or low in the atrial septum (ostium primum type). A persistent AV canal combines atrial and ventricular septal defects.

PATENT DUCTUS ARTERIOSUS (PDA)

- Connection between pulmonary artery and aorta
- Continuous "machine-like" murmur
- Indomethacin closes a PDA
- PGE keeps PDA open

The ductus arteriosus is a normal vascular channel of the fetus that connects the pulmonary artery to the aorta. Closure of the ductus usually occurs a few hours after delivery due to several factors, including a fall in pulmonary vascular resistance, a change in blood flow from right-to-left to left-to-right, increased blood levels of oxygen, and changes in prostaglandin metabolism (particularly decreased levels of PGE2). Persistence of a patent ductus arteriosus may occur, particularly in premature infants and in infants with respiratory distress syndrome at birth. If the PDA does not close, a shunt will remain between the high pressure of the aorta to the low pressure of the pulmonary circulation. This left-to-right shunting of blood produces a machinery-type murmur. With time a large PDA will result in pulmonary hypertension, which will reverse the flow of blood (Eisenmenger's syndrome).

Sometimes treatment with high oxygen atmosphere or inhibiting prostaglandin metabolism can induce the closure of a patent ductus. Indomethacin, aspirin, and other nonsteroidal anti-inflammatory drugs inhibit cyclooxygenase, and therefore inhibit the production of PGE2 and can close a PDA. (In some diseases it can be life-saving to have the ductus arteriosus patent, and in these individuals PGE2 may be given therapeutically.)

TETRALOGY OF FALLOT

- Pulmonary stenosis
- Ventricular septal defect
- Dextroposition (overriding) aorta
- Right ventricular hypertrophy
- Most common cause of congenital cyanotic heart disease

The tetralogy of Fallot (TOF) consists of the combination of obstruction to outflow of blood from the right ventricle (pulmonary stenosis), subaortic ventricular septal defect, dextroposition of the aorta (which overrides the septal defect), and right ventricular hypertrophy. These abnormalities produce a right-to-left shunt and *cyanosis*. The right ventricle becomes enlarged (hypertrophies) in response to the pulmonary stenosis and gives the heart a characteristic "boot-shaped" appearance. TOF is the most common cause of congenital cyanotic heart disease.

TRANSPOSITION OF THE GREAT VESSELS

- Aorta exits from right ventricle (anterior)
- Pulmonary artery exits from left ventricle (posterior)
- Not compatible with life unless shunt is present

In the most common type of transposition of the great vessels, the aorta arises from the right ventricle and the pulmonary artery arises from the left ventricle. This malformation is incompatible with survival after delivery unless there is a communication between pulmonic and systemic blood, such as with ASD, VSD, or patent ductus arteriosus. Clinical consideration should be given to keeping the ductus arteriosus open. At birth breathing will decrease pulmonary resistance and reverse the flow of blood through the ductus arteriosus. This oxygenated blood (flowing from the aorta into the ductus) inhibits prostaglandin production and closes the ductus arteriosus. Therefore, it may be necessary to give prostaglandin E2 to keep the ductus arteriosus open.

· C H A P T E R · 10 ·

GENETICS

INHERITED DISORDERS

Mendelian inheritance

- Autosomal dominant
- Autosomal recessive
- X-linked dominant
- X-linked recessive

Non-Mendelian inheritance

- Mitochondrial

Diseases frequently result from abnormalities involving genes, and sometimes these genes can be passed on from generation to generation (inherited). Disease may result from involvement of a single gene (monogenic disorders) or multiple genes (polygenic disorders). Examples of the latter include ischemic heart disease, hypertension, diabetes mellitus, and cleft lip and palate. These polygenic disorders result from complex processes that include genes and environmental influences.

Most diseases caused by a single abnormal gene are inherited in one of four Mendelian inheritance patterns. (The exceptions are diseases that are associated with DNA transmitted by maternal mitochondria.) Basically monogenic disorders are inherited in either a dominant or recessive fashion. Dominant inheritance refers to the finding that only one abnormal gene is necessary to cause disease. In contrast, recessive inheritance means that two abnormal genes, one on each chromosome, are necessary to cause disease. Additionally, the abnormal genes can be located on either an autosome or a sex chromosome. The combination of these two facts produces the four basic Mendelian inheritance patterns.

AUTOSOMAL DOMINANT INHERITANCE

- Disease produced in heterozygous state
- No skipped generations
- Father to son transmission possible
- Males and females affected equally
- Recurrence risk is 50%

Characteristics of autosomal dominant inheritance (AD) include: symptoms manifested in the *heterozygous* state (only one abnormal gene needs to be present), males and females affected equally, and vertical transmission. The latter term refers to the finding of successive generations affected (no skipped generations). Also, children with one affected parent have one chance in two (50%) of having the disease (Fig. 10-1). This is also the recurrence risk. Note that unaffected family members cannot transmit the disease.

With autosomal dominant inherited diseases, parents of affected children will have the disease unless it is the result of a new mutation, there is delayed age of onset, or the gene does not have complete *penetrance*. Reduced penetrance refers to the percent of individuals with the abnormal gene who express the abnormal trait. It is an "all or none" phenomenon. For example, a reduced penetrance of 50% indicates that 50% of those having the abnormal gene will express the abnormal trait. (In contrast to penetrance, variable expressivity means the degree of expression is different in different individuals with the abnormal gene.)

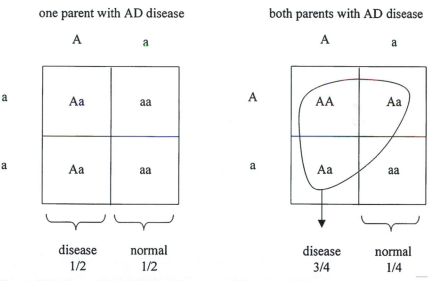

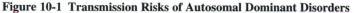

Figure 10-1 Transmission Risks of Autosomal Dominant Disorders
One way to examine the risk of transmission of autosomal disorders is to draw a Punnett square. In this Punnett square, "A" indicates an abnormal gene and "a" indicates a normal gene. A person with an autosomal dominant disorder will have at least one abnormal gene (AA or Aa), but most of the time will be heterozygous (Aa). If only one parent has the disease (most commonly), then 1/2 of their children will have the disease and 1/2 will be normal. In contrast, if both parents have the disease (rare), then 3/4 of their children will have the disease and 1/4 will be normal.

EXAMPLES OF AUTOSOMAL DOMINANT DISORDERS

Involve complex structural proteins

- Fibrillin → Marfan syndrome
- Collagen → Ehlers-Danlos syndrome and osteogenesis imperfecta
- Blood → hereditary spherocytosis

Involve regulatory proteins

- Familial hypercholesterolemia
- Von Willebrand's disease

Other

- Adult polycystic disease

Many disorders are transmitted as autosomal dominant disorders. For the most part these diseases involve structural or regulatory proteins, and the signs and symptoms are first manifested in adults.

AUTOSOMAL RECESSIVE INHERITANCE

- Disease produced in homozygous state
- Heterozygous individuals are carriers
- Skipped generations
- Father to son transmission possible
- Males and females affected equally
- Recurrence risk is 25%

Characteristics of autosomal recessive inheritance (AR) include: manifestations in the *homozygous* state, horizontal transmission, males and females affected equally, and complete penetrance is common. Horizontal transmission refers to finding the disease in siblings, not parents. That is, with autosomal recessive disorders, parents are usually heterozygous and are clinically normal, while symptoms occur in one-fourth of siblings. Also note that one-half of siblings are carriers (heterozygous) for the trait.

EXAMPLES OF AUTOSOMAL RECESSIVE DISORDERS

Storage diseases

- Glycogen storage diseases
- Lysosomal storage diseases
- Mucopolysaccharidoses
- Mucolipidoses
- Galactosemia

Blood disorders

- Sickle cell anemia
- Thalassemia

Amino acid disorders

- Hyperphenylalaninemia
- Alkaptonuria
- Albinism
- Maple syrup urine disease
- Hartnup's disease

Other

- Cystic fibrosis
- Wilson's disease
- Hemochromatosis
- Alpha-1-anitrypsin deficiency

In contrast to AD disorders, AR disorders are more likely to result from abnormality of proteins that function as enzymes. Enzyme deficiencies are usually not associated with AD inheritance, because decreased levels of enzymes usually can be compensated for. Also note that when compared to AD diseases, AR disorders tend to be more uniform in expression, and the age of onset is earlier in life. An example of the latter is the infantile form of polycystic renal disease, which has an AR inheritance, while the adult form of polycystic renal disease has an AD inheritance.

We have covered the majority of these AR disorders elsewhere. For example, we covered the storage diseases in the chapter dealing with cellular accumulations. Be sure to note that most, but not all storage disorders have an AR pattern of inheritance. For now we will briefly cover several important AR diseases that we have not previously discussed.

SICKLE CELL ANEMIA

- Replacement of glutamic acid by valine in the sixth position in the beta globin chain
- Abnormal hemoglobin causes red cells to sickle
- Chronic hemolysis of red cells
- Vascular occlusion
- Autosplenectomy
- Increased incidence of infections (encapsulated organisms and *Salmonella* osteomyelitis)
- Heterozygotes (sickle cell trait) resistant to malaria

Sickle cell anemia is a homozygous disorder characterized by the presence of sickled erythrocytes. The formation of these abnormally shaped red blood cells is due to the presence of sickle hemoglobin (hemoglobin S). Hemoglobin S (Hb S) is formed by the replacement of glutamic acid by valine in the sixth position in the beta chain. This replacement of a single amino acid is responsible for all of the signs and symptoms of patients with sickle cell anemia. On deoxygenation, Hb S polymerizes, which causes red cells to sickle. One of the most important factors affecting the amount of red cell sickling is the amount of hemoglobin S present and its interaction with the other hemoglobin chains in the cell. For example, patients who are heterozygous for Hb S (sickle cell trait, Hb AS) have about 45 percent Hb S and 55 percent Hb A. Because of the content of Hb A, erythrocytes sickle at low oxygen tension only, and symptoms are much milder than in sickle cell disease. Additionally, patients with large amounts of fetal hemoglobin (Hb F), which does not react with hemoglobin S, are asymptomatic. Newborns with sickle cell disease have large amounts of Hb F and are asymptomatic.

Patients with sickle cell disease have 60–90% of their hemoglobin composed of hemoglobin S; the remainder is hemoglobin F with a small portion of hemoglobin A2. Sickle cell disease is characterized by the triad of chronic hemolytic anemia, vascular occlusion, and increased vulnerability to infection. The severe chronic hemolytic anemia leads to chronic hyperbilirubinemia (jaundice), which is associated with the formation of pigment gallstones.

Vascular occlusion can produce leg ulcers, renal papillary necrosis, and multiple infarcts. Repeated splenic infarcts cause progressive fibrosis and splenic atrophy (autoinfarction). Most adults with sickle cell disease have a small, fibrotic spleen. The lack of splenic function along with defects in the alternate complement pathway predispose patients to infections, such as *Salmonella* osteomyelitis and pneumococcal infections. The vaso-occlusive disease can also lead to painful crises, hand-foot syndrome in children (the typical triad of fever, pallor, and symmetric swelling of hands and feet), and infarctive crises. In patients who have not yet undergone splenic autoinfarction (usually children), massive splenic sequestration (sequestration crisis) may lead to rapid splenic enlargement, hypovolemia, and shock.

The metabisulfite test is used to detect the presence of hemoglobin S. This test, however, does not differentiate heterozygous sickle cell trait from homozygous sickle cell disease. The test is based on the fact that erythrocytes with hemoglobin S will sickle in solutions of low oxygen content. Metabisulfite is a reducing substance that enhances the process of deoxygenation.

THALASSEMIA

Alpha thalassemia

- Silent carrier
- Alpha-thalassemia trait
- Hemoglobin H disease
- Hydrops fetalis

Beta thalassemia

- Beta-thalassemia minor
- Beta-thalassemia intermedia
- Beta-thalassemia major

The thalassemia syndromes are characterized by a decreased or absent synthesis of either the α or the β globin chain of hemoglobin A ($\alpha_2\beta_2$). α-Thalassemias result from reduced synthesis of α-globin chains, while β-thalassemias result from reduced production of β-globin chains. Therefore, α-thalassemias are associated with a relative excess production of non-α globin chains, while β-thalassemias are associated with a relative excess production of α-globin chains. In the fetus, the non-α globin chains are γ-globin chains (which form γ tetramers called hemoglobin Bart's), but in the adult the non-α globin chains are β-globin chains (which form β tetramers called hemoglobin H).

Most of the α-thalassemias result from deletions of one or more of the total of four α-globin genes (in contrast, β-thalassemias result from point mutations involving the β-globin gene). There are two α globin genes on each chromosome 16, and the normal genotype is αα/. On each chromosome, either or both of the α genes can be deleted. Deletion of both genes (--/) is called α thal 1. This genotype is found in individuals in Southeast Asia and the Mediterranean. In contrast, deletion of only one α gene on a chromosome (--α/) is called α thal 2 and is found in Africans. The severity of α-thalassemia depends on the number of α genes that are deleted. A deletion of only one gene (--α/αα) is seen in individuals who are silent carriers. These patients are completely asymptomatic, and all laboratory tests are normal. This clinical state can only be inferred from examination of a pedigree.

Deletion of two α genes results in α thal trait. There are two possibilities for deletion of two α genes, namely, the deletions may be on the same chromosome (-- --/αα, the *cis* type of deletion) or the deletions may be on different chromosomes (--α/--α, the *trans* type). The *cis* type of deletion, which is also called heterozygous α thal 1, is more common in Asians, while the *trans* type of deletion, which is also called α thal 2, is more common in Africans. Clinically this is quite important because the offspring of parents with the *trans* deletions cannot develop H disease or hydrops.

Deletion of three α genes (-- --/-- α) is called hemoglobin H disease. The name results from the fact that excess β chains postnatally form aggregates of β tetramers, called hemoglobin H. These aggregates form Heinz bodies, which can be seen with the crystal blue stain.

Finally, the most severe form of α-thalassemia, hydrops fetalis, results from deletion of all four α genes (-- --/-- --). In this disease, which is lethal in utero, no α chains are produced. Staining of the erythrocytes with a supravital stain will demonstrate numerous intracytoplasmic inclusions within the red cells that are aggregates of hemoglobin Bart's (γ4).

In patients with β thalassemia, a deficiency of β globins causes a deficiency of the hemoglobins that have β globin chains, and at the same time, there is an increase in hemoglobins that don't have β globin chains (due to the excess α chains present). These hemoglobins include hemoglobin A2 (α2δ2) and hemoglobin F (α2γ2).

Cooley's anemia (β thal major) is the most severe clinical form of β thalassemia. It is characterized by severe, transfusion-dependent anemia. Because of the need for repeated transfusions, over time these patients develop an accumulation of iron (hemosiderosis or hemochromatosis). Indeed, congestive heart failure due to iron deposition within the heart (a form of dilated cardiomyopathy) is the major cause of death. Individuals with β thal major have increased reticulocytes, increased hemoglobin A2, and markedly increased hemoglobin F (90%). In these patients, increased α chains produce intramedullary destruction ("ineffective erythropoiesis"). The resultant increased red marrow in the bone produces a "crew-cut" X-ray appearance of the skull and enlargement of the maxilla.

ABNORMALITIES INVOLVING TYROSINE METABOLISM

Phenylketonuria (PKU)

- Decreased phenylalanine hydroxylase (or tetrahydrobiopterin cofactor)
- Increased phenylalanine
- Mental deterioration soon after birth unless treated
- Restrict dietary phenylalanine (no Nutrasweet)
- Fair skin and musty body odor

Alkaptonuria

- Decreased homogentisic oxidase
- Increased homogentisic acid
- Black urine
- Black cartilage (arthritis)

Albinism

- Decreased tyrosinase or defective migration of neural crest cells
- Increased incidence of skin cancer

Phenylalanine and tyrosine are both dietary amino acids, but phenylalanine is normally converted to tyrosine by the liver enzyme phenylalanine hydroxylase. (It is important to note that at this step tetrahydrobiopterin, BH4, is reduced to quinoid dihydrobiopterin, qBH2.) Tyrosine is subsequently broken down into multiple substances including homogentisic acid, catecholamine, thyroxin, and melanin (Fig. 10-2). Blocks in this metabolic pathway can lead to several different diseases. For example, a deficiency of liver phenylalanine hydroxylase leads to phenylketonuria, while a deficiency of tyrosinase (involved in the synthesis of melanin from tyrosine) can lead to albinism. Also a deficiency of fumarylacetoacetate hydrolase can lead to the accumulation of tyrosine (tyrosinosis), while a deficiency of homogentisic oxidase is associated with alkaptonuria.

Phenylketonuria, PKU, is characterized by hyperphenylalaninemia, which leads to increased urinary levels of phenylpyruvate and phenylacetate. PKU most commonly results from a deficiency of the enzyme phenylalanine hydroxylase. Affected babies develop rising plasma phenylalanine level, which impairs brain development and causes the urine to have a "mousy" smell and the baby a musty body odor. Unless dietary restriction is started very early, irreversible mental damage can occur by six months of life. Dietary restriction consists of a low

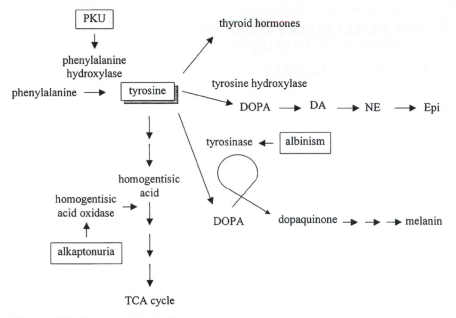

Figure 10-2 Tyrosine Metabolism
The amino acid tyrosine is involved in the formation of several important substances, including thyroid hormones, catecholamines, and melanin. Breakdown products of tyrosine also enter the TCA cycle. Abnormalities of these biochemical pathways lead to several autosomal recessive diseases, including phenylketonuria (PKU), albinism, and alkaptonuria. Realize that the enzyme tyrosinase, which is involved in the formation of melanin, is different from tyrosine hydroxylase, which converts tyrosine to DOPA in the catecholamine pathway.

phenylalanine diet. Nutrasweet must also be avoided. Very important: Pregnant women with hyperphenylalaninemia must have dietary restriction of phenylalanine since high levels of this amino acid are teratogenic during pregnancy. This form of PKU is called maternal PKU.

Alkaptonuria (ochronosis) is caused by the excess accumulation of homogentisic acid due to a deficiency of the enzyme homogentisic oxidase. Excess homogentisic acid causes the urine to turn dark upon standing for a period of time. Excess homogentisic acid also causes dark black discoloration of the sclera, tendons, and cartilage. After years, many patients develop a degenerative arthritis.

Albinism refers to a group of disorders characterized by an abnormality of the synthesis of melanin. Two forms of oculocutaneous albinism are characterized by the presence or absence of tyrosinase, the first enzyme in the conversion of tyrosine to melanin. Individuals with albinism are at a greatly increased risk for the development of squamous cell carcinomas in sun-exposed skin.

GALACTOSEMIA

- Decreased galactose-1-phosphate uridyl transferase (GALT)
- Increased galactose-1-phosphate
- Hepatomegaly with fatty change and cirrhosis
- Mental retardation
- Cataracts

Galactosemia can result from inherited enzyme deficiencies that impair the conversion of galactose to glucose. Two variants of galactosemia have been identified. The more common variant is a total lack of galactose-1-phosphate uridyl transferase (GALT); the much rarer variant arises from a deficiency of galactokinase. As a result of a deficiency of GALT, galactose-1-phosphate and other toxic metabolites, such as galactitol, accumulate in many locations. These locations include the liver, spleen, lens of the eye, kidney, heart muscles, cerebral cortex, and erythrocytes. Accumulation of galactose-1-phosphate in the liver causes a fatty liver, jaundice, and cirrhosis; accumulation in the CNS causes mental retardation.

Accumulation of galactitol can lead to the formation of cataracts. These symptoms can be explained by the sorbitol pathway. Normally this biochemical pathway converts glucose to sorbitol by the enzyme aldose reductase. Sorbitol is then converted to fructose by the enzyme sorbitol dehydrogenase. Galatose is converted to galactitol by aldose reductase, but galactitol cannot be converted by sorbitol dehydrogenase. The excess galactitol, an osmotically active substance, draws water in producing these signs and symptoms. This pathomechanism is analogous to the peripheral neuropathy, cataracts, and retinopathy associated with diabetes. Excess glucose stimulates aldose reductase and inhibits sorbitol dehydrogenase (by glycosylation). This leads to accumulation of the osmotically active substance sorbitol in certain tissues.

FRUCTOSE INTOLERANCE

- Decreased aldolase B (liver aldolase)
- Increased fructose-1-phosphate
- Inhibition of glycogenolysis and gluconeogenesis
- Severe hypoglycemia
- Cirrhosis

A hereditary deficiency of aldolase B results in fructose intolerance and the accumulation of fructose-1-phosphate. Patients with this disease tolerate milk, since the main carbohydrate of milk is lactose, but they have trouble with fruits and fruit juices, which have abundant free fructose. Normally fructose is absorbed in the gut and transported to the liver by the portal vein. Within the liver, fructose is phosphorylated to fructose-1-phosphate, which is then converted to glyceraldehyde and dihydroxyacetone phosphate (DHAP) by the liver enzyme aldolase B. Patients with a deficiency of this enzyme accumulate fructose-1-phosphate in their liver, which may produce cirrhosis. They also develop a decrease in the available phosphate, which in turn results in inhibition of glycogenolysis and gluconeogenesis. The end result is severe hypoglycemia. Treatment consists of dietary restriction of both fructose and sucrose (which consists of glucose and fructose).

X-LINKED DOMINANT INHERITANCE

- No skipped generations
- No male to male transmission
- Females affected twice as often as males

EXAMPLES OF X-LINKED DOMINANT DISORDERS

- Hypophosphatemic rickets
- Pseudohypoparathyroidism
- Incontinentia pigmenti type 1

X-linked disorders result if the abnormal gene resides on the X chromosome. The key point about X-linked disorders is that there is no male to male transmission. Note that in males, the terms *dominant* and *recessive* don't apply (since they have only one X chromosome). Also note that X-linked inheritance is different from sex-influenced autosomal dominant inheritance, an example of which is baldness.

Characteristics of X-linked dominant disorders (which are quite rare) include: no skipped generations (dominant inheritance) and no male to male transmission (X-linked inheritance). A key point is that females are affected twice as often as males. Affected females transmit the disease to 50% of their daughters and 50% of their sons. Affected males transmit the disease to all of their daughters and none of their sons.

X-LINKED RECESSIVE INHERITANCE

- Skipped generations
- No male to male transmissions
- Affected males more frequent than affected females

EXAMPLES OF X-LINKED RECESSIVE DISORDERS

Hematology disease

- Glucose-6-phosphate dehydrogenase deficiency
- Hemophilia A and B

Immunodeficiency diseases

- Bruton's agammaglobulinemia
- Chronic granulomatous disease
- Wiskott-Aldrich syndrome

Storage diseases

- Fabry disease
- Hunter's syndrome

Muscle diseases

- Duchenne muscular dystrophy
- Becker's muscular dystrophy

Metabolic diseases

- Diabetes insipidus
- Lesch-Nyhan syndrome

Other diseases

- Red-green color blindness
- Fragile X syndrome

Characteristics of X-linked recessive disorders include: an affected male does not transmit the disease to his sons (important); all daughters of affected males are carriers; sons of carrier females have a one in two chance of the disorder; all daughters are asymptomatic; and the trait occurs in maternal uncles and in male cousins descended from the mother's sisters (oblique transmission). Affected females are rare. They may be homozygous for the disease, or they may have an unfavorable Lyonization.

Examples of X-linked recessive disorders include a few hematology diseases, a few immunodeficiency diseases, a few, rare storage diseases, a few muscle diseases, rare metabolic diseases, and a few other diseases.

GLUCOSE-6-PHOSPHATE DEHYDROGENASE DEFICIENCY

- Glucose-6-phosphate dehydrogenase is rate-limiting enzyme in hexose monophosphate shunt
- Decreased NADPH in red blood cells
- Hemoglobin oxidized by certain drugs (antimalarials and antipyretics)
- Oxidized hemoglobin precipitates as Heinz bodies
- Drug-induced hemolytic anemia in African-American males
- Favism in Mediterranean region

A small portion of glucose is shunted to oxidative glycolysis through the hexose monophosphate shunt (pentose phosphate shunt). The end result of this pathway is to keep reduced glutathione (GSH) available to use as an antioxidant agent. Glucose-6-phosphate dehydrogenase (G6PD) is the first enzyme of the monophosphate shunt and converts glucose-6-phosphate to 6-phosphogluconate. This reaction maintains the levels of NADPH by converting NADP to NADPH. The NADPH can then maintain levels of reduced glutathione by converting oxidized glutathione (GSSG) back to GSH. A deficiency of G6PD results in a deficiency of reduced glutathione (GSH).

Glutathione normally protects hemoglobin from oxidative injury. If the erythrocytes are deficient in G6PD (G6PD deficiency) exposure to oxidant drugs, such as the antimalarial drug primaquine or sulfa drugs, denatures hemoglobin. This denatured hemoglobin then precipitates within erythrocytes as Heinz bodies. These cells become less deformable and are destroyed by the spleen (extravascular hemolysis). The gene for G6PD is located on the X chromosome, but it has considerable pleomorphism at this site. Two variants are the A- type (10% of African-Americans) and the Mediterranean type. The A- type is characterized by milder hemolysis of younger red cells. In contrast, the Mediterranean type is characterized by a more severe hemolysis of red cells of all ages. This Mediterranean type is also associated with hemolysis following ingestion of fava beans (favism).

LESCH-NYHAN SYNDROME

- Deficiency of hypoxanthine-guanine phosphoribosyl transferase (HGPRTase)
- Decreased salvage of guanine and hypoxanthine
- Increased uric acid
- Mental retardation
- Self-mutilation

Lesch-Nyhan syndrome is an X-linked recessive disorder that is caused by a deficiency of hypoxanthine-guanine phosphoribosyl transferase (HGPRT). This X-linked recessive disorder is characterized by gout (excess uric acid production), mental retardation, spasticity, self-mutilation, and aggressive behavior.

Y INHERITANCE

- Only males affected
- Only male to male transmission
- All males affected

Two final types of transmission are Y-transmission and mitochondrial transmission. Characteristics of the Y-transmission include: only males affected, only male to male transmission, and all males affected. An example of Y-inheritance is maleness itself.

MITOCHONDRIAL INHERITANCE

- Males and females affected
- Only females transmit the disease

Characteristics of mitochondrial transmission include: both males and females affected, but only females can transmit the disease. That is, offspring of males do not get the abnormal mitochondrial gene. We examined the mitochondrial disease in the chapter dealing with cell organelles.

CHROMOSOMES

- Haploid → number of chromosomes in germ cells (23)
- Diploid → number of chromosomes found in nongerm cells (46)
- Euploid → any exact multiple of the haploid number
- Aneuploid → any nonmultiple of the haploid number
- Triploid → three times the haploid number (69)
- Tetraploid → four times the haploid number (92)

The normal human karyotype consists of 23 pairs of chromosomes—22 pairs of homologous autosomes and one pair of sex chromosomes. The number of chromosomes found in germ cells (23) is called the haploid number (n), while the number of chromosomes found in all of the remaining cells in the body (46) is called the diploid number (2n). Any exact multiple of the haploid number (n) is called euploid. (Therefore, both haploid and diploid cells are euploid.) Any number that is not an exact multiple of n is called aneuploid. Chromosome numbers such as 3n and 4n are called polypoid; 3n is called triploid, 4n is called tetraploid. (Don't confuse triploid with trisomy. The latter refers to three copies of one chromosome, which produces a total of 47 chromosomes.)

Triploid karyotypes (69 chromosomes) are found in about 7% of miscarriages. Interestingly, they are also associated with abnormalities of the placenta, including cystic villi and partial hydatidiform moles (both of which produce large placentas). Triploid karyotypes are usually the result of double fertilization of a haploid ovum by two haploid sperm (that is, a total of 69 chromosomes, 46 of which are from the father).

AUTOSOMAL TRISOMIES
Trisomy 13 (Patau syndrome)

- Mental retardation
- Microcephaly and microphthalmia
- Holoprosencephaly
- Fused central face
- Cleft lip and palate
- Heart defects

Trisomy 18 (Edward syndrome)

- Mental retardation
- Micrognathia

- Heart defects
- Rocker-bottom feet
- Clenched fist with overlapping fingers

Trisomy 21 (Down syndrome)

- Mental retardation (most common familial cause)
- Oblique palpebral fissures with epicanthal folds
- Horizontal palmar crease
- Heart defects (endocardial cushion defect is most common)
- Acute lymphoblastic leukemia
- Alzheimer's disease
- Duodenal atresia

The three most common trisomies causing human disease are trisomy 13, 18, and 21. Trisomy 13, Patau syndrome, is characterized by forebrain and midline facial abnormalities. Patients have holoprosencephaly (fused frontal lobes with a single ventricle). Olfactory bulbs are absent. The midline facial abnormalities include cleft lip, cleft palate, nasal defects, and a single, central eye ("cyclops"). Other defects associated with Patau syndrome include polydactyly and congenital heart diseases.

Trisomy 18, Edward syndrome, is characterized by mental retardation, micrognathia (tiny jaw), low-set ears, rocker-bottom feet, and congenital heart diseases. Perhaps the most characteristic sign is a clenched fist with overlapping fingers (the index finger overlying the third and fourth fingers, the fifth finger overlapping the fourth). Edward syndrome is also associated with polyhydramnios and a single umbilical artery.

Trisomy 21, Down syndrome, is the most common chromosomal abnormality and is an important cause of mental retardation. Patients have characteristic facial features, which include a flat facial profile, oblique palpebral fissures, and epicanthal folds ("mongolism"). Patients also have a horizontal palmar (simian) crease. About one-third of these children have congenital heart defects (most commonly ventricular septal defects and AV canal defects). There is also a marked increase in the incidence of acute leukemia, usually acute lymphoblastic leukemia, in children with Down syndrome who are younger than 3 years of age.

The association of Down syndrome and Alzheimer's disease has been known for more than half a century. There is almost a 100% incidence of Alzheimer's disease in patients with Down syndrome by the age of 35. Changes in the brain of patients with Down syndrome that are similar to those seen in the brains of patients with Alzheimer's disease include senile plaques and neurofibrillary tangles. (Note: The gene for beta-2 amyloid protein is on chromosome 21, and other genes located at this site include the gene for superoxide dismutase.)

MECHANISMS PRODUCING TRISOMY 21

Nondisjunction during meiosis

- Maternal → associated with increasing maternal age
- Most common cause

Nondisjunction during meiosis (mosaicism)

- Nondisjunction early during somatic mitosis

Robertsonian translocation

- 14/21
- 21/21

Several mechanisms can produce trisomy 21, namely, nondisjunction and translocation. Nondisjunction is the failure of paired chromosomes or chromatids to separate at anaphase, either during mitosis or meiosis. Nondisjunction during the first meiotic division is responsible for producing trisomy 21 in the majority of patients with Down syndrome. The nondisjunction is maternal in origin and is associated with increasing maternal age. Nondisjunction during mitosis of a somatic cell early during embryogenesis results in mosaicism in about 1% of patients with Down syndrome.

In contrast to nondisjunction, translocation of an extra long arm of chromosome 21 causes about 5% of the Down syndrome cases. The type of translocation involved in the production of trisomy 21 is a special type of translocation called the Robertsonian translocation (centric fusion). This translocation involves two nonhomologous acrocentric chromosomes, and results in the formation of one large metacentric chromosome and a small chromosomal fragment (the latter is usually lost). Carriers of either a 14q21q Robertsonian translocation or a 21q21q translocation have 45 chromosomes, but are clinically normal. Because of the translocation, however, they can produce children with Down syndrome.

It is important to understand these different causes of Down syndrome in order to estimate the risk of recurrence to parents if they already have one child with Down syndrome. Overall, the recurrence risk of trisomy 21 is about 1%. If the karyotypes of the parents are normal, then the recurrence rate is dependent upon the age of the mother (because the trisomy was most likely due to nondisjunction during meiosis). The recurrence risk is different for a translocation-induced trisomy 21. A carrier of a Robertsonian translocation involving chromosomes 14 and 21 can theoretically produce six possible types of gametes (Fig. 10-3). In practice, about 15% of the progeny of mothers with this type of translo-

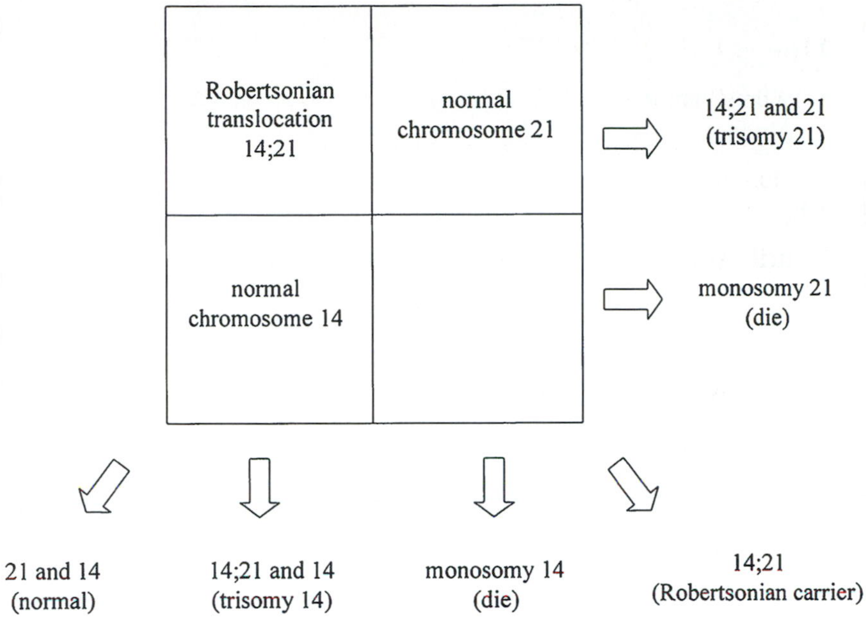

Robertsonian translocation 14;21	normal chromosome 21	⇨	14;21 and 21 (trisomy 21)
normal chromosome 14		⇨	monosomy 21 (die)

| 21 and 14 (normal) | 14;21 and 14 (trisomy 14) | monosomy 14 (die) | 14;21 (Robertsonian carrier) |

Figure 10-3 Gamete Formation in a Patient with 14;21 Robertsonian Translocation
One form of Robertsonian translocation involves chromosomes 14 and 21 and produces an abnormal 14;21 chromosome. A patient with this type of translocation has one 14 chromosome, one 21 chromosome, and one 14;21 translocated chromosome. During meiosis any two of these three chromosomes can pair together, leaving the third chromosome alone. This results in six possible combinations as demonstrated in this diagram.

cation and very few of the progeny of fathers with this type of translocation will develop Down syndrome. In contrast, carriers of a 21q21q translocation will produce gametes with either the translocated chromosome or lack any 21 chromosome. The progeny can have either trisomy 21 or monosomy 21, but since the latter is rarely viable, approximately 100% of their progeny will have Down syndrome.

CHROMOSOMAL DELETIONS

5p- (cri du chat)

- High-pitched cry
- Mental retardation
- Heart defects
- Microcephaly

11p-

- Wilms' tumor
- Absence of iris

13q-

- Retinoblastoma

15q-

1. Maternal deletion → Angelman syndrome
   - Stiff ataxic gait with jerky movements
   - Inappropriate laughter
2. Paternal deletion → Prader-Willi syndrome
   - Mental retardation
   - Short and obese
   - Small hands and feet
   - Hypogonadism

Several genetic diseases are characterized by a deletion of part of an autosomal chromosome. The 5p- syndrome is also called the cri du chat syndrome because affected infants characteristically have a high-pitched cry similar to that of a kitten. Additional findings include severe mental retardation, microcephaly, and congenital heart disease.

Two deletions associated with the formation of tumors involve chromosomes 11 and 13. The 11p- syndrome is characterized by the congenital absence of the iris (aniridia) and is often accompanied by Wilms' tumor of the kidney. (The WAGR syndrome is a combination of Wilms' tumor, aniridia, GU abnormalities, and mental retardation.) The 13q- syndrome is associated with the loss of the Rb suppressor gene and the development of retinoblastoma.

Deletions involving chromosome 15 (15q-) may result in either the Prader-Willi syndrome or the Angelman syndrome depending on whether the deletion involves the paternal or the maternal chromosome (genetic imprinting). Genetic imprinting refers to the finding that different diseases may result depending on whether a deletion involves the maternal or paternal chromosome. This finding is in sharp contrast to classic Mendelian inheritance, which states that the phenotype of a certain allele is independent of whether the chromosome is the maternal or paternal chromosome.

The best example of genetic imprinting involves deletions involving chromosome 15 (15q-). If the deletion involves the maternal chromosome, Angelman syndrome results, but if the deletion involves the paternal chromosome, the Prader-Willi syndrome results. Angelman syndrome is characterized by severe mental retardation, seizures, a stiff ataxic gait with jerky movements, and inappropriate laughter. Because of the combination of ataxic gait and inappropriate laughter, these patients are sometimes referred to as "happy puppets." The Prader-Willi syndrome is characterized by short stature, obesity, mild to moderate mental retardation, small hands and feet, and hypogonadism (characterized in males by cryptorchidism and micropenis, and in females by hypoplastic labia).

Because of genetic imprinting, loss of chromosome 15 can occur if two chromosomes 15 are inherited from the same parent. This condition is called uniparental disomy (normal is called biparental disomy). Inheritance of the same (duplicated) chromosome is called isodisomy, while inheritance of homologs from the same parent is called heterodysomy. To illustrate this concept, consider what paternal uniparental disomy of chromosome 15 means. This term refers to inheriting two paternal chromosome 15 and no maternal chromosome 15. Therefore, this is essentially the same as a deletion of maternal chromosome 15 and produces the Angelman syndrome.

ABNORMALITIES OF SEX CHROMOSOMES

Klinefelter's syndrome

- Male hypogonadism
- Most common genotype is 47XXY
- Testicular dysgenesis → small firm atrophic testes
- Decreased testosterone
- Increased FSH, LH, estradiol
- Decreased secondary male characteristics
- Tall, gynecomastia, and female distribution of hair

Turner syndrome

- Female hypogonadism
- Most common genotype is 45XO
- Ovarian dysgenesis → streak ovaries
- Decreased estrogen
- Increased LH, FSH
- Primary amenorrhea
- Decreased secondary female characteristics
- Skeletal abnormalities → short
- Web neck (cystic hygroma)

Abnormalities of the sex chromosomes can produce hypogonadism. Male hypogonadism (testicular dysgenesis) occurs with two or more X chromosomes and one or more Y chromosomes. This abnormality is called Klinefelter's syndrome and is classically associated with the karyotype 47,XXY. In most cases the extra X is from the mother and is associated with increased maternal age. (Note that these individuals have a single Barr body.) Klinefelter's syndrome is associated with decreased testosterone levels, lack of secondary male characteristics (eunuchoidism), increased breast tissue (gynecomastia), increased height (due to delayed fusion of the epiphysis), a high voice, and a female distribution of hair. Blood levels of follicle-stimulating hormone (FSH), luteinizing hormone (LH), and estradiol are all increased. Patients have small, firm, atrophic testes, which histologically reveal atrophy. Leydig cell hyperplasia, sclerosis of the tubules, and lack of sperm production. As a result, Klinefelter's patients are infertile. (Klinefelter's syndrome is an important cause of male infertility.) Patients have a slight decrease in intelligence, but they are not severely mentally retarded.

In contrast to Klinefelter's syndrome, XYY individuals, which most often results from nondisjunction at the second meiosis during spermatogenesis, are phenotypically normal except they may be tall and have severe acne (cystic acne). These individuals tend to have problems with motor and language development. The relationship of the extra Y to behavior is controversial.

Female hypogonadism can occur in individuals with the genotype XO, Turner syndrome. The lack of two functional X chromosomes precludes the development of normal ovarian tissue (ovarian dysgenesis). Instead, these XO individuals have atrophic ovaries that are devoid of ova and follicles and instead have fibrous strands ("streak ovaries"). Because of the hypoplasia of the ovaries, patients have decreased estrogen levels. Laboratory findings include decreased serum estradiol and increased gonadotropins (FSH and LH). Many of the clinical findings of patients with Turner syndrome are related to the low estrogen production. Patients are phenotypic females, but they fail to develop secondary characteristics at puberty. Turner syndrome is an important cause of primary amenorrhea. (Primary amenorrhea refers to the absence of menses by the age of 16 years.) Other characteristics include small stature (lack of a growth spurt during adolescence), a webbed neck (associated with lymphedema and dilated lymphatic channels, called a cystic hygroma), and multiple skeletal abnormalities (wide carrying angle of the arms with the elbow out, a "shield-shaped" chest, and a high-arched palate). Mental retardation is not associated with Turner syndrome.

SEXUAL EMBRYONIC DEVELOPMENT
Genetic XY

- Y chromosome produces testes determining factor (TDF)
- Sertoli cells produce Müllerian inhibiting factor (MIF)

- Leydig cells produce testosterone
- Testosterone forms Wolffian duct structures
- DHT forms prostate and external male genitalia

Genetic XX

- Two functional X chromosomes produce ovaries
- No testosterone causes Wolffian duct regression
- No MIF causes Müllerian duct development
- No DHT causes external female genitalia

Hypogonadism in females is also associated with abnormal sexual development. To understand the pathomechanism involved in this abnormal development we need to review normal embryonic sexual development (Fig. 10-4). In males (XY individuals) the presence of a Y produces testes determining factor (TDF), which causes the formation of testes. Sertoli cells within the testes secrete MIF (Müllerian inhibiting factor), which causes the Müllerian duct to regress. Leydig cells secrete testosterone, which causes the Wolffian ducts to develop the epididymis, vas deferens, and seminal vesicles. Testosterone is converted by the

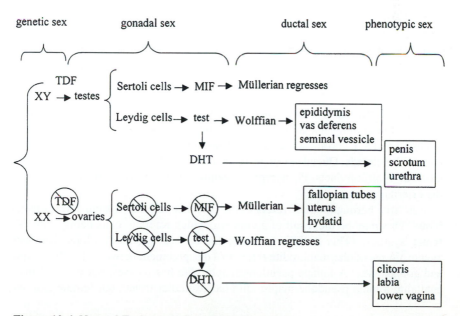

Figure 10-4 Normal Embryonic Sexual Development

enzyme 5α-reductase to dihydrotestosterone, which causes the formation of the prostate and external male genitalia, including the penis, scrotum, and urethra.

In females (XX individuals) the presence of 2 functional X chromosomes results in formation of ovaries. The lack of testosterone causes the Wolffian duct to regress; lack of MIF causes the Müllerian duct to form the fallopian tubes, uterus, and the hydatid. Without testosterone there is no formation of DHT, which causes the development of the clitoris, the labia, and the lower vagina.

AMBIGUOUS SEXUAL DEVELOPMENT

True hermaphrodite

* Ovaries and testes

Female pseudohermaphrodite

* Ovaries
* Male external genitalia
* Excess androgens → congenital adrenal hyperplasia

Male pseudohermaphrodite

* Testes
* Female external genitalia
* Decreased androgen effects → testicular feminization

Sexual ambiguity arises when there is disagreement between the various ways of determining sex (Fig. 10-4). Genetic sex is determined by the presence or absence of a Y chromosome. Gonadal sex is based upon the histologic appearance of the gonads. Ductal sex depends on the presence of derivatives of the Müllerian or Wolffian ducts. Phenotypic or genital sex is based on the appearance of the external genitalia.

A "true hermaphrodite" refers to the presence of both ovarian and testicular tissue. This may be the result of a chimera, which refers to cells being from different zygotes. (This is different from mosaicism, which develops from one zygote.) A pseudohermaphrodite refers to a disagreement between the phenotypic and gonadal sex. A female pseudohermaphrodite has ovaries, but external male genitalia; a male pseudohermaphrodite has testicular tissue, but female external genitalia. Female pseudohermaphroditism results from excessive exposure to androgens during early gestation, most often the result of congenital adrenal hyperplasia (see below). Male pseudohermaphroditism results from defective virilization of the male embryo, most commonly caused by complete androgen insensitivity syndrome. This syndrome results from an abnormality of androgen receptors (see below).

ABNORMAL SEXUAL DEVELOPMENT IN MALES
Androgen insensitivity syndrome (XY individual)

- Testicular feminization
- Müllerian duct regresses (due to MIF)
- Wolffian duct regresses (due to lack of testosterone receptors)
- Phenotypic female (due to lack of receptors for DHT)

Decreased 5 α reductase (XY individual)

- Testes form (due to presence of Y chromosome)
- Müllerian duct regresses (due to MIF)
- Wolffian duct develops (due to testosterone)
- Decreased DHT (due to lack of 5 α reductase)
- Variable external genitalia (due to decreased DHT)

The X-linked recessive disorder androgen insensitivity syndrome (testicular feminization) results from a defect involving androgen receptors (Fig. 10-5). Because the genotype is XY (male), testes form (most commonly in the inguinal canal), MIF is secreted, and the Müllerian regress. Testosterone is formed, but because of a lack of receptors, the Wolffian ducts regress, and the external genitalia remain female. DHT is formed from testosterone, but because of a lack of receptors, these individuals remain phenotypic female.

In an individual who is genetically XY, deficiencies of 5alpha-reductase result in decreased production of DHT (Fig. 10-5). Because of the presence of the Y chromosome, MIF is formed and the Müllerian duct regresses. The presence of testosterone results in development of the Wolffian duct. Recall that DHT (produced from testosterone by 5alpha-reductase) is specifically required in the male fetus for the differentiation of the prostate and the external genitalia (penis, penile urethra, and scrotum). In individuals with 5alpha-reductase deficiency, the internal genitalia are male and the external genitalia are variably ambiguous.

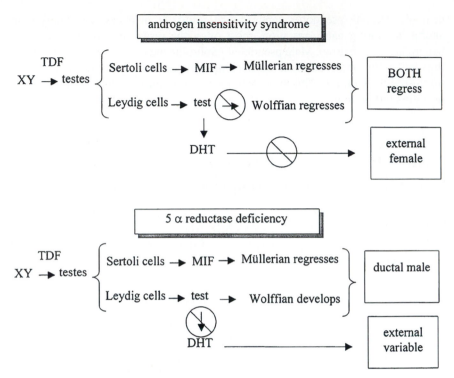

Figure 10-5 Abnormal Male Sexual Development

ABNORMAL SEXUAL DEVELOPMENT IN FEMALES

Turner syndrome (X0 individual)

- Streak gonads (due to lack of two X chromosomes)
- Müllerian duct develops (due to lack of MIF)
- Wolffian duct regresses (due to lack of testosterone)
- External female (due to lack of DHT)
- Decreased secondary female characteristics (due to decreased estrogen)

Congenital adrenal hyperplasia (XX individual)

- Ovaries develop (due to two X chromosomes)
- Müllerian duct develops (due to lack of MIF)
- Wolffian duct regresses (due to lack of local testosterone production)
- External male (due to excess systemic formation of DHT)

In an individual whose karyotype is X0 (Fig. 10-6), the lack of a Y chromosome results in Wolffian duct regression (no testosterone), Müllerian development (lack of MIF), and development of normal external female genitalia (lack of dihydrotestosterone). The lack of two functional X chromosomes precludes the development of normal ovarian tissue. Instead, these X0 patients with Turner syndrome have abnormal "streak ovaries."

In an individual whose karyotype is XX but who lacks the enzyme 21 hydroxylase in the adrenal cortex, the presence of 2 functional X chromosomes results in development of normal ovarian tissue, and the lack of MIF causes Müllerian duct development (Fig. 10-6). The deficiency of 21 hydroxylase causes excess adrenal secretion of sex steroids, which will result in excess and abnormal production of DHT in the peripheral tissue. This results in the development of malelike external genitalia in this genotypic female (ambiguous external genitalia). One might assume that the presence of excess testosterone would cause Wolffian duct development; however, this does not occur. The reason is that Wolffian duct development is dependent on local testosterone production and is not affected by systemic (adrenal) testosterone production. The end result is that

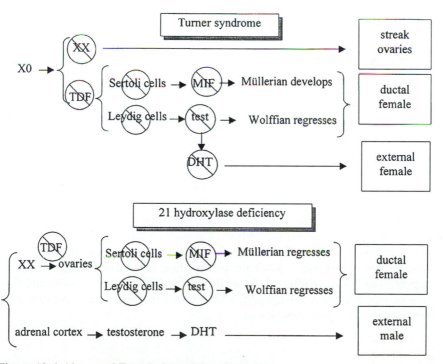

Figure 10-6 Abnormal Female Sexual Development

a female with 21 hydroxylase deficiency will have normal internal genitalia, but abnormal external genitalia. This condition is called congenital adrenal hyperplasia.

DISORDERS OF TRINUCLEOTIDE REPEATS

- Fragile X syndrome → CGG repeats
- Huntington's syndrome → CAG repeats
- Myotonic dystrophy → GCT repeats
- Spinal-bulbar muscular atrophy → CAG repeats

FRAGILE X SYNDROME

- Developmental delay
- Hereditary mental retardation (secondmost familial cause)
- Large everted ears with long face
- Large testes

Fragile X syndrome is one of four diseases characterized by long repeating sequences of three nucleotides. The fragile X syndrome, which is more common in males, is one of the most common causes of familial mental retardation. Additional clinical features include developmental delay, a long face with a large mandible, large everted ears, and large testicles (macro-orchidism).

Examination of the DNA from patients with fragile X syndrome reveals multiple tandem repeats of the nucleotide sequence CGG. Normally these repeats average up to 50 in number, but in patients with fragile X syndrome there are more than 230 repeats (full mutations). Normal transmitting males (NTM) and carrier females have between 50 to 230 CGG repeats (this process is called premutations). During oogenesis (but not spermatogenesis) premutations can be converted to mutations by amplification of the triplet repeats. This explains the much higher incidence of mental retardation in grandsons rather than brothers of normal transmitting males (Sherman paradox) as the premutation is amplified in females, but not in males. Since the premutation is not amplified in males, no daughters of NTM are affected. An additional finding associated with amplification of repeat units is anticipation, which refers to the fact that the disease is worse with subsequent generations.

· C H A P T E R · 11 ·

INFLAMMATION— PART ONE

INFLAMMATION

- Body's reaction to injury
- Cellular component
- Vascular component

INFLAMMATORY CELLS

Polymorphonuclear leukocytes

- Neutrophils
- Eosinophils
- Basophils and mast cells

Mononuclear leukocytes

- Monocytes and macrophages
- Lymphocytes
- Plasma cells

Inflammation is one of the major responses of the body to injury. Inflammation involves small blood vessels (vascular response) and cells (cellular response). The blood cells that participate in tissue inflammatory reactions are the white blood cells (leukocytes). These inflammatory cells include neutrophils, monocytes, lymphocytes, plasma cells, eosinophils, and basophils.

NEUTROPHILS

- Polymorphonuclear leukocytes (multiple lobes)
- Phagocytic cells
- Short-lived (cannot divide)
- Primary (azurophilic) granules
- Secondary (specific) granules
- Acute inflammatory responses (first cells to arrive)

Neutrophils are white blood cells that have nuclei with three to five lobes. This morphologic feature gives rise to their other name, polymorphonuclear leukocytes (PMNs or "polys" for short). Neutrophils are phagocytic cells (important) that contain cytoplasmic granules. Neutrophils have two main types of granules. The larger primary (azurophil) granules contain many different substances. One of these, myeloperoxidase (MPO), is used clinically in the diagnosis of acute leukemia. The smaller secondary (specific) granules also contain many different substances. Rather than memorize all of these different compounds, be aware of the clinical significance of two: alkaline phosphatase and NADPH oxidase. Leukocyte alkaline phosphatase (LAP) is a laboratory test that is used to differentiate a reactive increase in neutrophils in the peripheral blood (a leukemoid reaction) from chronic leukemia. NADPH oxidase is an enzyme complex found in the membrane of lysosomes that helps to destroy ingested bacteria. (Abnormalities of this enzyme complex produce a disease called chronic granulomatous disease.)

MONOCYTES

- Mononuclear cells
- Phagocytic cells (mononuclear phagocytic system)
- Long-lived (can divide)
- Chronic inflammatory responses

Monocytes are a type of leukocyte that give rise to many different types of cells, collectively known as the mononuclear phagocytic system (MPS). Sometimes this same system is called the reticuloendothelial system (RES). Cells of the MPS include macrophages, microglia of the central nervous system, Kupffer cells of the liver, and alveolar macrophages within the lung. Macrophages are monocytes that have left the blood, entered the tissues, and transformed into larger phagocytic cells. Essentially monocytes and macrophages are the same type of cell. In the blood it's called a monocyte, while in the tissue it's called a macrophage. Macrophages are the central figure in chronic inflammation.

Macrophages are phagocytic cells, but they can synthesize and release a tremendous number of substances (called *monokines*). There are far too many monokines to memorize. (A small list of the monokines includes oxygen metabolites, chemotactic factors, complement factors, coagulation factors, arachidonic acid metabolites, nitric oxide, growth factors, fibrosis factors, and angiogenic factors.) Given any substance associated with inflammation, it probably could be synthesized by monocytes or macrophages.

LYMPHOCYTES

* B lymphocytes differentiate into plasma cells (secrete immunoglobulins)
* T lymphocytes process antigens and secrete lymphokines

Lymphocytes are active in both inflammatory and immune reactions. There are two basic subtypes of lymphocytes: B lymphocytes and T lymphocytes. Lymphocytes can be activated and then can release numerous substances. B lymphocytes mature into plasma cells that secrete immunoglobulins, while T lymphocytes can secret lymphokines. We will examine lymphocytes in much greater detail in the chapter dealing with immunology, but for now we will examine how lymphocytes characteristically respond to certain inflammatory reactions.

CARDINAL SIGNS OF INFLAMMATION

* Rubor → red
* Calor → hot
* Tumor → swollen
* Dolor → pain

Now that we have briefly looked at the cells of inflammation let's turn to the processes involved in inflammatory reactions. Think about what happens when you get a splinter in your finger and it becomes infected. Your finger will become red, hot, swollen, and painful. These are the cardinal (classic) signs of acute inflammation. (Sometimes a fifth cardinal sign is added to this list, namely, loss of function.)

VASCULAR COMPONENT OF INFLAMMATION

Arterioles

* Constriction (transient)
* Dilation
* Increased blood flow

Postcapillary venules

* Increased permeability of blood vessels
* Formation of exudate

Basically the cardinal signs of inflammation result from the steps that are involved in acute inflammation. We previously mentioned that inflammation involves a cellular component and a vascular component. Simply put, the steps of acute inflammation involve blood vessels first (vasodilation and increased permeability) and cells second (neutrophil margination to the sides of blood vessels and then migration into tissue). The first step of acute inflammation is vasoconstriction of arterioles. This effect is the result of a reflex that involves the autonomic nervous system and lasts a few seconds. This vasoconstriction is transient and is quickly followed by dilation of these same arterioles. Vasodilation increases blood flow and produces the cardinal signs of heat and redness. (Increased flow of hot blood produces calor, while increased numbers of red cells associated with increased blood flow produces rubor.)

INFLAMMATORY EDEMA

* Change in permeability of postcapillary venules
* High protein content
* Abundant cellular debris
* Specific gravity of >1.020

Along with vasodilation of arterioles, the vascular component of inflammation consists of increased permeability of postcapillary venules. This "leakiness" is due to endothelial cells being pulled apart. As a result, a protein-rich fluid enters the tissues. Excess fluid in the interstitial tissue or serous cavities is called *edema*. There are in fact two types of edema. One is the result of inflammation (inflammatory edema) and one is the result of abnormalities of pressure (noninflammatory edema). Inflammatory edema is called an exudate and is characterized by extravascular fluid having a high protein content, cellular debris, and a specific gravity of >1.020. The inflammatory edema is responsible for the cardinal sign of swelling (tumor). A special type of inflammatory edema contains numerous leukocytes and cellular debris and is called a purulent exudate (pus).

CELLULAR COMPONENT OF INFLAMMATION

Intravascular phase

- Margination
- Rolling
- Adhesion

Migration

- Diapedesis
- Chemotaxis

Activation

- Arachidonic acid metabolites
- Respiratory burst
- Secretion of lysosomal enzymes

Killing

- Phagocytosis
- Destruction

The goal of the cellular component of acute inflammation is for inflammatory cells (neutrophils) to arrive at the sites within tissue where they are needed. The basic steps of this cellular component involve an intravascular phase, where leukocytes marginate to the sides of blood vessels and attach to the endothelial cells, and an extravascular phase, where leukocytes migrate to the site of inflammation and kill organisms.

Who do the neutrophils marginate to the sides of blood vessels? The loss of fluid from the blood vessels into the tissue causes the blood left in the vessels to have an increased viscosity. This increased viscosity slows the flow of blood and produces stasis. Normally both red blood cells (erythrocytes) and white blood cells (leukocytes) travel in the center of blood vessels (central axial flow). As stasis develops leukocytes begin to travel at the sides of blood vessels (margination) where they bump into the endothelial cells and bind to them (Fig. 11-1).

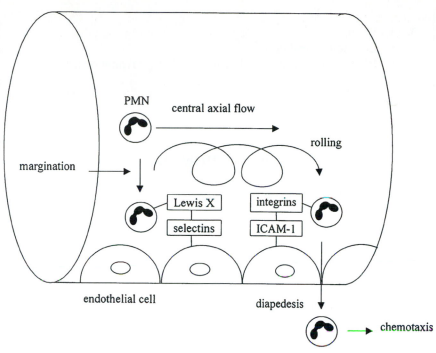

Figure 11-1 Cellular Component of Inflammation

The intravascular cellular phase of inflammation begins with margination of neutrophils (PMNs), followed by a weak binding to selectins expressed on the surface of endothelial cells. This binding results in rolling of the PMNs along the endothelial surface. This is followed by strong binding of integrins on the surface of neutrophils to ICAM-1 on the surface of endothelial cells. Following this strong binding PMNs leave the blood vessels and enter the interstitial tissue.

CELL ADHESION MOLECULES

Selectins

1. E-selectin
   - Location → endothelial cells
   - Binds → Lewis X on leukocytes
2. P-selectin
   - Location → endothelial cells and platelets
   - Binds → Lewis X on leukocytes

3. L-selectin
   • Location → leukocytes
   • Binds → high endothelial venules (HEV) in lymph nodes

Immunoglobulin family

1. ICAM-1
   • Location → endothelial cells
   • Binds → CD11a/CD18 and CD11b/CD18
2. VCAM
   • Binds beta-1 integrin

Integrins

1. Beta-2 integrins → CD18 plus one of the following:
   a. Cd11a (LFA-1)
      • Binds → ICAM-1 and ICAM-2
   b. CD11b (MAC-1 or complement receptor 3)
      • Binds → ICAM-1 and C3bi
   c. CD11c (complement receptor 4)
      • Binds → C3bi

The initial binding of neutrophils to endothelial cells is due to P-selectins and E-selectins on endothelial cells binding to carbohydrate ligands on neutrophils (sialyl Lewis X). This selectin binding is relatively weak and transient. This allows the leukocytes to roll and skip along the sides of the blood vessels.

The next intravascular phase of inflammation involves the tight binding of neutrophils to endothelial cells. This strong adhesion involves the expression of integrins on the surface of leukocytes. The integrins LFA-1 and MAC-1 bind to ICAM-1 on endothelial cells. Rare genetic diseases, leukocyte adhesion deficiency (LAD) diseases, are characterized by recurrent bacterial infections and impaired leukocyte adhesion. Patients with LAD type I have a deficiency of the beta chains of LFA-1 and MAC-1 integrins. These patients have severe recurrent bacterial infections and decreased wound healing (which can manifest itself early by delayed separation of the umbilical cord). Since the neutrophils cannot adhere to the endothelial cells, they cannot leave the blood vessels and enter the tissue. Patients with LAD type I have increased numbers of neutrophils in their blood during infections, but there will be decreased numbers of neutrophils at the actual sites of infection.

CHEMOTAXIS

1. Unidirectional migration of cells
2. Chemotactic factors
    *   Bacterial products
    *   C5a
    *   5-HETE and LtB4

Once the neutrophils adhere to endothelial cells they migrate across the wall of the blood vessels and enter the tissue. This process is called *diapedesis* and occurs mainly within venules (Fig. 11-1). Once within the tissue, the neutrophils must find the source of inflammation. To do this certain substances attract the neutrophils and cause them to move. This process is called *chemotaxis*. The most significant chemotactic agents for neutrophils include bacterial products, complement components (particularly C5a), products of the lipoxygenase pathway (5-HETE and leukotriene B4), and cytokines. These chemotactic factors function through the Gq second messenger system. Binding of a substance (in this case the chemoattractant) to a receptor bound to Gq activates phospholipase C and leads to the hydrolysis of PIP2 in the plasma membrane to IP3 and DAG. The increased IP3 in turn releases calcium from endoplasmic reticulum stores. This is the pivotal point in chemotaxis. Increased cytoplasmic calcium stimulates the contractile elements in the cytoplasm of the neutrophils (actin and myosin), and this causes them to move.

LEUKOCYTE ACTIVATION

*   Production of arachidonic acid metabolites
*   Activation of the respiratory (oxidative) burst
*   Secretion of lysosomal enzymes

Once they have arrived at the sites where they are needed, neutrophils must be activated. What substances are responsible for activating leukocytes? The same chemotactic factors that cause chemotaxis also cause leukocyte activation. This makes the neutrophils ready to perform their killing functions. Components of leukocyte activation include stimulation of archidonic acid metabolism, activation of the respiratory burst, and increased synthesis of adhesion molecules.

PHAGOCYTOSIS

1. Recognition → needs opsonins
    - Fc portion of IgG → binds to Fc receptor
    - C3 → binds to complement receptors 1, 2, 3, and 4
2. Engulfment
    - Phagosome
    - Phagolysosome
3. Degradation

Phagocytosis is the process by which certain leukocytes engulf and degrade foreign material (Fig. 11-2). Phagocytosis involves several steps: recognition of foreign substance, engulfment, and degradation. The first step in phagocytosis involves recognition by the inflammatory cell that a substance is foreign. Most microorganisms are not recognized until they are coated with special substances called *opsonins*. Two major opsonins are the Fc portion of immunoglobulin and

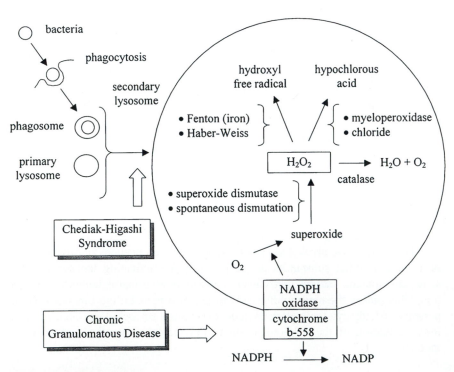

Figure 11-2 Phagocytosis

complement factors C3b and iC3b. Once attached to their surface, the neutrophils engulf and eat the bacteria. First the cytoplasmic membrane of the leukocyte surrounds the bacteria and forms a cytoplasmic vacuole that is called a phagosome. This vacuole then fuses with another cytoplasmic vacuole, the primary lysosome, to form a secondary lysosome (phagolysosome). This process is essentially the process of heterophagy.

INTRACELLULAR MICROBIAL DESTRUCTION

Oxygen-dependent mechanisms

- Hydrogen peroxide
- Hydroxyl radical
- Hypochlorous acid

Oxygen-independent mechanisms

- Lysozyme
- Hydrolases
- BPI (bacteria permeability increasing protein)
- Defensins

Now that the bacteria is within the lysosomes of neutrophils, they must be destroyed. Neutrophils have two major mechanisms to destroy bacteria: oxygen-dependent mechanisms and oxygen-independent mechanisms. Oxygen-dependent mechanisms are the major mechanisms and are illustrated in Figure 11-2. These oxygen-dependent mechanisms are also called the respiratory burst because oxygen is involved in the process. Not only do chemoattractants cause chemotaxis of neutrophils, but they also activate neutrophils. One of the results of this activation is the stimulation of the respiratory burst by activation of the NADPH oxidase enzyme complex. This complex is a group of enzymes that are located on the membrane of the secondary lysosome. Activation of NADPH oxidase causes reduced NADPH to be oxidized to NADP within the cytoplasm while O_2 is converted to superoxide ion within the secondary lysosome. NADPH oxidase is composed of cytoplasmic proteins and a membrane cytochrome complex (cytochrome b-558). Superoxide is then converted within the lysosome to hydrogen peroxide by either spontaneous dismutation (the major way) or by superoxide dismutase. Hydrogen peroxide can then be converted into powerful killing compounds, such as the hydroxyl free radical or certain acids. Hydrogen peroxide may react with myeloperoxidase (a very important enzyme in neutrophil granules) in the presence of a halide (usually chloride) to form an acid (usually hypochlorous acid). This system is called the peroxide-myeloperoxidase-halide system. (Interestingly, hypochlorous acid is responsible for the greenish tint of pus.) Hydrogen peroxide may also form the highly reactive hydroxyl radical; this is called the Haber-Weiss reaction. It usually proceeds slowly at physiologic pH, but occurs much more rapidly in the presence of Fe++. This latter reaction is called the Fenton reaction.

DEFECTS IN LEUKOCYTE FUNCTION
Familial defects

- Leukocyte adhesion deficiency
- Chediak-Higashi syndrome
- Chronic granulomatous disease
- Myeloperoxidase deficiency

Acquired defects

- Overwhelming infections
- Diabetes mellitus
- Severe trauma or burns

CHÉDIAK-HIGASHI SYNDROME

- Autosomal recessive disorder
- Defective polymerization of microtubules
- Giant lysosomes in leukocytes
- Recurrent infections
- Albinism

Several disorders result from acquired or inherited defects in leukocyte function. Chédiak-Higashi syndrome is an autosomal recessive disorder that is characterized by defects in microtubule polymerization. Microtubules are important components of the fusion of phagosomes with primary lysosomes to form secondary lysosomes. In neutrophils, decreased fusion of lysosomes with phagosomes (Fig. 11-2) results in the fusion of the primary azurophilic granules to each other. This forms giant granules (giant lysosomes) and inhibits the normal neutrophil response necessary in acute inflammation. Interestingly, these individuals with Chédiak-Higashi syndrome also have albinism because the formation of melanin pigment in melanocytes is dependent upon microtubule polymerization and is also defective.

CHRONIC GRANULOMATOUS DISEASE

- Defective NADPH oxidase
- Recurrent infections with catalase-positive organisms
- Abnormal nitroblue tetrazolium dye test

Chronic granulomatous disease of childhood (CGD) is characterized by a failure of the production of hydrogen peroxide by neutrophils during phagocytosis. This failure is due to inherited defects involving components of NADPH oxidase (Fig. 11-2). The most common form is an X-linked defect involving production of the membrane-bound cytochrome. Patients with CGD have recurrent infections, especially catalase-positive organisms, such as *Staphylococcus aureus*. Why are these patients prone to infections with catalase-positive organisms? Most of the hydrogen peroxide produced from superoxide in the secondary lysosomes is broken down by the enzyme catalase into water and O_2, while some is also destroyed by the enzyme glutathoine oxidase. The neutrophils of patients with CGD produce a small amount of hydrogen peroxide, but this small amount is quickly broken down by the catalase produced by catalase-positive bacteria.

CHEMICAL MEDIATORS OF INFLAMMATION

- Vasoactive amines
- Cytokines
- Arachidonic acid metabolites
- Complement cascade
- The kinin system

VASOACTIVE AMINES

Histamine and serotonin

- Preformed and stored in mast cells
- Dilation of arterioles (constricts large arteries)
- Increased permeability of small veins

We have discussed in depth the vascular and cell components of acute inflammation. But how does this process actually start, and how is it controlled? Inflammation is controlled by a complex system of substances and chemicals, many of which are released by white blood cells. One of the more important chemicals that controls the response of blood vessels is histamine (a vasoactive amine). Histamine is mainly released from mast cells, which are located in the connective tissue around blood vessels and lymphatics. Histamine is preformed and stored in mast cells, basophils, and platelets. (Serotonin is a similarly acting vasoactive amine.) Because it is preformed it can be released quickly, and its actions are seen early in the inflammatory response. Receptors for histamine causes dilation of arterioles and increased vascular permeability of venules. These actions produce two of the cardinal signs of inflammation, rubor (redness) and tumor (edema). To reiterate, histamine is an important chemical that is responsible for the early vascular changes of inflammation.

CYTOKINES

- Interleukin-1 and tumor necrosis factor
- Nitrous oxide
- Platelet activating factor

INTERLEUKIN-1 AND TUMOR NECROSIS FACTOR

1. Stimulate acute phase reactants
   - Acute phase proteins (C-reactive proteins, alpha-1-antitrypsin, alpha-2-macroglobulin, haptoglobin)
   - Prostaglandin E2 in anterior hypothalamus → fever
   - Increased neutrophils in peripheral blood (neutrophilia)
2. Stimulate endothelial cells
   - Increased leukocyte adherence
   - Increased procoagulation effects
   - Decreased anticoagulation effects
3. Stimulate fibroblasts
   - Increased proliferation
   - Increased synthesis

Cytokines are products of cells that affect the function of other cells (a vague definition indeed). These effects can be on the same cell that produced the cytokines (autocrine effect), on cells in the immediate vicinity (paracrine effect), or on cells systemically (endocrine effect). There are many different types of cytokines including many different types of interferons and many different types of interleukins. There are so many that it is quite difficult to memorize them all (and besides new substances seem to be discovered every day).

Four of the more important cytokines that participate in inflammatory responses are interleukin-1 (IL-1), tumor necrosis factor (TNF), nitrous oxide, and platelet activating factor. IL-1 and TNF have many similar functions and are often lumped together. IL-1 is produced by numerous cell types, including macrophages, lymphocytes, and vascular endothelial cells. Many of the systemic effects associated with acute inflammation are the result of the actions of IL-1 and TNF. Some examples include fever, decreased appetite, and altered sleep patterns. IL-1/TNF cause fever by inducing the synthesis of prostaglandin E2 (PGE2) in the anterior hypothalamus. Aspirin is effective in treating fever because it inhibits the synthesis of PGE2. IL-1/TNF also increase the numbers of cells and amounts of certain substances within the blood during acute inflammation. Increased numbers of neutrophils in the peripheral blood are called neutrophilia, while increased proteins during acute inflammation are called acute phase proteins. Examples of the latter include C-reactive protein, α-1-antitrypsin, haptoglobin, and α2-macroglobulin.

An interesting abnormality that results from the prolonged (chronic) secretion of IL-1 is a specific form of anemia associated with chronic inflammatory processes. This anemia, called anemia of chronic disease (AOCD), is characterized by trapping iron within the macrophages of the bone marrow. Normally the macrophages of the bone marrow give iron to developing red cell precursors (erythroblasts). In a patient with AOCD a bone marrow biopsy that is stained with Prussian blue will reveal an increased amount of stainable iron, but it will be mainly within macrophages instead of erythroblasts (sideroblasts). AOCD results from chronic increased levels of IL-1 stimulating the release of lactoferrin from neutrophils. The lactoferrin takes iron to the macrophages in the bone marrow and traps it there.

NITROUS OXIDE

- Stimulates Gt receptors
- Increases intracellular cGMP
- Vasodilation
- Treatment of angina
- Excess secretion produces shock

Nitrous oxide (NO) is an important substance that is found in endothelial cells, macrophages, and the brain. Nitrous oxide is one of the few substances that functions by increasing the intracellular concentration of cGMP. Nitrous oxide relaxes the smooth muscle in the walls of blood vessels. This effect produces vasodilation and increased blood flow. Substances that are metabolized to nitrous oxide (such as nitroglycerin) are beneficial in the treatment of chest pain (*angina*) caused by decreased blood flow to the heart. Too much nitrous oxide, however, is a bad thing. Excess secretion of nitrous oxide is important in the development of shock.

PLATELET ACTIVATING FACTOR

- Stimulates platelets to release histamine
- Vasoconstriction
- Bronchoconstriction

Platelet activating factor (PAF) is synthesized from membrane phospholipids (mainly basophils and mast cells) by the activation of phospholipases (phospholipase A2). PAF stimulates platelets to release histamine and serotonin. The end result is vasoconstriction and bronchoconstriction. Platelet activating factor also causes increased permeability of venules and increased leukocyte adhesion by causing the redistribution of selectin and increased integrin binding.

ARACHIDONIC ACID

Leukotrienes

1. Leukotriene B4
   - Chemotaxis
   - Leukocyte aggregation and adhesion
2. Leukotrienes C4, D4, and E4
   - Increased vascular permeability
   - Vasoconstriction

Prostaglandins

1. Prostaglandin E2
   - Fever
   - Vasodilation
2. Prostaglandin F2
   - Vasoconstriction
   - Bronchoconstriction

3. Prostaglandin I2 (prostacyclin)
    • Inhibits platelet aggregation
    • Vasodilation
    • Bronchodilation
4. Thromboxane
    • Stimulates platelet aggregation
    • Vasoconstriction
    • Bronchodilation

We have previously examined in depth the metabolism of arachidonic acid. To review briefly, arachidonic acid (AA) is formed by the actions of phospholipase A2 and can be metabolized by one of two pathways. The enzyme cyclooxygenase converts arachidonic acid into prostaglandins, while lipoxygenase converts arachidonic acid into leukotrienes. All of these metabolites of arachidonic acid are important in the pathophysiology of inflammatory processes, such as vasodilation, vasoconstriction, bronchoconstriction, and increased vascular permeability.

COMPLEMENT CASCADE

Initiators

1. Classic pathway → immune complexes
    • IgM
    • IgG
2. Alternate pathway
    • Bacterial endotoxins and lipopolysaccharide (shock)
    • Aggregated IgA (Berger's disease)
    • Cobra venom
    • C3 nephritic factor (membranoproliferative glomerulonephritis type II)

Products

• C3b → opsonin
• C5a → chemotaxis and leukocyte activation
• C3a, C4a, C5a → anaphylatoxins
• C5-9 → membrane attack complex

As involved as the metabolism of arachidonic acid is, the complement cascade is even more complicated (Fig. 11-3). It's very easy to get lost in the complement system. Basically, the complement system is a group of plasma proteins whose function is to do one of three things: attract leukocytes to sites of inflammation, activate leukocytes, and directly destroy cells. The central player in the complement cascade is C3. The key step is the conversion of C3 into C3a and C3b. The substance that converts C3 into C3a and C3b is appropriately named C3 convertase. Unfortunately there are two complement pathways and two C3 convertases.

These two pathways are the classic pathway and the alternate pathway. The classic pathway is initiated by binding of an antigen-antibody complex to a com-

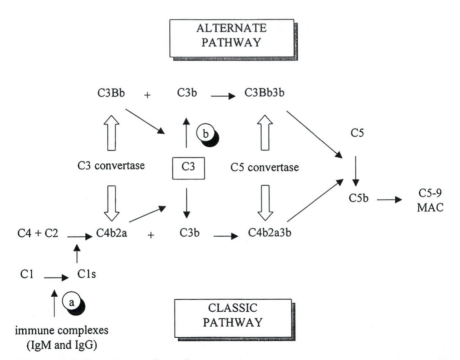

Figure 11-3 Complement Cascade
Two different complement pathways converge at the complement component C3. The alternate pathway is illustrated in the upper half of the diagram, the classic pathway in the lower half. The classic pathway can be initiated by immune complexes composed of antigen plus IgM or IgG (letter "a"). The alternate pathway can be initiated by endotoxin, aggregated IgA, and C3 nephritic factor (letter "b").

plement component called C1. The antibodies that can activate the classic complement system are IgM and IgG. Activated C1 then cleaves C4 and C2 to form a complex called C4b2a. This complex is the C3 convertase of the classic pathway. The C3b in turn forms a complex with C4b2a (which is C4b2a3b). This complex is called C5 convertase because it converts C5 into C5a (which leaves) and C5b. Note the similarity of C5 convertase and C3 convertase. Just as there are two C3 convertases, there are two C5 convertases: one for the classic pathway and one for the alternate pathway. C5b then combines with C6 and C7 to form a C5b67 complex that binds to C8 and C9. This last step produces C5b-9, which is the membrane attack complex (MAC).

The individual proteins formed during the activation of the complement cascade have different functions. The main products of the complement pathway are C3b, the anaphylatoxins, and the membrane attack complex (MAC). The anaphylatoxins are C3a, C4a, and C5a. They are called anaphylatoxins because their actions (stimulating smooth muscle contraction and increasing vascular permeability) produce some of the signs seen with anaphylaxis. These substances accomplish this by stimulating histamine release from mast cells and platelets. C3b is a potent opsonin, while C5a is an important chemotactic factor for leukocytes. Finally, the membrane attack complex can be inserted into the plasma membrane of cells forming transmembrane channels that directly destroy cells.

What about the alternate pathway? First note the similarities of this pathway to the classic pathway. Both paths have complexes that convert C3 and C5, and both paths end with the production of MAC. In contrast to the classic complement pathway, the alternate complement pathway can convert C3 directly by substances such as lipopolysaccharide (LPS), bacterial endotoxins, aggregated immunoglobulins (mainly IgA), and strange substances like cobra venom. Why is this clinically important? Think about how this alternate pathway is different from the classic pathway. Diseases that are associated with the production of IgG and IgM can activate the classic pathway, while diseases associated with the production of IgA can activate the alternate pathway. This is an important concept. Whenever a disease is associated with the production of IgA, look for activation of the alternate complement pathway.

Furthermore, when the complement cascade system is activated some components are produced and increase in amount (or are deposited in tissue), while others are used and decrease in amount. For example, with activation of the complement cascade, serum levels of C3 decrease and levels of C3b increase. Activation of the classic complement pathway can decrease levels of the early complement components, namely C1, C4, and C2. In contrast, activation of the alternate complement pathway, which bypasses these early complement components, can produce decreased levels of C3, but the levels of the early factors would remain within normal levels.

DEFICIENCIES OF THE COMPLEMENT CASCADE COMPONENTS

- Deficiency of C3 and C5 → recurrent pyogenic bacterial infections
- Deficiency of C6, C7, and C8 → recurrent infections with *Neisseria* species
- Deficiency of C1 esterase inhibitor → hereditary angioedema
- Deficiency of decay accelerating factor → paroxysmal nocturnal hemoglobinuria

Since the complement system is capable of massive destruction, it is important that the body has mechanisms that regulate and control this system to keep it from cascading out of control. Factors that control the complement system include substances that bind to and inhibit complement components (such as C1 esterase inhibitor) and substances that increase the breakdown of activated factors (such as decay accelerating factor). C1 esterase inhibitor obviously binds to C1 esterase, while decay accelerating factor (DAF) breaks down the C3 convertase complex.

Inherited deficiency of C1 esterase inhibitor results in recurrent nonpitting edema of soft tissues, especially around the face. This type of edema is called *angioedema*, and this disease is called hereditary angioedema. Patients with this disease also develop severe abdominal pain and cramps from edema of the gastrointestinal tract. To understand how a deficiency of C1 inhibitor can cause vascular-produced edema (angioedema), you have to know that not only does C1 esterase inhibitor inhibit C1 esterase, but it also inhibits other pathways, such as the conversion of kininogen to bradykinin. Therefore, a deficiency of C1 esterase inhibitor leads to excess production of bradykinin. It is the uncontrolled activation of bradykinin that produces the angioedema. (One of the actions of bradykinin is to increase vascular permeability.)

Since decay accelerating factor (DAF) increases the breakdown of the C3 convertase complex, a deficiency of DAF results in excessive activation of the C3 convertase complex, and this leads to excessive activation of the complement system. DAF is found on cell surfaces, such as red blood cells and white blood cells. With a deficiency of DAF these cells have an increased chance of being destroyed by the activation of complement. The complement system can be activated by acidic conditions, such as sleep (slow breathing causes CO_2 retention). Therefore patients with a deficiency of DAF are at risk for destroying their red blood cells during sleep. Since the destruction of red blood cells (hemolysis) can produce hemoglobin in the urine and since individuals normally sleep at night, the disease caused by a deficiency of DAF is called paroxysmal nocturnal hemoglobinuria.

COMPONENTS OF THE KININ SYSTEM

Activated factor XII (Hageman factor)

- Activates intrinsic clotting cascade
- Converts prekallikrein to kallikrein

Kallikrein

- Converts high molecular weight kininogen to bradykinin
- Converts plasminogen to plasmin
- Activates Hageman factor

Bradykinin

- Increases vascular permeability
- Dilates blood vessels
- Contracts smooth muscle
- Pain

The kinin system is involved in the production of the vasoactive peptide bradykinin. This system is initiated by the activation of Hageman factor (coagulation factor XII), a very important coagulation factor to understand because it links several major cascade systems. In addition to the kinin system, Hageman factor participates in the clotting cascade, the fibrinolytic cascades, and the complement cascade. Activators of Hageman factor include negatively charged surfaces such as basement membrane material, bacterial lipopolysaccharides, and endotoxin. Activated factor XII activates the intrinsic clotting cascade, which eventually produces the conversion of fibrinogen to fibrin by thrombin. Activated factor XII also converts plasma prekallikrein into kallikrein, which in turn cleaves both high molecular weight kininogen (HMWK) into bradykinin and plasminogen into plasmin. Kallikrein is also a potent activator of Hageman factor (positive feedback). Bradykinin is a peptide that increases vascular permeability, dilates blood vessels, contracts smooth muscle, and causes pain when injected into the skin. Plasmin causes fibrin degradation, producing fibrin-split products. It may also cause the production of the anaphylatoxins C3a and C5a.

CHEMICAL MEDIATORS OF INFLAMMATORY RESPONSES

Vasodilation

- Histamine
- Prostaglandins
- Bradykinin
- PAF

Vasoconstriction

- Thromboxane
- Leukotrienes
- PAF

Increased vascular permeability

- Histamine/serotonin
- Prostaglandins
- Leukotrienes
- Bradykinin
- PAF

Chemotaxis

- C5a
- Prostaglandins
- Leukotrienes

Opsonins

- C3b

Pain

- Bradykinin

Take a look at the chart above. It lists all of the main chemical mediators of inflammation that we have discussed in a different way, but the information is the same. (It's always a good idea to look at information in more than one way.) This should serve as a good short review of the mediators of inflammation.

· C H A P T E R · 12 ·

INFLAMMATION—
PART TWO

·

·   ·   ·   ·   ·   ·   ·   ·   ·   ·   ·   ·

TYPES OF INFLAMMATORY REACTIONS

Acute inflammation

- Sudden onset
- Short duration
- Usually involves polymorphonuclear leukocytes (neutrophils)
- Peripheral neutrophilia
- Systemic signs → fever and leukocytosis

Chronic inflammation

- Insidious onset
- Longer duration
- Usually involves mononuclear leukocytes (monocytes, lymphocytes, and plasma cells)
- systemic signs → fever (low grade), weight loss, and anemia
- Viral infections

Inflammation is subdivided into two basic types based on the length of time the inflammatory response has been present. Acute inflammation has a short duration; chronic inflammation has a long duration. There are several other basic differences between these two types of inflammation, but two of the most important basic concepts are the type of leukocytes involved in the inflammatory response and the type of infections that are present.

For the first basic concept, recall that the blood cells that participate in tissue inflammatory reactions are the white blood cells (leukocytes). These inflammatory cells include neutrophils, monocytes, lymphocytes, plasma cells, eosinophils, and basophils. Acute inflammation of tissue is characterized by an infiltrate of neutrophils, while chronic inflammation is associated with an infiltrate consisting of monocytes and lymphocytes. Therefore, neutrophils are acute inflammatory cells, while monocytes and lymphocytes are chronic inflammatory cells. (Eosinophils and basophils respond to special situations, such as allergies and parasitic infections, and will be covered separately.)

During inflammation these leukocytes are not only increased in number in the tissues, they are also increased in number in the peripheral blood. For example, neutrophils are increased in number in the peripheral blood of patients with acute inflammation. One of the reasons for this increased number of neutrophils (neutrophilia) is that the bone marrow is releasing more neutrophils and their precursors (bands) from the marrow. The increased number of bands in the peripheral blood is called a "left shift" and is a sign of acute inflammation. Additionally, not only are the neutrophils increased in number, but they have changes that indicate they are reacting to some inflammatory process. Characteristics of reactive neutrophils include toxic granulations (intracytoplasmic granules that are darker than normal), Döhle bodies (large blue intracytoplasmic inclusions composed of aggregates of rough endoplasmic reticulum), and cytoplasmic vacuoles.

Acute appendicitis is a classic example of an acute inflammation process that illustrates many of the characteristic features of acute inflammation. Acute appendicitis, a disease found predominantly in adolescents and young adults, is characterized histologically by acute inflammatory cells, neutrophils, within the mucosa and muscular wall of the appendix. Clinically patients with acute appendicitis develop right lower quadrant abdominal pain (at the McBurney point, which is 2/3 of the distance from the umbilicus to the anterior iliac spine), nausea, vomiting, a mild fever, and leukocytosis in the peripheral blood.

Similar symptoms can be found in older patients with acute inflammation of outpouchings of the colon. These outpouchings are called diverticula, and acute inflammation of these outpouchings is called diverticulitis. Most colonic diverticula are found in older patients and are found in the sigmoid region (left side) in a double vertical row along the antimesenteric taenia coli. They are thought to be formed because of increased intraluminal pressure in the colon that results from decreased dietary fiber. Most diverticula are asymptomatic (diverticulosis), but they may become acutely inflamed in a manner that is analogous to acute inflammation of the appendix. Patients with acutely inflamed diverticula present with fever, leukocytosis, and left-sided abdominal pain ("left-sided appendicitis").

In contrast to peripheral neutrophilia, increased numbers of lymphocytes in the peripheral blood (lymphocytosis) may be seen together with increased numbers of monocytes (monocytosis) in chronic inflammatory states or in viral infections (viral hepatitis or infectious mononucleosis). This leads us to our second basic concept: The inflammatory cells that respond to bacterial infections are neutrophils (acute inflammatory cells), while the cells that respond to viral infections are lymphocytes (chronic inflammatory cells). Therefore, bacterial infections cause peripheral neutrophilia, while viral infections cause peripheral lymphocytosis. This fact is of paramount importance, but there are exceptions. Make a mental note that whooping cough, caused by *Bordetella pertussis*, is associated with a peripheral lymphocytosis rather than the expected neutrophilia.

INFECTIOUS MONONUCLEOSIS

- Young adults
- Fever
- Sore throat
- Lymphadenopathy
- Caused by EBV infection (B lymphocytes)
- T lymphocytes proliferate (atypical lymphocytes)
- Positive heterophil reaction

An important characteristic of the body's response to viral infections is the presence of atypical lymphocytes in the peripheral blood. These cells are called atypical because they have abundant deep blue cytoplasm (which may be indented by adjacent erythrocytes). They are described as having a "ballerina-skirt" appearance. The presence of numerous atypical lymphocytes in the peripheral blood is characteristic of patients with infectious mononucleosis. The triad of fever, sore throat, and lymphadenopathy (enlarged lymph nodes), especially in a young adult, is highly suggestive of infectious mononucleosis (IM). This disease most commonly is caused by an infection of B lymphocytes by the Epstein-Barr virus (EBV). This virus infects B lymphocytes because they have a particular cell surface receptor (called CD21). The virus causes the B lymphocytes to proliferate (*polyclonal* proliferation), but this proliferation is stopped by activated cytotoxic T lymphocytes. These proliferating T cells are the atypical lymphocytes that appear in the peripheral blood. The proliferation of these same T lymphocytes in the paracortical (T-cell) regions of lymph nodes can produce enlargement of lymph nodes (lymphadenopathy). Additional findings of IM include splenomegaly, a positive heterophil reaction (Monospot test), and *petechiae* on the soft palate.

COMPARING ACUTE AND CHRONIC INFLAMMATORY PROCESSES

Infectious diseases

- Bacterial and viral pneumonia
- Bacterial and viral meningitis
- Bacterial and viral myocarditis

Gastrointestinal

- Acute and chronic cholecystitis
- Acute and chronic pancreatitis
- Acute and chronic gastritis

Genitourinary

- Acute and chronic endometritis
- Acute and chronic prostatitis
- Acute and chronic pyelonephritis

Let's now examine several specific inflammatory processes to illustrate the differences between acute and chronic inflammation. Let's first look at infectious diseases and the types of inflammation they produce.

INFECTIONS OF THE LUNG

Typical pneumonia → bacterial infections

- Bronchopneumonia (lobular pneumonia)
- Lobar pneumonia

Atypical pneumonia

- Viral infections
- Mycoplasma

The classification of infections of the lung (pneumonia) can be based on either the etiologic agent or the anatomic distribution of the infection. Bacteria typically cause inflammation within the alveoli ("alveolitis"), while viruses (and mycoplasma) cause inflammation within the interstitial tissue between alveoli ("pneumonitis"). The intra-alveolar inflammation of bacterial pneumonia consists of neutrophils; the interstitial inflammation of viral pneumonia consists of lymphocytes. Viral and mycoplasmal pneumonias are sometimes called "primary atypical pneumonia." The "atypical" refers to the lack of the alveolar acute inflammatory exudate that is seen in the bacterial pneumonias. Clinically the onset of bacterial pneumonia is sudden, with *malaise* (feeling bad), shaking chills, fever, and a peripheral leukocytosis. In contrast, the symptoms of atypical pneumonia usually are mild and nonspecific.

Bacterial pneumonia produces either a patchy (focal) infiltrate that involves only a portion of the lobe (lobular pneumonia), or a much larger infiltrate that involves a large portion of the lobe (lobar pneumonia). Lobular pneumonia is usually an extension of a preexisting bronchitis and is confined to the area around a bronchus or a bronchiole. As such it is sometimes called bronchial pneumonia. Lobar pneumonia is usually produced by a virulent organism. Over 90% of the cases are due to *Streptococcus pneumoniae.*

INFECTIONS OF THE MENINGES

Bacterial infections

- Increased neutrophils and protein in CSF
- Decreased glucose in CSF
- Life threatening

Viral infections

- Increased lymphocytes in CSF
- Normal glucose in CSF

BACTERIAL MENINGITIS

AGE	ORGANISM
Neonates	*Escherichia coli*
6 months to 6 years	*Haemophilus influenzae*
6 years to 16 years	*Neisseria meningitidis* (meningococcus)
Older than 16 years	*Streptococcus pneumoniae*
Epidemics	*Neisseria meningitidis*

Infections of the central nervous system (CNS) may affect either the meninges (meningitis), the parenchyma of the brain (encephalitis), or the spinal cord (myelitis). Meningitis, inflammation of the arachnoid and the CSF, may be divided into acute pyogenic, aseptic, or chronic meningitis. Acute pyogenic meningitis is usually caused by bacteria. The most frequent causes of bacterial meningitis vary according to age. Clinical symptoms produced by acute bacterial meningitis include fever and signs of meningeal irritation (including headache, vomiting, and a stiff neck). Bacterial meningitis can cause death by producing cerebral edema and increasing the intracerebral pressure. The CSF in acute bacterial meningitis is grossly cloudy and has increased pressure, increased neutrophils, increased protein, and decreased glucose.

Aseptic meningitis is usually caused by viruses (viral meningitis). In contrast to bacterial meningitis (which is life-threatening), viral meningitis is usually a mild, self-limited infection. (Note that viral meningitis is not the same thing as viral encephalitis, which is infection of the brain parenchyma.) Examination of the CSF will reveal increased numbers of lymphocytes, slightly elevated protein, and normal sugar content. Histologically the meninges are infiltrated by monocytes, lymphocytes, and plasma cells.

INFECTIONS OF THE HEART

Bacterial infection

- Neutrophil infiltrate within the myocardium

Viral infections

- Lymphocyte infiltrate within the myocardium

Inflammation of the myocardium (myocarditis) has numerous causes, but lymphocytic myocarditis is usually the result of viral infection (viral myocarditis), most commonly Coxsackie or influenza virus. Sections of the heart histologically reveal patchy or diffuse interstitial infiltrates composed of T lymphocytes and macrophages. Patients with viral myocarditis usually develop symptoms a few weeks after a viral infection elsewhere. Most patients recover from the acute myocarditis, but some patients may die from congestive heart failure or arrhythmias.

In contrast to viral infections, bacterial infections of the myocardium (bacterial myocarditis) produce multiple foci of inflammation composed mainly of neutrophils. The heart can also be damaged from bacterial toxins rather than as a direct infection of the heart itself. The myocardial inflammation in patients with diphtheria is the result of an exotoxin.

INFLAMMATION OF THE GALLBLADDER

Acute inflammation

- Right upper quadrant pain that does not subside
- Fever
- Peripheral neutrophilia
- Palpable mass
- Neutrophils in wall of gallbladder

Chronic inflammation

- Intermittent cramps in right upper quadrant
- No fever, peripheral neutrophilia, or palpable mass
- Lymphocytes in thickened wall of gallbladder

Now that we have seen several examples that illustrate the differences between the inflammatory response produced by bacteria and viruses, let's look at several clinical examples of diseases that illustrate the differences between the acute inflammatory response and the chronic inflammatory response. For example, inflammation of the gallbladder may occur quickly (acute cholecystitis), or it may occur over a prolonged period of time (chronic cholecystitis). Histologic examination of the gallbladder in a patient with acute cholecystitis reveals an acute inflammatory response (neutrophils) along with edema and vascular congestion. Acute cholecystitis in the majority of cases is caused by impaction of a gallstone in the neck of the gallbladder or cystic duct (calculous acute cholecystitis). Patients more often are older, obese females. In contrast, the remaining cases that have no stones (acalculous acute cholecystitis) occur more often in older males and children. Acalculous acute cholecystitis may be associated with prolonged fasting, which makes the bile become thick like "sludge." Acute cholecystitis usually presents with right upper quadrant pain that does not subside, and many times is a surgical emergency. Patients develop typical signs of acute inflammation including fever and a peripheral leukocytosis (neutrophilia). Physical examination may reveal a palpable mass in the right upper quadrant of the abdomen.

Chronic cholecystitis is almost always associated with a gallstone (cholelithiasis) and is seen most often in middle-aged and older, obese females. The histologic changes are extremely variable and include chronic inflammation (lymphocytes), fibrosis of wall of the gallbladder, and invaginations of mucosa into the muscularis (Rokitansky-Aschoff sinuses). Patients with chronic cholecystitis develop intermittent biliary-type pain, that is, cramping pain in the right upper quadrant. The pain develops very rapidly and then subsides over several hours. In contrast to acute cholecystitis, patients with chronic cholecystitis do not develop fever, peripheral neutrophilia, or a palpable mass in the right upper quadrant. This latter physical finding is quite important clinically in the differentiation between obstruction of the bile ducts caused by chronic gallbladder disease with obstruction caused by cancer of the pancreas.

INFLAMMATION OF THE PANCREAS

Acute inflammation

- Severe constant epigastric pain
- Pain may radiate to the back
- Fever, nausea, and vomiting
- Increased serum amylase and lipase
- Systemic complications (ARDS and DIC)

Chronic inflammation

- Severe constant or intermittent epigastric pain
- Signs of malabsorption
- Local complications (pseudocyst and cancer)

Inflammation of the pancreas (pancreatitis) may be either acute or chronic. Acute pancreatitis may be clinically mild (interstitial or edematous pancreatitis) or severe (acute hemorrhagic pancreatitis). Most cases of acute pancreatitis are associated with either biliary tract disease (gallstones) or alcoholism. Other less frequent associations include hypercalcemia (which stimulates the activation of trypsinogen in the pancreatic duct), hyperlipidemias, shock, infections (CMV and mumps), and drugs.

Acute pancreatitis usually presents as a medical emergency. Symptoms of acute pancreatitis include abdominal pain that is localized to the epigastrium and may radiate to the back, vomiting, and shock. The latter is the result of hemorrhage and kinin release into the blood. In severe pancreatitis there may be hemorrhage in the subcutaneous tissue around the umbilicus (Cullen's sign) or in the flanks (Turner's sign). Activation of the plasma coagulation cascade may lead to disseminated intravascular coagulation (DIC). Laboratory diagnosis of pancreatitis involves the initial finding of elevated serum amylase levels, and rising lipase levels over the next several days. Other pancreatic enzymes, such as trypsin, chymotrypsin, and carboxypeptidases are not useful for diagnosis. (One reason is that substances within the blood can inhibit their activity. For example, alpha-1-antitrypsin can obviously inhibit trypsin activity.) Many patients with pancreatitis also have liver damage (from alcoholism) or gallstone disease. Enzymes that detect liver damage include aspartate aminotransferase (AST) and gamma-glutaryl transpeptidase (GGT).

The signs and symptoms of acute pancreatitis are the result of activation of pancreatic enzymes. For example, the release of lipase results in local and systemic fat necrosis. This local change, seen grossly as focal chalky white areas, is one of the characteristic features of acute pancreatitis. It produces the formation of calcium soaps and decreases the blood levels of calcium. Hypocalcemia in a patient with acute pancreatitis is a bad prognostic finding. Fat necrosis releases fat globules into *ascites* fluid and gives it the appearance of "chicken broth." Lipase activation in the lungs interferes with the functioning of surfactant and can lead to the development of adult respiratory distress syndrome (ARDS). Both trypsin and chymotrypsin activate many enzymes and serum factors, including phospholipase (cell membrane injury), elastase (vascular injury and hemorrhage), Hageman factor (disseminated intravascular coagulation, DIC), and complement and kinins (acute inflammation). The combination of all of these factors can produce shock. (Note that amylase, although used clinically as a laboratory test to diagnose pancreatitis, does not itself contribute to the symptoms of acute pancreatitis.)

In contrast to acute pancreatitis, chronic pancreatitis is characterized histologically by chronic inflammation, atrophy of the acini, and irregular fibrosis. Grossly the pancreas is hard with focal areas of calcification. Stones (pancreatic calculi) may be found within the ducts. It can be quite difficult to differentiate chronic pancreatitis grossly from cancer of the pancreas.

In adults the major cause of chronic pancreatitis is chronic alcoholism, while in children the major cause is cystic fibrosis. Hypercalcemia and hyperlipidemia predispose patients to chronic pancreatitis because they are causes of acute pancreatitis, and recurrent attacks of acute pancreatitis can produce chronic pancreatitis. In a significant number of patients, recurrent pancreatitis is associated with pancreas divisum. This condition refers to the finding that the accessory duct becomes the major excretory duct of the pancreas. Chronic ductal obstruction may be a cause of chronic pancreatitis and may be associated with gallstones. (It is better, however, to associate gallstones with acute ductal obstruction and acute pancreatitis rather than chronic disease.)

Chronic pancreatitis can present as repeated attacks of abdominal pain, or persistent abdominal and back pain. These attacks may be precipitated by alcohol abuse, overeating, or the use of certain drugs. Other symptoms of chronic pancreatitis may be produced by decreased functioning of the exocrine pancreas. The absence of lipase (essential for fat digestion) leads to greasy, bulky, light-colored stools (*steatorrhea*). In contrast, although pancreatic amylase and trypsin are important for carbohydrate and protein digestion, patients with pancreatic insufficiency seldom present with maldigestion of carbohydrates and protein because other enzymes in gastric and intestinal juice can compensate for their loss. Other symptoms of chronic pancreatitis include malabsorption of fat-soluble vitamins, vitamin B12 deficiency (pancreatic enzymes are needed to degrade the normal complex of B12 and its binding protein), and weight loss. Complications of chronic pancreatitis include pseudocyst formation and an increased risk of developing pancreatic carcinoma.

INFLAMMATION OF THE STOMACH
Acute gastritis

1. Mucosal erosions (hemorrhages)
2. Causes
   - Drugs (alcohol, NSAIDs, chemotherapy)
   - Ischemia or shock
   - Burn injury → Curling's ulcers
   - Brain injury → Cushing's ulcers

Chronic gastritis

1. Lymphocytes in mucosa (plus neutrophils = active chronic gastritis)
2. Types
   a. *Helicobacter pylori* gastritis (active chronic gastritis)
   b. Reflux gastritis
   c. Atrophic (metaplastic) gastritis
      - Type A → autoimmune gastritis (pernicious anemia)
      - Type B → environmental gastritis

Gastritis is a nonspecific term that describes any inflammation of the gastric mucosa. Gastritis may be either acute or chronic. Based on our previous discussions, you should expect acute gastritis to be characterized by acute inflammatory cells (neutrophils). Unfortunately, most rules have exceptions, and inflammation of the stomach is one of the exceptions to the rule about neutrophils and acute inflammation. In the stomach, the presence of neutrophils is described as being "active" inflammation and not "acute" inflammation. Instead, the term "acute gastritis" is used to refer to erosions of the gastric mucosa. (*Erosions* involve only the most superficial portion of the mucosa, in contrast to mucosal ulcers, which involve the full thickness of the mucosa.) Acute gastritis is also known as hemorrhagic gastritis or acute erosive gastritis. It is associated with the use of nonsterodial anti-inflammatory drugs (aspirin, ibuprofen, and corticosteroids), alcohol, chemotherapy, ischemia, and severe stress. (Curling's ulcers are seen in patients with severe burns, while Cushing's ulcers are seen in patients with intracranial lesions.) Grossly there are multiple, scattered, punctate (less than 1 cm) hemorrhagic areas in the gastric mucosa. This is a helpful sign to differentiate them from peptic ulcers, which tend to be solitary and larger. Microscopically the gastric mucosa from a patient with acute gastritis is likely to reveal mucosal erosions (obviously), scattered neutrophils, edema, and possibly *hemorrhage*.

In contrast, chronic gastritis is characterized histologically by the presence of lymphocytes and plasma cells. Again it is important to realize that the presence of neutrophils within the glandular epithelium indicates active inflammation. Neutrophils may be the main type of inflammatory cell that is present (acute gastritis), or they may be combined with more numerous chronic inflammation (active chronic gastritis). Chronic gastritis is divided into subgroups based on etiology, location, histopathology, and clinical features. The basic types of chronic gastritis include *Helicobacter pylori* gastritis, chemical (reflux) gastritis, and metaplastic atrophic gastritis.

HELICOBACTER PYLORI

- Location → stomach
- Produces urease (raises stomach pH)
- Active chronic gastritis
- Peptic ulcers of stomach and duodenum
- Treatment is antibiotics combined with bismuth agents

Helicobacter pylori gastritis is associated (obviously) with *Helicobacter pylori*, a small, curved, gram-negative rod that is present in about 20% of the general population. These bacteria are found in the mucus overlying the surface epithelium. This type of gastritis affects primarily the antral mucosa and is associated with active chronic gastritis.

Reflux gastritis is usually seen following partial gastrectomy and refers to the reflux of duodenal contents and bile back into the stomach. It is actually a misnomer because the inflammatory response is minimal. Instead histologically there is foveolar hyperplasia, edema, and congestion of the mucosa.

Atrophic gastritis (decreased numbers of parietal cells) is associated with intestinal metaphasia and is also called metaplastic atrophic gastritis. There are two types of atrophic gastritis, type A and type B. Autoimmune gastritis, type A atrophic gastritis, is characterized by the presence of parietal cell antibodies or intrinsic factor antibodies. This is the type of gastritis that is associated with pernicious anemia. Type B (environmental) gastritis is associated with intestinal metaplasia of the antrum. This type of gastritis is not associated with autoimmune antibodies, and there is a questionable association with *H. pylori*.

INFLAMMATION OF THE ENDOMETRIUM

Acute inflammation

- Neutrophils in endometrium (not menstrual endometrium)
- Bacterial infections following delivery or a miscarriage

Chronic inflammation

- Plasma cells in the endometrium

The endometrium and myometrium are relatively resistant to infections. As a result, inflammation of the endometrium (endometritis) is rare. The diagnosis of endometritis depends on finding inflammatory cells within the endometrium that are not normally present during the normal menstrual cycle. Polymorphonuclear leukocytes (neutrophils) are normally present during menstruation, and there is usually a stromal lymphocytic infiltrate at other times of the menstrual cycle. Lymphoid aggregates and lymphoid follicles may also be seen in normal endometrium. Acute endometritis, usually caused by bacterial infections following delivery or a miscarriage, is characterized by the presence of neutrophils in endometrial tissue that is not menstrual endometrium. The most common organisms causing acute endometritis are *Staphylococcus aureus* and *Streptococcus* species.

Chronic endometritis may be seen in patients with intrauterine devices (IUDs), pelvic inflammatory disease (PID), retained products of conception (postpartum), or tuberculosis (caseating *granulomas* with giant cells). These are secondary causes of chronic endometritis. In a significant number of cases, no underlying cause is found. The histologic diagnosis of chronic endometritis depends on finding plasma cells within the endometrium. All it takes is *one* plasma cell to make this diagnosis.

INFLAMMATION OF THE PROSTATE

Acute inflammation

1. Acute bacterial prostatitis
   - *Escherichia coli*

Chronic inflammation

1. Chronic bacterial prostatitis
   - Recurrent urinary tract infections
2. Chronic abacterial prostatitis
   - *Chlamydia trachomatis*
   - *Ureaplasma urealyticum*

Inflammation of the prostate (prostatitis) is related to bacterial infection of the prostate. This is the case for acute prostatitis, but unfortunately some cases of chronic prostatitis are also associated with bacterial infections (another exception to the general rule). This divides chronic prostatitis into three groups: acute bacterial, chronic bacterial and chronic abacterial prostatitis.

Bacterial prostatitis is caused by the same organisms that commonly cause urinary tract infections (UTI). *E. coli* is the most common etiology. In acute prostatitis the organism reaches the prostate by direct extension from the posterior urethra or the bladder. In chronic bacterial prostatitis the bacteria are protected from antibiotics (most antibiotics do not penetrate the prostate). Chronic prostatitis is associated with recurrent UTIs with the same organism. Sometimes bacteria can be found in the prostatic secretions of patients with chronic prostatitis, but there are increased numbers of leukocytes. These cases are called chronic abacterial prostatitis and are the most common form of prostatitis. They are thought to be caused by *Chlamydia trachomatis* or *Ureaplasma urealyticum*. Histologically acute prostatitis reveals edema, congestion, and acute inflammation (neutrophils). Chronic prostatitis reveals numerous lymphocytes, plasma cells, and macrophages.

The diagnosis of prostatitis depends on combining clinical signs and symptoms with laboratory cultures. Symptoms of acute and chronic prostatitis include low back pain, *dysuria* (pain and burning with urination), *frequency* (voiding small amounts of urine at frequent intervals) and *urgency* (the feeling of having to urinate immediately). Fever, chills, and malaise can also be present in acute infections, but finding increased numbers of leukocytes in prostatic secretions is needed to make the diagnosis. Clinical examination reveals marked tenderness with rectal examination.

INFLAMMATION OF THE KIDNEY

Acute inflammation

1. Glomeruli (glomerulonephritis)
   - Nephritic syndrome
   - Red blood cells and red blood cell casts in urine
2. Tubules and interstitium (acute pyelonephritis)
   - Bacterial infection (gram-negative enteric bacilli)
   - Ascending infection from urinary bladder
   - High fever, chills, and flank pain
   - White blood cells and white blood cell casts in urine

Chronic inflammation

1. Glomeruli (chronic glomerulonephritis)
2. Tubules and interstitium (chronic pyelonephritis)
   - Chronic reflux or obstruction
   - U-shaped scars
   - "Thyroidization"

Inflammation of the kidneys may affect primarily the glomeruli (glomerulonephritis) or the tubules and the interstitium (pyelonephritis). Glomerular diseases are broadly classified as producing either the nephritic syndrome or the nephrotic syndrome. The nephrotic syndrome is characterized by the massive loss of protein in the urine (proteinuria), while the nephritic syndrome is mainly caused by inflammatory glomerular diseases. In contrast to the nephrotic syndrome, the nephritic syndrome is associated with hematuria (blood in the urine). Red blood cell casts may be present. These patients may lose protein in the urine, but it is generally less severe than in patients with the nephrotic syndrome. Patients also retain salt and water, and this can lead to hypertension and peripheral edema. The major causes of the nephritic syndrome involve immune-related processes with electron-dense deposits. We will discuss these diseases in the chapter dealing with immunology.

Acute pyelonephritis is characterized histologically by the presence of acute inflammation (neutrophils) in the renal tubules and interstitium. Most cases of acute pyelonephritis are the result of bacterial infection of the kidneys. Patients present with the sudden onset of high fever, chills, and flank pain. Examination of the urine reveals mild proteinuria with neutrophils, bacteria, and white cell casts. The presence of white cell casts helps to differentiate acute pyelonephritis and bacterial infection of the urinary bladder (in which no white cell casts are formed). In fact, the presence of white cell casts in the urine is pathognomonic for acute pyelonephritis.

The bacteria that cause acute pyelonephritis are usually gram-negative enteric bacilli. The bacteria may reach the kidney via the bloodstream (hematogenous route), but more often they ascend to the kidneys from the urinary bladder. Factors that predispose individuals to acute pyelonephritis include renal stones (calculi), diabetes mellitus, urinary obstruction, vesicoureteral reflux, catheterization, and a short urethra (females). Complications of acute pyelonephritis include gram-negative sepsis, pyonephrosis (pus in a dilated renal pelvis), perinephric abscess, and renal papillary necrosis (diabetes mellitus).

Chronic pyelonephritis results from chronic infection of the kidney and is related to chronic obstruction or chronic reflux from the bladder. Clinically patients develop hypertension, chronic renal failure, pyuria (neutrophils in the urine), mild proteinuria, and bacteriuria. Grossly the kidneys develop deep U-shaped scars overlying deformed calyxes. These scars cause the kidneys to become asymmetrically contracted. These U-shaped cortical scars contrast with the V-shaped scars produced by vascular disease (blood vessel occlusion). Histologic examination of the kidneys in patients with chronic pyelonephritis reveals interstitial fibrosis with chronic inflammatory cells (lymphocytes and plasma cells). Many of the glomeruli are fibrotic (global sclerosis); many of the tubules are dilated and contain amorphic, eosinophilic material. This histologic change is called "thyroidization" of the kidney. This refers to a vague histologic resemblance to the follicles of the thyroid and is not the result of a metaplastic process.

MORPHOLOGIC PATTERNS OF INFLAMMATION
Classic acute inflammation

* Bacterial infections
* Tissue necrosis

Suppurative (purulent) inflammation

* Pyogenic bacteria

Serous inflammation

* Skin blisters
* Burns
* Effusions

Fibrinous inflammation

- Fibrinous pericarditis

Catarrhal inflammation (coryza)

- Common cold (rhinovirus)
- Allergy

Membranous (pseudomembranous) inflammation

- Larynx
- Colon

Abscess

- Lung abscess
- Brain abscess

Granulomatous inflammation

- Caseating granulomas
- Noncaseating granulomas

Ulcer

- Peptic ulcers
- Ulcerative colitis

Inflammatory reactions can be divided into several morphologic patterns based on their histologic appearance. Classic acute inflammation reveals numerous neutrophils along with the possible deposition of fibrin or destruction of tissue. This appearance can be seen with acute tissue necrosis or bacterial infections and is illustrated by all of the above clinical examples. Suppurative (purulent) inflammation is a term used to describe the production of pus, which consists of the combination of edema, necrotic tissue, and neutrophils (liquefactive necrosis).

In addition to the classic appearance, there are other morphologic patterns of inflammation, including serous inflammation, fibrinous inflammation, catarrhal inflammation, pseudomembranous inflammation, and abscesses. Serous inflammation refers to the production of a clear fluid, such as within skin blisters or body cavities. With serous inflammation, there is not enough fibrinogen present to form fibrin. In contrast, fibrinous inflammation is seen with more severe injuries and is associated with the deposition of fibrin in body cavities or spaces (such as the pericardial cavity). Histologically fibrin is seen as amorphic eosinophilic material.

PERICARDITIS

Acute pericarditis

- Serous pericarditis → rheumatic fever, systemic lupus erythematosus, uremia
- Fibrinous pericarditis → more severe serous pericarditis, viruses, myocardial infarction
- Purulent (suppurative) pericarditis → bacteria
- Hemorrhagic pericarditis → carcinoma and tuberculosis

Chronic pericarditis

- Adhesive pericarditis
- Constrictive pericarditis

Fibrinous inflammation within the pericardial cavity (fibrinous pericarditis) produces a characteristic "bread and butter" appearance grossly. It is one type of pericarditis. Inflammation of the pericardium (pericarditis) may be acute or chronic. Patients develop severe retrosternal chest pain that is typically worse with deep inspiration or coughing. Physical examination reveals a characteristic pericardial friction rub. Acute pericarditis may be subdivided into serous, fibrinous, purulent (suppurative), or hemorrhagic types. Chronic pericarditis can be adhesive or constrictive. Adhesive pericarditis is the result of fibrous plaques and causes cardiac dilation and hypertrophy. In contrast, constrictive pericarditis produces decreased cardiac output and increased jugular venous pressure, but there is no cardiac dilation or hypertrophy.

Catarrhal (phlegmonous or coryza) inflammation refers to excessive mucous secretions, such as seen with a runny nose or allergies. We will discuss the pathomechanisms of allergies in depth in the chapter dealing with immunology.

Pseudomembranous inflammation refers to the formation of necrotic membranes on mucosal surfaces. Two classic infections that are associated with pseudomembrane formation are *Clostridium difficile* and *Corynebacterium diphtheria*. *C. difficile* infection produces a characteristic "mushroom-shaped" pseudomembrane in the colon of people who are taking broad-spectrum antibiotics. In contrast, *C. diphtheria* produces a pseudomembrane in the larynx of individuals with diphtheria. *Corynebacterium diphtheria* secretes an exotoxin that causes the inactivation of EF-2 (elongation factor 2) by transferring ADPR to EF-2. In this process, NAD is converted to nicotinic acid. The mechanism of this toxin is the same as in exotoxin A produced by *Pseudomonas aeruginosa*.

An *abscess* is a localized collection of neutrophils and necrotic debris. Essentially an abscess is a localized form of suppurative inflammation. *Staphylococcus aureus* classically produce abscesses, because these bacteria are coagulase-positive, and the coagulase helps to produce fibrinous material that localizes the infection. Two examples of localized abscess formation are lung abscesses and brain abscesses. A lung abscess may be the result of aspiration of food or gastric material, or it may be a complication of a bacterial pneumonia. Aspiration more often produces a right-sided single abscess, because the right-sided airways are more vertical, while bacterial pneumonia produces multiple abscesses. Clinically a patient with a lung abscess may develop a prominent cough with copious amounts of foul-smelling purulent sputum. Changes in the patient's position can produce paroxysms of coughing. Patients also have fever and malaise.

Brain abscess usually occurs secondary to other diseases, such as chronic suppurative infections of the middle ear, the mastoid air spaces, the paranasal sinuses, the heart (infective endocarditis), or the lung. Grossly a brain abscess is a mass within the brain that has a liquefied center filled with pus. Symptoms are the result of the mass effect produced by the abscess itself and include headache, vomiting, and papilledema.

INFLAMMATION OF THE COLON
Ulcerative colitis

- Crypt abscesses (microabscesses) and crypt distortion
- Disease begins in rectum and extends proximally (no skip lesions)
- Doesn't involve small intestines
- Superficial mucosal involvement (not transmural)
- Risk of colon cancer and toxic megacolon

Crohn's disease

- Granulomas
- Segmental involvement (skip lesions)
- May involve small intestines (regional enteritis or ileitis)
- Transmural involvement → fissures, fistulas, and obstruction

The term *inflammatory bowel disease* (IBD) is used to describe two diseases that have many similar features—Crohn's disease and ulcerative colitis. Histologically both of these diseases produce destruction and distortion of the normal architecture of the colon crypts. Abnormalities of the colonic crypts themselves help to differentiate IBD from infectious colitis. Both Crohn's disease and ulcerative colitis produce acute and chronic inflammation of the colonic mucosa. Lymphocytes and plasma cells are increased in number in the lamina propria. Neutrophils may be seen within the colonic epithelium, and if present as aggregates within the lumens of the crypts are called *crypt abscesses*. This latter change, however, is more commonly associated with ulcerative colitis. One important way to differentiate between these two inflammatory bowel diseases is to examine the portion of intestines that is involved by the inflammatory process. Crohn's disease may affect any portion of the GI tract, but most commonly there is involvement of the terminal ileum (regional enteritis) or the proximal portion (right side) of the colon. GI involvement is segmental, that is, normal intestine may be found between inflamed intestine (skip areas). In contrast, almost all cases of ulcerative colitis involve the rectum, and the inflammation extends proximally (left side) without skip lesions (diffuse involvement).

Crohn's disease is classically described as being a granulomatous disease; but granulomas are not present in every case. Classically, the inflammation of the intestines in patients with Crohn's disease is transmural and can form fistulas and sinuses. This deep inflammation produces deep longitudinal, serpiginous ulcers that impart a "cobblestone" appearance to the mucosal surface of the colon. Additionally, the mesenteric fat wraps around the bowel surface and produces what is called "creeping fat." The thickened bowel wall narrows the lumen and produces a characteristic "string sign" on X-ray.

In contrast to Crohn's disease, ulcerative colitis affects only the colon, and the disease involvement is continuous. The rectum is involved in all cases, and the inflammation extends proximally. Since ulcerative colitis involves the mucosa and submucosa but not the wall of the colon, fistula formation and wall thickening is absent (but toxic megacolon may occur). Grossly the mucosa displays diffuse hyperemia with numerous superficial ulcerations. The regenerating, nonulcerated mucosa appears grossly to be "pseudopolyps."

INFLAMMATION OF BLOOD VESSELS
Large vessels
- Giant cell arteritis
- Takayasu's arteritis

Medium vessels

- Kawasaki's syndrome
- Polyarteritis nodosa

Small vessels

- Microscopic polyarteritis nodosa
- Hypersensitivity angiitis
- Buerger's disease

Vasculitis refers to inflammation and necrosis of blood vessels. Inflammatory vascular disorders may be systemic diseases, or they may affect particular types of blood vessels. For example, large to medium-sized arteries are typically involved in patients with giant cell arteritis (temporal arteritis) and Takayasu's arteritis. Medium-sized blood vessels (medium-sized arteries and smaller arteries) are typically affected in patients with classic polyarteritis nodosa and Kawasaki's disease. Smaller blood vessel involvement is seen in patients with microscopic polyarteritis, Wegener's granulomatosis, Churg-Strauss syndrome, and cutaneous leukocytoclastic angiitis.

LARGE VESSEL VASCULITIS

Temporal arteritis

- Granulomatous inflammation with giant cells
- Unilateral headache
- Risk of blindness

Takayasu's arteritis

- "Pulseless" disease
- Stenosis of aortic arch and proximal great vessels
- Decreased pulse and blood pressure in upper extremities
- Affects young Asian females

Giant cell arteritis most commonly affects the temporal artery (temporal arteritis). Microscopically the affected artery may show granulomatous inflammation with giant cells, fragmentation of the internal elastica, and intimal thickening with *thrombosis*. Visual symptoms may be present and progress to permanent blindness unless treated with corticosteroids. Patients also develop painful, tender nodules in the temporal area.

Takayasu's arteritis ("pulseless disease") is a disorder that is seen in young women. The disease affects large and medium arteries, especially the aortic arch and its larger branches. This abnormality decreases the pulse and blood pressure in the upper extremities and may produce ocular problems because of decreased blood flow.

MEDIUM VESSEL VASCULITIS

Kawasaki's disease (mucocutaneous lymph node syndrome)

- Infants and young children (Japan)
- Oral erythema
- Skin rash
- Lymphadenitis
- Inflammatory aneurysms of coronary arteries

Classic (macroscopic) polyarteritis nodosa (PAN)

- Multisystem disorder (renal and visceral vessels)
- Thrombosis and infarction of visceral organs

Kawasaki's disease (mucocutaneous lymph node syndrome) predominantly affects children (boys under the age of four) and is characterized by high fever, skin rash, conjunctival and oral erythema, lymphadenitis, and coronary artery aneurysms. The latter may rupture or produce a myocardial infarction.

The classic form of polyarteritis nodosa (macroscopic PAN) is a systemic multisystem disease. Classic PAN involves the renal and visceral vessels, but spares the pulmonary vessels. Involvement of medium-sized vessels may lead to thrombosis and infarction of visceral organs. Biopsies of affected vessels reveal a combination of acute changes (fibrinoid necrosis and thrombosis) and chronic changes (fibrous and focal aneurysmal dilation).

SMALL VESSEL VASCULITIS
Microscopic PAN

- Affects smaller vessels of lungs and kidneys
- p-ANCA positive

Hypersensitivity angiitis

- Fragmented neutrophils ("leukocytoclastic vasculitis")
- Subtype is Henoch-Schönlein purpura

Buerger's disease

- Thromboangiitis obliterans
- Associated with smoking
- Produces gangrene of extremities

In contrast to classic macroscopic PAN, which involves larger vessels and produces macroscopic infarcts, microscopic PAN and hypersensitivity angiitis involve smaller vessels (arterioles, venules, and capillaries). Microscopic PAN may affect the smaller vessels of the lungs and kidneys, and produce signs of *hemoptysis* and hematuria. These patients are often ANCA (anti-neutrophil cytoplasm antibody) positive, mainly p-ANCA.

Hypersensitivity angiitis also affects smaller blood vessels and may be limited to the skin (cutaneous vasculitis). Histologically fragmented neutrophils are seen surrounding blood vessels (leukocytoclastic vasculitis). The stimulating antigen for this reaction may be drugs (aspirin or penicillin) or microorganisms (*streptococci*). One special subtype of small vessel vasculitis is Henoch-Schönlein *purpura*. This disease is seen in children who present with hemorrhagic *urticaria* and hematuria following an upper respiratory infection. The pathology of this disease involves the deposition of IgA immune complexes in small vessels of the skin. Because the antibody is IgA, the alternate complement pathway is activated in these patients.

Buerger's disease (thromboangiitis obliterans) is a disease that is related to cigarette smoking and is typically seen in young adult males. It is characterized histologically by blood vessels with acute inflammation involving the entire vessel wall, thrombosis (with microabscesses), and obliteration of vessel lumens by intimal proliferation.

GRANULOMATOUS INFLAMMATION

Caseating granulomas

- Tuberculosis

Noncaseating granulomas

- Sarcoidosis
- Fungal infections
- Foreign-body reaction

A distinctive and very important type of chronic inflammation is called granulomatous inflammation. *Granulomas* are small collections of activated macrophages called *epithelioid cells*, so called because they have abundant cytoplasm that is somewhat similar to the abundant cytoplasm of epithelial cells (such as squamous epithelial cells). These epithelioid macrophages define granulomatous inflammation. Other types of cells may be present in granulomas, including lymphocytes, plasma cells, and giant cells. Giant cells, which are formed by the fusion of epithelioid cells, are large cells with abundant cytoplasm and many nuclei.

TUBERCULOSIS

Types

1. Primary tuberculosis → Ghon complex
2. Secondary tuberculosis → apex of lungs
3. Progressive tuberculosis
   - Cavitary tuberculosis → apex of lungs
   - Miliary tuberculosis → hematogenous spread
   - Pott's disease → tuberculosis of spine
   - Scrofula → tuberculosis of lymph nodes

Signs and symptoms

- Fever
- Weight loss
- Night sweats

Sometimes there is a peculiar type of necrosis in the center of the granuloma. These granulomas are called caseating granulomas because grossly tissue with caseating granulomas has the appearance of cheese. This type of inflammation is quite characteristic of infection with *mycobacterium tuberculosis*. The giant cells in the caseating granulomas of tuberculosis occasionally have nuclei arranged at the periphery of the cytoplasm (creating a horseshoe pattern). This type of giant cell is called a *Langhans' giant cell*. (Don't confuse Langhans' giant cells with *Langerhans' cells* of the skin or the islets of Langerhan in the pancreas.)

There are several clinical forms of infection with tuberculosis. For the most part, tuberculosis infection occurs either as a primary infection or a secondary infection (reactivation or reinfection). The initial infection of primary infection, the *Ghon complex*, consists of a subpleural lesion near the fissure between the upper and lower lobes and enlarged caseous lymph nodes that drain the pulmonary lesion. In contrast, the pulmonary lesions of secondary tuberculosis are usually located in the apex of one or both lungs. Why is this? It is basically the result of tuberculosis growing best in areas of higher PO_2 levels, which in the normal lung are located at the apex. In a healthy individual who is standing, gravity pulls the lungs down, which causes the pleural pressure to be more negative at the apex and more positive at the base. This causes the alveoli in the apex to be more expanded, but because lung compliance is greater at lower lung volumes (the base), ventilation is greater to the lower lobes. Additionally, because the pulmonary blood flow system is a low-pressure system, gravity causes increased blood flow in the bases of the lung (gravity causes the arterial pressure to be less in the apex and therefore the flow will be less). Note that blood flow and ventilatory flow are both greater in the bases than the apex, but the change in ventilation is less than the change in blood flow. This fact results in higher ventilation/perfusion ratios (V/Q) in the apex and lower ratios in the bases, which in turn results in higher alveolar PO_2 levels (PAO_2) in the apex.

Other rare forms of tuberculosis (progressive pulmonary tuberculosis) include cavitary fibrocaseous tuberculosis, miliary tuberculosis, or tuberculous bronchopneumonia. Miliary tuberculosis refers to the finding of multiple small yellow-white lesions scattered throughout the entire lung. These lesions result from hematogenous spread of tuberculosis, which is the result of a caseating granuloma eroding into a blood vessel.

Symptoms of patients with tuberculosis include malaise, anorexia, weight loss, fever, night sweats, cough and hemoptysis (coughing up blood). The clinical diagnosis of tuberculosis depends upon the identification of *mycobacterium tuberculosis*. Mycobacteria have special characteristics that make them stain with special stains (acid-fast stains).

MYCOBACTERIA OTHER THAN TUBERCULOSIS
Mycobacterium avium-intracellulare
- Important cause of infection in patients with AIDS

Mycobacterium marinum

- Disease associated with swimming pools and aquariums

Mycobacterium leprae

- Tuberculoid leprosy
- Lepromatous leprosy

It is important to remember that there are mycobacteria other than tuberculosis (and these mycobacteria are sometimes called MOTT, which stands for mycobacteria other than tuberculosis). These mycobacteria are separated into different classes—Runyon classes—based on several characteristics (such as pigment production, colony morphology, and rate of growth). Examples of MOTT include *M. avium-intracellulare*, *M. marinum*, and *M. leprae* (the cause of leprosy). *M. avium-intracellulare* is an important cause of infection in patients with AIDS. Histologic sections of infected tissue from these immunosuppressed patients do not reveal granulomas, but numerous organisms can be seen with special stains. *M. marinum* inhabits marine organisms and grows in water. It can cause superficial disease (skin and subcutaneous disease), and infections are associated with aquariums and swimming pools.

Leprosy, caused by *mycobacterium leprae* (which cannot be cultured), is divided into two clinical types, tuberculoid leprosy and lepromatous leprosy. Tuberculoid leprosy is characterized by flat, erythematous plaques. Histologic sections from involved areas of skin reveal noncaseating granulomas with few bacilli. In contrast, lepromatous leprosy is characterized by extensive macules, papules, and nodules. Severe infection of the face produces an appearance that is similar to a lion ("lion facies"). Histologic sections from involved skin reveal no granulomas, but there are numerous foamy macrophages filled with many bacilli. These macrophages are called foam cells or leprae cells.

SARCOIDOSIS

Histologic changes

- Noncaseating granulomas
- Inclusion in giant cells

Abnormal immunity

- Cutaneous anergy
- Decreased circulating helper T lymphocytes
- Increased circulating cytotoxic T lymphocytes
- Polyclonal hyperactive B lymphocytes

Lung changes

- Interstitial fibrosis (restrictive lung disease)
- Bilateral enlarged hilar lymph nodes

Blood changes

- Hypercalcemia (increased activation of vitamin D by epithelioid cells)
- Increased angiotensin-converting enzyme

Granulomas that lack the central necrosis of caseating granulomas are called noncaseating granulomas. Examples of diseases characterized by noncaseating granulomatous inflammation include sarcoidosis, fungal infections, and foreign body reactions. Sarcoidosis is a unusual disease that is characterized by noncaseating granulomas in multiple areas of the body (especially the lymph nodes of the hilum of the lung). The giant cells within these granulomas may contain inclusions, such as asteroid bodies and Schaumann bodies. The former are stellate bodies composed of products of lipoprotein metabolism; the latter are concentric laminated, calcified bodies. The epithelioid cells of these granulomas also produce vitamin D, and this leads to increased serum level of calcium (hypercalcemia).

Patients with sarcoidosis have abnormal immune responses, including cutaneous *anergy*, which is the failure of immune cells to react to normal antigens. This anergy is the result of decreased cell-mediated immunity. There are also decreased numbers of circulating CD4 cells, increased numbers of circulating CD8 cells, and hyperactive B cells, which produce a polyclonal immune response.

The diagnosis of sarcoidosis depends upon finding noncaseating granulomas in commonly affected sites. The majority of patients with sarcoidosis have bilateral hilar lymphadenopathy or lung involvement. These changes can be seen by chest X-ray or transbronchial biopsies. The eye and skin are next most commonly affected, so that both conjunctival biopsies and skin biopsies are clinical possibilities. Noncaseating granulomas may be found in multiple infectious diseases, such as fungal infections, but sarcoidosis is not caused by any known organism. Therefore, before the diagnosis of sarcoidosis can be made, cultures must be taken from affected tissues, and there must be no growth of any organism that can produce granulomas. Also in patients with sarcoid, blood angiotensin-converting enzyme (ACE) levels are increased, and this may be used as a clinical test. In the past, the Kveim skin test was used to assist in the diagnosis, but since it involves injecting into patients extracts of material from humans, it is no longer used.

FUNGAL INFECTIONS

* Superficial mycoses → limited to the outermost skin and hair
* Cutaneous mycoses → involves entire epidermis, hair, and nails
* Subcutaneous mycoses → dermis and subcutaneous tissue
* Systemic mycosis → systemic organ involvement

Noncaseating granulomas can be seen histologically with fungal infections (mycoses). The mycoses can be divided into superficial mycoses, cutaneous mycoses, subcutaneous mycoses, and systemic mycoses. For the most part granulomas can be found in the subcutaneous and systemic mycoses. The superficial mycoses infect the outermost skin and hair and can produce tinea nigra and tinea (pityriasis) versicolor. The latter is caused by *Malassezia furfur (Pityrosporum orbiculare)* and is characterized by hyperpigmented or hypopigmented lesions of the trunk. These lesions fluoresce under a Wood's light, and examination with KOH (potassium hydroxide) reveals characteristic "spaghetti and meatball" shapes.

The cutaneous mycoses infect deeper into the epidermis, the hair, and the nails. The organisms are called dermatophytes and include three genera: microsporum (spindle-shaped macroconidia with rough thick wall and few microconidia), trichophyton (few, smooth wall, cigar-shaped macroconidia and many microconidia), and epidermophyton (club-shaped macroconidia with thin smooth walls and no microconidia). The different types of dermatophyte infections, called tinea ("ringworm") infections, are often named according to the site of infection, such as tinea capitis (scalp), tinea corporis (trunk), tinea cruris (groin), and tinea pedis (feet). The most common cause of these infections is *Trichophyton rubrum*, which is a major cause of athlete's foot and nail infections.

Two organisms that produce subcutaneous mycotic infections (dermis and subcutaneous tissue) include *Sporothrix schenckii* and chromoblastomycosis. The former is a dimorphic fungus that is a mold in the soil and a yeast in the body. *Sporothrix* is inoculated into the skin from thorns and splinters, so individuals at risk for developing sporotrichosis are gardeners (rose growers). Infection produces a local pustule or ulcer and histologic sections reveal round or cigar-shaped yeast that are surrounded by an eosinophilic, spiculated zone (asteroid body). Chromoblastomycosis is characterized by verrucous (cauliflower-like) lesions. Microscopic sections reveal brown pigmented organisms having an appearance of "copper pennies."

SYSTEMIC MYCOSES

Candidiasis

- *Candida albicans*
- Pseudohyphae
- White plaques (thrush)

Histoplasmosis

- *Histoplasma capsulatum*
- Found within the cytoplasm of macrophages
- Bird droppings
- Ohio and Mississippi valleys

Aspergillosis

- *Aspergillus* species
- Septate hyphae with acute-angle branching
- Fruiting bodies
- Fungas ball

Blastomycosis

- Blastomyces dermatitidis
- Broad-based budding

Coccidiomyocosis

- *Coccidioides immitis*
- Large spherules filled with many small endospores
- Southwest United States (San Joaquin Valley)

Cryptococcosis

- *Cryptococcus neoformans*
- CNS infection in immunosuppressed patients

- Mucicarmine-positive capsule
- India ink stain of CSF

Mucormycosis

- Nasal infection in diabetic patients
- Broad, nonseptate hyphae with right angle branching

There are numerous causative agents of the systemic mycoses (Fig. 12-1). Candida species grow as yeast, or elongated chains of yeast without *hyphae* (pseudohyphae). Canidida infections frequently produce white plaques called thrush.

Histoplasma capsulatum, a dimorphic fungus, causes a granulomatous reaction, and multiple small yeast surrounded by clear zones may be found within the cytoplasm of macrophages. The source for histoplasma is soil contaminated by

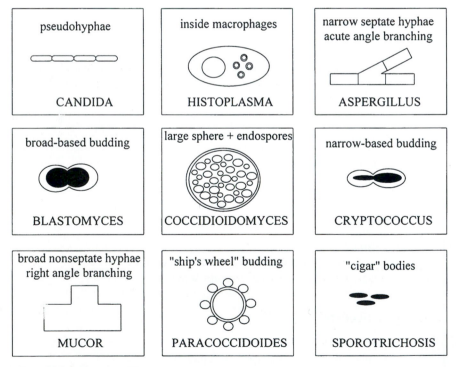

Figure 12-1 Fungi in Tissue

bird droppings (starlings and chickens) and bats (think of caves). The typical location for individuals to develop histoplasmosis is the Ohio and Mississippi Valley areas.

Aspergillus species produce several clinical disease states, including allergic apsergillosis, systemic aspergillosis, and aspergilloma. Typically, aspergillus is seen in tissue as acute-angle branching septate hypae. However, aspergillus may form fruiting bodies in cavities, such as cystic cavities within the lungs. Within these pulmonary cavities, aspergillus may form a large mass called a fungus ball or aspergilloma.

Blastomycosis is a chronic granulomatosis disease that is caused by a dimorphic fungus, *Blastomyces dermatitidis*, which in tissues is seen as a thick-walled yeast having broad-based budding (without the budding, *Blastomyces* may be mistaken as cryptococcosis). The infection, known also as Gilchrist disease, is seen in individuals living in the Ohio and Mississippi Valley areas and is usually confined to the lungs.

Coccidiomycosis is a mycotic infection caused by inhalation of the arthrospores of the dimorphic fungus *Coccidioides immitis*. Within the lung the spores enlarge to form large spherules (sporangia), which become filled with many small endospores. The cyst ruptures, releasing the endospores. Unruptured spherules incite a granulomatous reaction, while the endospores cause a neutrophilic response. *Coccidioides immitis* grows as a mold in the soil in areas with little rainfall, such as the southwestern United States (San Joaquin Valley fever).

Paracoccidiomycosis (South American blastomycosis) is a chronic granulomatous infection caused by *Paracoccidioides brasiliensis*, a dimorphic fungus seen in tissues as a large central organism having peripheral oval budding (having the appearance of a mariner's wheel).

Cryptococcosis is caused by *Cryptococcus neoformans*, an encapsulated yeast (not dimorphic) that infects the CNS, primarily in immunocompromised patients. The capsule can be seen with a mucicarmine stain, or it can be negatively stained using India ink. Do not confuse cyptococcus with cryptosporidium. *Cryptosporidium parvum* is a protozoan parasite that may cause a transient diarrhea in immunocompetent individuals or a chronic diarrhea in patients with AIDS. Histologically sporozoites may be found attached to the surface of intestinal epithelial cells. They are best seen with an acid-fast stain.

Mucormycosis (zygomycosis) is a disease caused by "bread mold fungi" that typically occurs in neutrophenic patients or diabetic patients. One form of the disease, found in diabetic patients, is called rhinocerebral mucormycosis and is characterized by facial pain, headache, changing mental status, and a blood-tinged nasal discharge. Tissue sections reveal characteristic broad, nonseptate, right-angle branching hyphae.

· C H A P T E R · 13 ·

REPAIR AND REGENERATION

·

- Healing
- Stages of Lobar Pneumonia
- Steps in Scar Formation
- Granulation Tissue
- Components of Repair
- Growth Factors
- Extracellular Matrix
- Collagen
- Collagen Types
- Abnormalities of Collagen Deposition
- Scurvy
- Decreased Vitamin D
- Synthesis of Abnormal Collagen
- Excessive Deposition of Collagen

- Idiopathic Pulmonary Fibrosis
- Cirrhosis
- Elastin and Fibrillin
- Marfan Syndrome
- Basement Membranes
- Diabetes Mellitus
- Alport's Syndrome
- Factors Involved in Wound Healing
- Healing of the Skin
- Healing of the Myocardium
- Healing of the Central Nervous System
- Healing of the Gastrointestinal Tract

· · · · · · · · · · · ·

HEALING
- Repair of damaged tissue
- Removal of inflammatory debris
- Restoration to normal state
- Regeneration of cells

> ## STAGES OF LOBAR PNEUMONIA
> - Congestion
> - Red hepatization
> - Gray hepatization
> - Resolution

Inflammation damages tissue, and damaged tissue needs to be repaired. The principal object of repair is to restore damaged tissue to its normal preinflammatory state. The first step in this process involves the removal of the inflammatory and cellular debris. If there is little debris to be removed and only a few cells are destroyed, it is likely that the tissue can be restored to normal. This is the best possible outcome of inflammation and is called resolution. One of the best examples of this process of resolution is healing of the lung damaged by pneumococcal infection. *Streptococcus pneumoniae* typically produces a lobar pneumonia. Four classic stages are involved in the healing of *Streptococcus pneumoniae* lobar pneumonia. The initial stage, *congestion*, is characterized by a rapid proliferation of bacteria. The alveoli contain edema fluid, scattered neutrophils, and numerous bacteria. In the next stage, red hepatization, the alveoli are packed with neutrophils, red cells, and precipitated fibrin. Grossly the lungs have a congested liverlike appearance. With consolidation, the gray hepatization stage, there is progressive destruction of the leukocytes and red cells with continued accumulation of fibrin in the alveoli. The final stage is resolution, in which the exudate within the alveoli is removed.

Notice that the expected outcome of pneumococcal pneumonia is resolution with restoration of the tissue to its normal preinjury stage. Resolution is not the same as *organization*, a term that describes the deposition of collagen. Organizing pneumonia is a complication of bacterial pneumonia that is characterized by the deposition of loose fibrous tissue within the alveoli (organizing exudates). This same histologic appearance can be seen in the lungs of patients with bronchiolitis obliterans-organizing pneumonia (BOOP), a nonspecific reaction to multiple infectious or inflammatory lesions of the lungs. Patients present with cough and dyspnea, and their chest X-ray reveals interstitial infiltrates. Patients usually improve gradually, but steroid therapy may be necessary.

If there is significant loss of tissue cells, tissue repair must involve the regeneration of cells, and this depends upon the ability of the cells of the organ to divide and proliferate. Recall that the cells of the body are divided into three groups: labile, stable, and permanent cells. Labile cells have a short G0 phase and continue proliferating throughout life. Stable cells have a long G0 phase and generally don't divide. They can, however, rapidly proliferate if they need to. Permanent cells, in contrast, cannot replicate. The regeneration process is different for these different groups of cells. The healing of tissue composed of labile cells tends to be rapid with a complete regeneration of cells. Examples of this include regeneration of bone marrow cells (red cells or platelets) and regeneration of the endometrium. This process requires some cells present that are capable of dividing. For example, destruction of the stem cells of the bone marrow can produce aplastic anemia. Another example is the Asherman syndrome in which numerous (and too aggressive) dilatation and curettages (D&Cs) of the endometrium for excessive bleeding (*menorrhagia*) remove the stratum basalis, and no glandular epithelium remains. This can lead to an inability of the endometrium to regenerate and results in lack of menstruation and infertility.

Healing of tissues that are composed of stable cells, such as the kidneys and the liver, is rapid and complete provided that viable cells remain that are capable of regeneration and there is an intact framework. For example, destruction of the renal tubular cells (acute tubular necrosis) can be repaired by the regeneration and proliferation of surviving renal tubular epithelial cells provided the renal tubular framework remains intact. If this framework is destroyed (as with renal infarction), the regeneration cannot take place, and the tissue forms a scar. This is analogous to the regeneration of the liver. If the basic framework is not intact, regeneration of the tissue cannot take place and massive scar tissue is formed. We will examine this process (cirrhosis) in depth below.

Healing of tissues that are composed of permanent cells is different in that regeneration of the parenchymal cells is not possible and the loss of cells is irreversible. Examples of this include infarcts of the heart and the brain. We will examine these abnormalities in depth below.

STEPS IN SCAR FORMATION

- Removal of inflammatory debris
- Formation of granulation tissue
- Formation of scar (collagen deposition)

GRANULATION TISSUE

- Proliferating small blood vessels (angiogenesis)
- Proliferating fibroblasts

When resolution or regeneration of tissue is not possible, repair is likely to form a scar, which is a mass of collagen. This process is characterized by the ingrowth of *granulation tissue*, which consists of proliferating capillaries and fibroblasts. (Important note: Although the names sound similar, granulation tissue is quite different from granulomas, which are aggregates or activated macrophages.) Histologic examination of granulation tissue reveals numerous endothelial cells and fibroblasts with large and prominent nuclei. Mitoses can also be numerous. These histologic signs indicate the cells are metabolically active and are rapidly proliferating. Grossly granulation tissue is soft, pink, and granular ("fleshy") because of the numerous proliferating capillaries. The formation of excessive amounts of granulation tissue that protrudes above the surrounding tissue and is not lined by epithelium is sometimes called proud flesh, because of the "fleshy" appearance of granulation tissue. More commonly small masses composed of excessive granulation tissue are called pyogenic granulomas. These common tumors are misnamed because they are not pyogenic, and they have nothing to do with granulomas. (Note again the confusion of the terms *granulomas* and *granulation tissue*.) Pyogenic granulomas are composed of proliferating capillaries, proliferating fibroblasts, and interspersed inflammatory cells. The collagen deposition in these lesions is minimal.

COMPONENTS OF REPAIR

- Growth factors
- Growth-inhibiting factors
- Extracellular material

GROWTH FACTORS

- Platelet-derived growth factor (PDGF) → stimulates endothelial cells, smooth muscle cells, and fibroblasts
- Epidermal growth factor (EGF) → stimulates epidermal cells and fibroblasts
- Fibroblast growth factor (FGF) → stimulates fibroblasts and endothelial cells
- Transforming growth factors (TGF) → similar to EGF

Many mechanisms are involved in repair and scar formation. They include growth factors, cell-to-cell and cell-to-matrix interactions, the synthesis of extracellular material. One of the first steps in repair of an injury involves the formation of a plug to stop bleeding. We will examine this process in depth in another chapter, but for now it is important to note that this plug is composed of activated platelets that release two important growth factors, platelet-derived growth factor (PDGF) and transforming (tumor) growth factor-beta (TGF-beta). These growth factors cause the proliferation of many types of cells, including fibroblasts, endothelial cells, and smooth muscle cells. Other growth factors include epidermal growth factor and fibroblast growth factor.

These growth-promoting factors are balanced by factors that inhibit the growth of cells. Examples of these growth-inhibiting factors includes tumor necrosis factor (TNF), TGF-beta, and chalones. TGF-beta can act as either a growth stimulator or a growth inhibitor. In low concentrations it causes the synthesis and secretion of PDGF, but in high concentrations it is a growth inhibitor due to the inhibition of the PDGF receptors. Chalones are ill-defined substances secreted by mature cells that inhibit the division of neighboring cells.

EXTRACELLULAR MATRIX

- Collagen
- Elastin
- Adhesive glycoproteins (fibronectin and laminin)
- Proteoglycans

The extracellular matrix surrounds stromal cells and lies beneath endothelial and epithelial cells (where it forms basement membranes). The extracellular matrix is composed of collagen, elastin, glycoproteins, and proteoglycans. Two important glycoproteins are fibronectin and laminin. The major function of the glycoproteins is to link the components of the extracellular matrix to each other and to cells. Fibronectin is produced by fibroblasts, monocytes, and endothelial cells and binds to other components of the extracellular matrix and to cells via integrin receptors. Fibronectin is chemotactic for fibroblasts and is important in the formation of the capillaries in granulation tissue. Laminin is the most abundant glycoprotein in basement membranes. It is a cross-shaped structure that binds to cells and matrix components such as collagen type IV and heparan sulfate. The proteoglycans consist of glycosaminoglycans (such as dermatan sulfate, keratin sulfate, and heparan sulfate) and are important in regulating the permeability of the connective tissue. Their structure allows them to retain water and act as interstitial "shock absorbers."

COLLAGEN

- Glycoprotein composed of three polypeptide chains (triple helix)
- Every third amino acid is glycine
- Hydroxylated proline and lysine (needs vitamin C)
- Decreased vitamin C (scurvy) produces poor collagen formation
- Cross-linked by lysyl oxidase

One of the most important components of the extracellular matrix is colla-gen. This protein is made up of three separate polypeptide chains (α chains), every third amino acid being glycine. Important points to remember about the synthesis of collagen include the hydroxylation of proline and the oxidation of lysine. The former reaction is dependent on ascorbic acid and is necessary to hold the three α chains to the rough endoplasmic reticulum (RER). The latter reac-tion results in the cross-linking between α chains and gives collagen its structural stability.

COLLAGEN TYPES

Fibrillar collagens

- Type I → skin, bones, tendons, mature scars
- Type II → cartilage
- Type III → embryonic tissue, blood vessels, pliable organs, immature scars

Amorphous collagens

- Type IV → basement membranes
- Type VI → connective tissue

There are at least 19 types of collagen, and these types have different char-acteristics. Types I, II, and III are the interstitial or fibrillar collagens. These col-lagens form strong cable-like fibrils and bundles that provide the tensile strength of tissues. For example, type I collagen is the major collagen of bone, skin, ten-don, and mature scars. Type II collagen is the major collagen in cartilage. Type III collagen, the first collagen deposited in wound healing, is abundant in embry-onic tissues and in pliable organs in adults. Collagen types IV and VI are amor-phous and found in interstitial tissue and basement membranes. Type IV collagen is the network-forming collagen and is found exclusively in basement mem-branes. This type of collagen has characteristic interruptions in the three amino acid sequences of collagen that allow it to bend. Type VI collagen is a filamen-tous fibril type of collagen that is prevalent in most connective tissue.

Scars result from the tissue deposition of collagen. The term *fibrous tissue* also refers to the deposition of collagen. (Note that although they sound similar, fibrous and fibrinous do not refer to the same process. Fibrinous refers to the deposition of material that is similar to fibrin.) Histologically, using routine stains (hematoxylin and eosin) collagen appears as pink material. With a trichrome stain collagen appears blue.

Collagen fibers are somewhat flexible, but because they are inelastic they provide much of the tensile strength of scar tissue. There are several reasons why scars increase in strength with time. These reasons include increased amounts of collagen, changing the type of collagen in the scar (from type III to type I), and increased cross-linking between collagen molecules. Also important is the fact that with time scars tend to contract and become smaller.

ABNORMALITIES OF COLLAGEN DEPOSITION

• Decreased synthesis
• Synthesis of abnormal collagen
• Excessive deposition of collagen (fibrosis)

SCURVY

• Decreased vitamin C (ascorbic acid)
• Decreased collagen synthesis
• Impaired wound healing
• Fragile blood vessels
• Perifollicular hemorrhages

Abnormal deposition of collagen can involve too little synthesis, too much synthesis of collagen, or synthesis of an abnormal form of collagen. Vitamin C (ascorbic acid) is a water-soluble vitamin that is important for many body functions including the synthesis of collagen. Vitamin C functions as a cofactor for the hydroxylation of proline and lysine and for the formation of the triple helix of tropocollagen. In patients with decreased vitamin C (scurvy) there is abnormal synthesis of connective tissue due to abnormal synthesis of collagen. This leads to impaired wound healing (previous wounds may reopen) and fragile blood vessel formation. The latter leads to bleeding gums and tooth loss, subperiosteal hemorrhage, and perifollicular petechial skin hemorrhages. Decreased vitamin C also leads to decreased synthesis of osteoid (unmineralized bone) and increased calcification of the cartilage. The bone of patients with scurvy has a decreased layer of osteoid on the surface of the bone trabeculae.

DECREASED VITAMIN D

Adults → osteomalacia

- Increased osteoid
- Decreased mineralized bone
- Bone pain

Children → rickets

- Increased osteoid at growth centers (epiphyses)
- Soft bones
- Craniotabes and frontal bossing
- Bowing of legs

It is important to compare the bone changes of decreased vitamin C with the bone changes of decreased vitamin D. In the latter disorder the osteoblasts in the bone continue to synthesize osteoid, but this material is not mineralized (because of the lack of calcium and phosphorous). This results in increased amounts of osteoid and decreased mineralized bone (the opposite of scurvy). In adults this produces osteomalacia and bone pain. Histologically, the bone osteoid seams increase markedly in thickness. In children this produces rickets, which is characterized by increased osteoid at normal growth centers of bone. This produces wide epiphyses at the wrists and knees, which leads to growth retardation.

Children with rickets develop other characteristic changes, which include craniotabes (pushing in the skull results in it popping back), frontal bossing (prominent frontal areas), "rachitic rosary" (increased osteoid at the costochondral junction), pigeon-breast (anterior protrusion of the sternum), Harrison's groove (a transverse line across the lower rib cage that is the result of the inward pull of the diaphragm on the abnormal chest), and bowing of the legs (secondary to the bones being unmineralized and soft).

SYNTHESIS OF ABNORMAL COLLAGEN

Ehlers-Danlos syndrome

- Defective collagen synthesis or synthesis of abnormal collagen
- Fragile and hyperextensible skin ("India rubber man" appearance)
- Hypermobile joints (contortionists)

- Many different types depending upon defect present
- Type I associated with diaphragmatic hernia
- Type IV associated with blood vessel rupture
- Type VI associated with retinal detachment and corneal rupture

Osteogenesis imperfecta

- Abnormal type I collagen
- Brittle bones
- Blue sclera
- Hearing loss

Ehlers-Danlos syndrome is a group of disorders that are characterized by defective synthesis of collagen. There are many different types, which result from different abnormalities of collagen synthesis. In general the skin is fragile and hyperextensible, while the joints are hypermobile. In contrast, osteogenesis imperfecta results from the synthesis of an abnormal form of collagen type I. Because this type of collagen is a major component of bone, these patients have abnormally brittle bones and develop multiple fractures. Type I collagen is also found in the sclera of the eye. In patients with osteogenesis imperfecta the sclera is abnormally thin, and the color of the pigmented uvea underneath the thin sclera imparts an abnormal blue color to the normally white sclera.

EXCESSIVE DEPOSITION OF COLLAGEN

- Skin → keloids
- Abdominal wall → desmoids
- Lung → interstitial fibrosis
- Bone marrow → myelofibrosis
- Liver → cirrhosis

Excess deposition of collagen can occur at many different sites in the body. Excess collagen deposition (scar formation) in the skin can result in the formation of a keloid. Histologically keloids are characterized by broad eosinophilic bands within the dermis that are formed by the excessive accumulation of collagen. Keloids are more common in African-American individuals, a typical site being the earlobes (following ear piercing). Excessive deposition of collagen in the abdominal wall is characteristic of desmoids (aggressive fibromatosis). They are characteristically found in the abdominal wall of women who have had previous C-sections.

IDIOPATHIC PULMONARY FIBROSIS

- UIP = usual interstitial pneumonitis
- DIP = desquamative interstitial pneumonitis
- LIP = lymphoid interstitial pneumonitis
- GIP = giant cell interstitial pneumonitis
- PIP = plasma cell interstitial pneumonitis

Excessive deposition of collagen in the interstitial tissue of the lungs produces interstitial fibrosis. This disease process is known by many different names, including interstitial pneumonitis, Hamman-Rich syndrome, and diffuse fibrosing alveolitis. The classification of interstitial fibrosis depends on the histologic appearance of the lung and the type of inflammatory cells that are present. The most common (usual) type is called usual interstitial pneumonitis (UIP). The etiology of UIP is unknown (idiopathic), but the pathophysiology involves damage to type I pneumocytes with the subsequent proliferation of type II pneumocytes. By some mechanism the alveolar macrophages are activated and produce PDGF, which stimulates fibroblasts to proliferate and produce collagen. The result is interstitial fibrosis (a restrictive lung disease). Symptoms of patients with UIP include progressive dyspnea, cough, and clubbing of the fingers. UIP is a very serious disorder that has a steady downhill course and ultimately ends in respiratory failure. (The most rapidly progressive form of interstitial fibrosis is called Hamman-Rich syndrome.) DIP is an important variant of pulmonary fibrosis because the disease may respond to steroid treatment (immunosuppression). Histologically DIP has sheets of cells within the alveoli in addition to fibrosis in the interstitium. The endstage lung disease in all forms of idiopathic pulmonary fibrosis characteristically is markedly fibrotic lungs with large cysts ("honeycomb" lung).

CIRRHOSIS

1. Diffuse fibrosis of liver with regenerating liver nodules
2. Types
   - Micronodular cirrhosis → usually chronic insult (alcohol)
   - Macronodular cirrhosis → usually acute insult (viral or drugs)
3. Results
   - Portal hypertension → varices, ascites, splenomegaly
   - Jaundice
   - Encephalopathy
   - Increased risk of hepatocellular carcinoma

---

4. Etiology
- Alcohol
- Hemochromatosis
- Wilson's disease
- Alpha-1-antitrypsin deficiency

Excessive deposition of collagen in the liver produces cirrhosis, which refers to fibrosis of the liver involving both central veins and portal triads. This fibrosis is the result of liver cell necrosis and regenerative hepatic nodules. There is distortion of the normal lobular architecture by these nodules, which consists of hyperplastic hepatocytes (with enlarged, atypical nuclei), irregular hepatic plates, and distorted vasculature. These changes are not focal and diffusely involve the entire liver. It is thought that the fibrosis is the result of fibril-forming collagens being released by hepatic lipocytes (cells of Ito). Normally, interstitial collagens (types I and III) are found in portal tracts, while the collagen framework between hepatocytes is formed by type IV collagen within the space of Disse. In cirrhosis, types I and III collagen produced by the Ito cells are found throughout the entire lobule. These Ito cells are stimulated by such factors as platelet-derived growth factor and transforming growth factor-beta.

Cirrhosis used to be classified as being either micronodular (less than 3 mm nodules) or macronodular (greater than 3 mm nodules), but this classification is no longer used since it does not correlate with the etiology of the cirrhosis. In fact with time some cases of macronodular cirrhosis become micronodular. Instead cirrhosis is classified according to the etiology, such as alcoholic (Laennec's cirrhosis), viral, immune, or idiopathic (cryptogenic).

ELASTIN

- Returns to original shape after stretching
- Rich in proline and lysine (not hydroxylated)
- Protected from degradation by anti-elastases (α1-antitrypsin)
- Degenerated in cystic medial necrosis of aorta

FIBRILLIN

- Glycoprotein produced by fibroblasts
- Provides scaffolding for elastin
- Abnormal in Marfan syndrome

Elastin is a protein of the extracellular matrix that has elastic properties. That is, after it is stretched it returns to its original shape. In tissue elastic fibers (the central core of which is formed by elastin) have the appearance of eosinophilic wavy fibers. (In the media of arteries they form sheetlike structures.) *Fibrillin* is a glycoprotein produced by fibroblasts that provides the scaffolding for elastin in the connective tissue.

MARFAN SYNDROME

- Abnormal fibrillin gene
- Large skeleton
- Arachnodactyly
- Subluxed lens
- Prolapse of mitral valve
- Cystic medial necrosis

Abnormalities involving the gene that codes for fibrillin are the basis for Marfan syndrome. This syndrome is characterized by specific changes involving the skeleton, the eyes, and the cardiovascular system. Skeletal changes seen in patients with Marfan syndrome include arachnodactyly (spider fingers), and a large skeleton that causes an increase in height. (Marfan patients are more often tall females; however, some people speculate that Abraham Lincoln had a form of Marfan syndrome.) The eyes in patients with Marfan syndrome may have a subluxed lens (ectopia lentis). The cardiovascular lesions that can be found in patients with Marfan syndrome include prolapse of the mitral valve and a particular type of degeneration of the aorta called systic medial necrosis.

Cystic medial necrosis is somewhat of a misnomer because this abnormality is neither cystic nor necrotic. It does involve the media of the aorta, though. Cystic medial necrosis results from the focal loss of elastic and muscle fibers in the media of vessels. This degeneration predisposes the aorta to dissection of blood lengthwise through the media. Aortic dissection occurs in two types of patients—older men with hypertension and patients with Marfan syndrome. Most cases of dissecting aneurysms have a transverse tear in the intima that is located in the ascending aorta, just above the aortic ring. The tear allows blood to enter the wall of the aorta and dissects along its length. The pain caused by an aortic dissection is similar to the pain caused by a myocardial infarction—a sudden tearing pain in the chest that can radiate to the back—but this pain can extend into the abdomen as the dissection progresses. Untreated, aortic dissection has a very high mortality.

BASEMENT MEMBRANES

- Collagen type IV
- Laminin
- Heparan sulfate

Basement membranes are specialized areas of the extracellular matrix that typically separate epithelial or endothelial cells from the underlying extracellular matrix. Histologically basement membranes stain a pale eosinophilic color with routine stains. They also stain positively with the periodic acid-Schiff (PAS) stain because of their high carbohydrate content. The main components of basement membranes include laminin, collagen type IV, and heparan sulfate. Basement membranes have many functions. One important function is ultrafiltration by the basement membranes of the blood in capillaries. This is a very important function of the capillaries of the renal glomeruli and is due in large part to the anionic charge of the basement membrane. This negative charge repels negatively charged proteins, such as albumin, but allows small molecular weight uncharged (neutral) proteins to pass through. This negative charge is mainly due to the proteoglycan heparan sulfate, which is found in the lamina rara interna and externa.

Loss of this negative charge is seen in patients with minimal change disease (MCD), a disease that is characterized by the loss of protein in the urine (proteinuria). This proteinuria is selective because not all types of proteins are found in the urine. Albumin is selectively found in the urine rather than globulins. Minimal change disease is associated with decreased polyanions (mainly heparan sulfate) in the glomerular basement membrane. These polyanions normally block the filtration of the small, but negatively charged albumin molecules.

DIABETES MELLITUS

- Decreased insulin production
- Hyperglycemia
- Nonenzymatic glycosylation of proteins
- Increased thickness of basement membranes
- Small blood vessel disease
- Nodular glomerulosclerosis (Kimmelstiel-Wilson disease)

Several other important renal diseases involve abnormalities of the basement membrane within the glomerulus. One of the more important is thickening of the basement membrane in patients with diabetes mellitus. Patients with diabetes have increased blood levels of glucose (hyperglycemia) due to a deficiency of the normal functions of insulin. The major complications of hyperglycemia are related to two mechanisms, nonenzymatic glycosylation of proteins and abnormalities in polyol pathways. Nonenzymatic glycosylation involves the attachment of glucose to proteins, which forms unstable Schiff bases. These compounds may then rearrange to form more stable Amadori-type products, which in turn can form advanced glycosylation end products (AGE). These glycosylated end products are formed in the basement membranes of endothelial cells and can bind albumin and IgG. This produces an increase in the thickness of basement membranes and interferes with their normal functioning, resulting in abnormal function of small blood vessels, a major factor in the pathogenesis of the long-term complications of diabetes. In the glomerulus this is seen as either diffuse or nodular (Kimmelstiel-Wilson) glomerulosclerosis.

ALPORT'S SYNDROME

- Defective synthesis of glomerular basement membrane
- Recurrent hematuria
- Progressive hearing loss
- Cataracts

In contrast to the thick basement membranes seen in patients with diabetes, a thin glomerular basement membrane is characteristic of Alport's syndrome. This disease results from defective synthesis of the glomerular basement membrane and causes an absence of the globular region of the alpha 3 chain of type IV collagen. Alport's syndrome is characterized by glomerular injury (producing recurrent hematuria), progressive hearing loss (especially to high frequencies), and ocular abnormalities (cataracts and dislocated lens). Alport's syndrome is particularly common in the Mormon population. The region of the glomerular basement membrane that is abnormal in patients with Alport's syndrome is the same portion of the basement membrane that patients with Goodpasture's syndrome develop auto-antibodies against. We will discuss Goodpasture's syndrome along with other immune diseases that affect the glomerulus in the chapter dealing with immune disease.

FACTORS INVOLVED IN WOUND HEALING

Local factors

- Infection
- Adequate blood supply
- Foreign bodies

Systemic factors

- Nutrition
- Hematologic abnormalities
- Diabetes mellitus
- Steroid use

It is important to realize that all of the repair processes that we will discuss below depend upon many factors. Normal processes must be working properly for healing to occur. For example, there must be an adequate blood supply to provide for the cells and the nutrients that are necessary for the repair process. Additionally, abnormal processes, such as foreign bodies or infections, can severely impede or prevent healing.

HEALING OF THE SKIN

Healing by primary intention

- Clean surgical incision
- Cut surfaces brought together
- Little dermal granulation tissue
- Little fibrosis

Healing by secondary intention

- Larger defect
- More granulation tissue
- More fibrosis
- Contraction of scar

We now turn our attention to specific examples of tissue repair. We will use these examples to illustrate the basic concepts of healing in general. A classic example is the healing of wounds of the skin. There are two basic types of wound healing in the skin: healing by primary union and healing by secondary union. These two types are differentiated by the severity of the skin injury. Primary union involves less severe wounds, secondary union involves more severe wounds (the edges of the wound cannot be brought together).

An example of healing by primary union (primary intention) is a clean sutured surgical incision. Within 24 hours the defect in the epidermis is sealed by clotted blood, and within 48 hours regenerating epidermal cells close the defect.

In the dermis an acute inflammatory exudate is found. The inflamed tissue is rapidly removed in a couple of days because there is not much of this inflammatory tissue present. By the third day neutrophils are replaced by macrophages. About this time fibroblasts begin to proliferate, and new blood vessels are formed. This combination of proliferating fibroblasts and proliferating small blood vessels is called granulation tissue. Sutures are typically removed from a surgical wound about the end of the first week. The tensile strength of the wound increases with time as the granulation tissue is replaced by a scar with abundant collagen (fibrous tissue).

Healing by secondary intention differs from healing by primary intention in that it involves more initial tissue damage. Therefore there is a greater inflammatory response, and it takes longer to clear away the debris. Surgery may be necessary to help remove dead tissue and any foreign material (debridement). Additionally, granulation tissue is formed, and more collagen is produced by fibroblasts. Collagen can contract, and because of the greater amount of collagen, healing by secondary intention is often complicated by contraction of the scar.

HEALING OF THE MYOCARDIUM

	GROSS	LIGHT
0–12 hours	none	usually none (? wavy fibers)
12–24 hours	pallor	coagulative necrosis
1–3 days	hyperemic (red) border	above + neutrophils
4–7 days	pale-yellow	above + macrophages
7–14 days	red-purple border	above + granulation tissue
>2 weeks	gray-white scar	fibrosis (scar)

Areas of infarcted myocardial tissue reveal typical changes of ischemic coagulative necrosis. The dead myocardial tissue heals by the usual inflammatory and repair processes. These produce a characteristic sequence of gross and histologic changes on the days that follow the *infarction*. For the first 12 hours no gross abnormalities can be seen. By 12 to 24 hours there is pallor in the area of infarction, due to the trapped blood in the area. Over the next few days, the necrosis becomes surrounded by a hyperemic area consisting of vascularized granulation tissue. Over the next few weeks (to months) the area of necrosis changes to a white fibrotic scar.

The earliest histologic changes are the formation of wavy fibers, formed by pulling on the dead fibers by adjacent viable fibers. Histologic features of coagulation necrosis are seen at about 12 to 14 hours. These changes consist of a loss of cross-striations, increased cytoplasmic eosinophilia, and pyknosis of the nuclei. An acute inflammatory response (neutrophils) is most prominent on days

2 to 3, while macrophages predominate during days 5 to 10. Vascularized granulation tissue predominates on days 7 to 14. This is important because granulation tissue has little collagen and is structurally weak. Therefore the risk of perforation is greatest when the amount of granulation tissue is greatest. Lastly, the necrotic tissue is replaced by the deposition of eosinophilic collagen (fibrosis).

In contrast to light microscopy, electron microscopy (EM) can reveal changes in infarction in the first few minutes. In the first half hour signs of reversible injury to myocardial cells can be seen. These changes include swelling of the mitochondria and distortion of their cristae. Signs of irreversible injury can be seen after about one hour and consist of disruption of the plasma membrane, margination of the nuclear chromatin, and formation of amorphous densities in the mitochondria (flocculent densities).

HEALING OF THE CENTRAL NERVOUS SYSTEM

First 24 hours

* Ischemic neuronal change (red neurons)
* Liquefactive necrosis
* Demyelination

First several days

* Increased neutrophils and macrophages
* Edema
* Increased numbers of glial cells (astrocytes)

Weeks to months

* Cavity surrounded by dense gliosis

A good exercise is to compare the changes seen during repair of an infarction of the myocardium with the changes seen during repair of an infarction of the central nervous system. It is very important to realize that infarction of the myocardium produces coagulative necrosis, while infarction of the brain produces liquefactive necrosis. Many of the gross and microscopic differences between these two types of infarctions are based on the differences between coagulative necrosis and liquefactive necrosis. The microscopic changes of a cerebral infarction are first seen at about 24 hours and are characterized by ischemic neuronal change, liquefaction, loss of glial cells, and demyelination. After several days there are increased numbers of leukocytes (neutrophils and macrophages), edema, liquefactive necrosis, and the beginning of a glial reaction. After several weeks to months a cavity surrounded by dense gliosis forms. (This can be incredibly difficult to differentiate histologically from a neoplastic proliferation of glial cells, such as an astrocytoma.)

HEALING OF THE GASTROINTESTINAL TRACT

Peptic ulcers

- Gross → round, regular with punched-out straight walls
- Microscopic → inflamed necrotic tissue on surface, granulation tissue at base
- Location → proximal duodenum and antrum of stomach
- Associations → *Helicobacter pylori*, hypersecretion of acid or gastrin, smoking, and NSAIDs

---

Gastric peptic ulcers by definition penetrate the muscularis mucosa and extend into the submucosa and deeper tissue. This is in contrast to acute gastric (stress) ulcers, which are really erosions and not true ulcers (because they are confined to the superficial layers of the mucosa). Grossly benign peptic ulcers are round and regular with punched-out straight walls. The margins are only slightly elevated, and rugae radiate outward from the ulcer itself. Histologically the surface of the ulcer has acute inflammation and necrotic fibrinoid debris, while the base has granulation tissue that overlies a fibrous scar. The gastric epithelium adjacent to the ulcer is reactive and is characterized by numerous mitoses and epithelial cells with prominent nucleoli. These gross and microscopic characteristics help to differentiate benign peptic ulcers from malignant ulcers produced by gastric cancers. In contrast to benign ulcers, malignant ulcers grossly have an irregular shape with raised irregular margins.

The pathomechanisms involved in the formation of peptic ulcers are complex. There is a strong association between peptic ulcers and infections with *Helicobacter pylori*. Additionally, the formation of peptic ulcers requires gastric acid and the actions of pepsin. Hypersecretion of gastric acid is associated with the formation of peptic ulcers in the duodenum (not the stomach). Additional factors associated with the formation of peptic ulcers include ingestion of NSAIDs, smoking, and hypersecretion of gastrin (seen in patients with the Zollinger-Ellison syndrome).

Because the formation of peptic ulcers involves the actions of acid (Fig. 13-1), treatment involves trying to decrease the effects of gastric acid. These methods include the use of certain drugs, such as cimetidine and omeprazole. Because food relieves the typical epigastric pain (food neutralizes acid within the

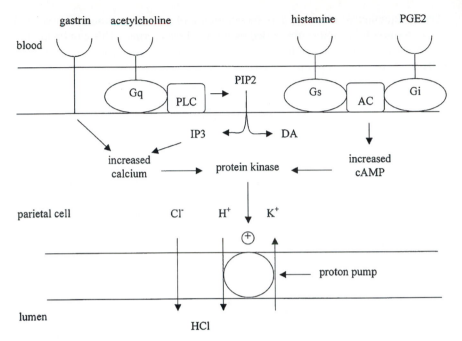

Figure 13-1 Normal Functioning of the Gastric Parietal Cell
There are many factors that stimulate acid production by parietal cells of the stomach, such as acetylcholine, gastrin, and histamine. Drugs that inhibit these factors can be used to treat peptic ulcer disease by decreasing the production of acid. For example, the muscarinic receptor can be inhibited by atropine or pirenzepine; the histamine receptor (H2) can be inhibited by cimetidine; and the proton pump can be inhibited by omeprazole. Note that aspirin increases the production of acid by inhibiting the production of PGE2.

stomach), patients are advised to eat frequent small meals. Additional therapeutic measures include abstaining from substances or actions that increase gastric acid production, such as coffee, alcohol, and prostaglandin inhibitors (aspirin, indomethacin, ibuprofen, and smoking).

· C H A P T E R · 14 ·

FLUIDS AND
HEMODYNAMICS

·

- Edema
- Cerebral Edema
- Brain Herniations
- Exudates
- Triple Response of Lewis
- Transudates
- Congestive Heart Failure
- Portal Hypertension
- Nephrotic Syndrome
- Causes of the Nephrotic Syndrome
- Minimal Change Disease
- Focal Segmental Glomerulosclerosis
- Clinical Examples Comparing Transudates and Exudates
- Pulmonary Edema
- Pleural Effusions
- Pericardial Effusions
- Hyperemia and Congestion
- Shock

· · · · · · · · · · · · ·

EDEMA

- Anasarca → generalized edema
- Pleural effusion → fluid in the pleural cavity
- Ascites → fluid in the peritoneal cavity
- Pericardial effusion → fluid in the pericardial cavity
- Spongiosis → intraepidermal edema
- Angioedema → edema in the deep dermis

Edema is the accumulation of excess fluid in the intercellular (interstitial) tissue spaces or body cavities. Generalized accumulation of edema fluid in the body is sometimes called anasarca. Fluid can accumulate in the pleural cavity (hydrothorax or pleural effusion), the peritoneal cavity (ascites), or the pericardial cavity (hydropericardium or pericardial effusion). We will examine each of these accumulations after we have discussed the basic mechanisms involved in the production of edema.

Edema can be demonstrated clinically in the skin by the presence of pitting, which refers to producing a depression in the skin by pressing on it with a finger (typically demonstrated in the anterior shin). Pitting edema is caused by fluid accumulating within the dermis. This is also the site of the edema fluid produced by urticaria and angioedema. The edema of urticaria is in the perivascular spaces of the superficial dermis, while with angioedema the fluid is deeper in the dermis and may extend into the subcutaneous adipose tissue. This is in contrast to edema within the epidermis (intraepidermal edema), which is called *spongiosis*. This type of edema is characteristic of acute (eczematous) dermatitis.

CEREBRAL EDEMA

Vasogenic edema

- Hypertension
- Toxins

Cytotoxic edema

- Anoxia
- Hypoglycemia

Interstitial edema

- Fluid escaping from ventricles

Cerebral edema refers to accumulation of fluid within the cranium that is outside of the vascular compartment ("water in the brain"). It can be secondary to increased vascular permeability (vasogenic edema), altered cell regulation of fluid (cytotoxic edema), or fluid escaping from the ventricles (interstitial edema). Cerebral edema causes increased intracranial pressure, which can cause swelling of the optic nerve (papilledema), headaches, vomiting, or herniation of part of the brain into the foramen magnum or under a portion of the dura.

BRAIN HERNIATIONS

Subfalcine herniation

- Compression of anterior cerebral artery

Tentorial herniation

- Compression of cranial nerve III (oculomotor nerve)
- Compression of cerebral peduncles

Tonsillar herniation

- Compression of medulla
- Compression of respiratory centers

Brain herniations are classified according to the portion of the brain that is herniated. Subfalcine herniations are caused by herniation of the medial aspect of the cerebral hemisphere (cingulate gyrus) under the falx. Transtentorial herniation occurs when the medial part of the temporal lobe (uncus) herniates over the free edge of the tentorium. Masses in the cerebellum may cause herniation of the cerebellar tonsils into the foramen magnum (tonsillar herniation). This may compress the medulla and respiratory centers of the midbrain and cause death. This tonsillar herniation may also occur if an LP (lumbar puncture) is performed in a patient with increased intracranial pressure. Before performing an LP it is therefore necessary to check the patient for the presence of papilledema.

EXUDATES

Composition

- Increased protein
- Increased cells
- Specific gravity >1.020

Cause

- Inflammation
- Increased blood vessel permeability

Two basic mechanisms are involved in the production of excess fluid in the interstitium or body cavities (Fig. 14-1). Edema may result from either inflammatory damage to blood vessels (inflammatory edema) or abnormalities of the normal hydrostatic or oncotic pressures affecting blood vessels (noninflammatory edema). Edema fluids produced by inflammation are called exudates, while edema fluids produced by noninflammatory mechanisms are called transudates.

Recall that edema is one of the cardinal signs of inflammation (tumor). Inflammatory edema is the result of acute inflammation, which causes blood vessels to have increased permeability. This results in fluid entering the tissue from the blood vessels. This edema fluid, which has increased protein and cells and a specific gravity of >1.020, is called an exudate.

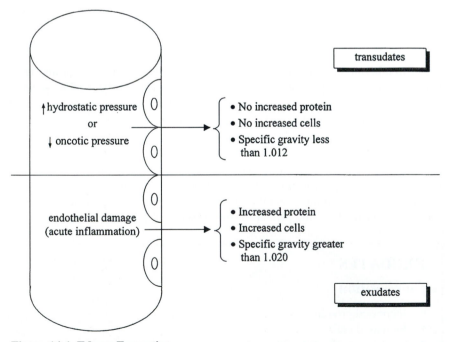

Figure 14-1 Edema Formation

TRIPLE RESPONSE OF LEWIS

- Dull red line → vasodilation at site of injury
- Red flare → vasodilation in surrounding tissue
- Wheal → increased endothelial permeability of capillaries and venules

You can produce a small exudate in your skin if you scratch it. A scratch produces the following series of changes: first a dull red line, next a red halo (flare), and finally swelling (wheal). This response is the classic triple response of Sir Thomas Lewis. The flare response is the result of a local axonal reflex, while the red line and wheal formation are the result of vasoactive mediators of acute inflammation. Lewis demonstrated that the same response (red line and wheal) could be produced by injecting histamine into the skin (Lewis's "H substance").

TRANSUDATES

Composition

- No increased protein
- No increased cells
- Specific gravity <1.012

Cause

1. Increased hydrostatic (venous) pressure
   - Congestive heart failure
   - Portal hypertension
2. Decreased oncotic pressure
   - Liver disease
   - Renal disease (nephrotic syndrome)
3. Lymphatic obstruction
   - Tumors
   - Surgery
   - Filaria

In contrast to inflammatory edema, noninflammatory edema (transudates) are formed by abnormalities of the normal Starling forces that affect the transfer of fluid between the tissues and the blood vessels (Fig. 14-1). The opposing effects of intravascular hydrostatic pressure (which pushes fluid out of blood vessels) and plasma colloid osmotic pressure (which pulls fluid into blood vessels) are the main factors in the formation of noninflammatory edema. Increased hydrostatic pressure or decreased plasma oncotic pressure are the main causes of transudates. Increased hydrostatic pressure producing edema is usually associated with increased venous pressure. Locally this may be due to venous obstruction caused by thrombosis of the veins; systemically it is most often caused by congestive heart failure. Increased pressure in the portal vein (portal hypertension) can produce ascites.

Plasma oncotic pressure is mainly due to the effect of plasma proteins, and the major plasma protein is albumin. Therefore, the main cause of decreased plasma oncotic pressure is decreased protein within the blood (hypoproteinemia), and the main cause of hypoproteinemia is decreased levels of albumin (hypoalbuminemia). Decreased albumin levels result from either decreased synthesis (liver disease) or increased excretion (kidney disease).

Finally, noninflammatory edema may result from lymphatic obstruction. Causes of lymphatic obstruction include tumors, surgical resection, and certain infections. Infection by the filaria *Wucheria bancrofti* results in a type of localized lymphedema called elephantiasis.

CONGESTIVE HEART FAILURE

Left heart failure

- Pulmonary congestion
- Pulmonary edema
- Prerenal azotemia
- Right heart failure

Right heart failure

- Increased jugular venous pressure
- Chronic passive congestion of liver
- Splenomegaly
- Ascites
- Pedal edema

The most common cause of generalized (systemic) edema is congestive heart failure. This basic concept is very important. When the right ventricle fails, all the tissues in the body are affected (although the pathogenesis of this can be complicated). The most common cause of right heart failure is left heart failure. Left ventricle (LV) failure produces symptoms related to the effects of forward failure (decreased cardiac output) and backward failure (increased blood in the venous system). The effects of LV failure are seen mainly in the lungs as pulmonary congestion and edema. An increase in LV and left atrial (LA) pressure is reflected back to the lungs as an increase in the pulmonary capillary pressure, which causes fluid to move into the interstitial tissue (pulmonary edema). In the alveoli, hemoglobin may be released from erythrocytes and subsequently phago-cytized by macrophages, producing hemosiderin-laden macrophages (heart fail-ure cells). Pulmonary symptoms produced by this LV failure include dyspnea (breathlessness), *orthopnea* (dyspnea upon lying), cough, and paroxysmal noc-turnal dyspnea. With LV failure there is also decreased cardiac output that decreases renal blood flow (forward failure). This activates the renin-angiotensin-aldosterone system and causes the retention of salt and water (increasing intersti-tial and blood volumes). This can lead to renal failure (prerenal azotemia).

Right-sided heart failure is usually the result of left-sided failure. Therefore pulmonary symptoms of left-sided failure may coexist with symptoms of right-sided failure. Pure right-sided failure can occur secondary to intrinsic diseases of the lung (cor pulmonale). The major difference between the symptoms of right-sided failure and left-sided failure is that forward failure (pulmonary congestion) with right-sided failure is minimal, but backward failure (systemic and portal congestion) is extensive. The right ventricle failure is reflected backwards as an increase in the right atrial pressure. This can be seen clinically as an increase in the jugular venous pressure (increased distention of the neck veins). There is prominent congestion in the centrilobular areas of the liver, which produces a gross "nutmeg" appearance. This liver congestion is called chronic passive con-gestion, and if long-standing can produce fibrosis (cardiac sclerosis). Increased pressure can occur in the portal system and can produce an enlarged spleen (con-gestive splenomegaly) or ascites (fluid within the peritoneal cavity). Effusions may also occur in the thoracic cavity. Peripheral edema may occur in the depen-dent portions of the body (pedal edema).

PORTAL HYPERTENSION
Cause

- Prehepatic → portal vein thrombosis
- Intrahepatic → cirrhosis
- Posthepatic → right heart failure, Budd-Chiari syndrome, hepatic veno-occlusive disease

Results

- Ascites
- Portosystemic venous shunts
- Congestive splenomegaly
- Hepatic encephalopathy

Portal hypertension is defined as elevated pressure in portal circulation. The causes of portal hypertension can be divided into prehepatic, intrahepatic, and posthepatic causes. Prehepatic causes include obstruction of main portal vein (usually due to thrombosis). Posthepatic causes include right heart failure, obstruction of the hepatic veins (Budd-Chiari syndrome), and hepatic veno-occlusive disease. Intrahepatic causes are usually the result of cirrhosis. Despite all of these possible causes, portal hypertension means cirrhosis until proven otherwise. Cirrhosis obstructs the flow of blood through the liver sinusoids and increases the blood pressure within these sinusoids. This increased pressure is transmitted back to the portal vein and beyond.

The consequences of portal hypertension include ascites, shunts between the portal and systemic venous systems (portocaval shunting), splenomegaly, and hepatic encephalopathy. Ascites refers to excess fluid in the peritoneal cavity. The pathogenesis of ascites involves increased pressure in the sinusoids causing increased flow into the lymphatic vessels. This excess lymphatic flow results in leakage of lymphatic fluid into the peritoneal space. Portosystemic (portocaval) shunting refers to the shunting of blood into areas where systemic and portal circulations are connected. These sites include veins around the rectum (producing hemorrhoids), the cardioesophageal junction (producing esophageal varices), the retroperitoneum, the falciform ligament of the liver, and around the umbilicus. Dilated vessels around the umbilicus produce a clinical appearance called "caput medusae." Splenomegaly caused by chronic splenic congestion resulting from portal hypertension may lead to hypersplenism. Clinically this results in anemia and thrombocytopenia.

NEPHROTIC SYNDROME

1. Marked proteinuria
   - Hypoalbuminemia
   - Edema
2. Increased cholesterol
   - Oval fat bodies in the urine
3. Nonproliferative glomerular disease
   - Minimal change disease
   - Focal segmental glomerulosclerosis
   - Membranous glomerulonephropathy
   - Diabetes mellitus

One of the important causes of generalized edema is decreased oncotic pressure that is due to the loss of albumin in the blood. Albumin can be lost in the urine in patients with a particular clinical type of renal disease called the nephrotic syndrome. Basically glomerular diseases of the kidney can produce one of two major clinical syndromes: the nephrotic syndrome and the nephritic syndrome. The key feature that characterizes the nephrotic syndrome is marked loss of protein in the urine (proteinuria), while the key feature of the nephritic syndrome is hematuria. A somewhat confusing fact is that patients with the nephritic syndrome may have proteinuria, but massive proteinuria (greater than 3.5 g/day) is only characteristic of the nephrotic syndrome. Because of this proteinuria, patients with the nephrotic syndrome lose albumin (hypoalbuminemia) and develop peripheral edema. For some obscure reason the hypoalbuminemia is a stimulus for the liver to produce more cholesterol, and this causes increased lipids in the serum (hyperlipidemia). The cholesterol is carried within LDL (low-density lipoprotein) and spills into the urine (lipiduria), where it can be seen microscopically as fatty casts and oval fat bodies. The latter are renal tubular epithelial cells or macrophages that have excess cholesterol in their cytoplasm. Polarization of this excess cholesterol produces characteristic Maltese crosses.

CAUSES OF THE NEPHROTIC SYNDROME

Abnormalities of the epithelial cells

- Minimal change disease
- Focal segmental glomerulosclerosis

Abnormalities of the basement membrane

- Diabetes mellitus
- Amyloidosis
- Multiple myeloma

Abnormalities of both the epithelial cells and the basement membranes

- Membranous glomerulonephropathy

Most of the causes of the nephritic syndrome involve the activation of the immune system and the deposition of immune complexes within the glomerulus. In contrast, the majority of the causes of the nephrotic syndrome do not involve deposition of immune complexes (the most important exception being membranous glomerulonephropathy, a disease that we will discuss in detail with the other immune disorders). The nephrotic syndrome can result from abnormalities involving either the epithelial cells (podocytes) or the basement membrane (Fig. 14-2).

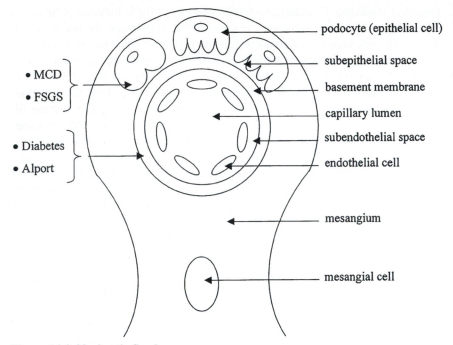

Figure 14-2 Nephrotic Syndrome
This is a highly stylized schematic of the renal glomerulus. It is important to understand the relationship of the epithelial cells and endothelial cells to the basement membranes, because they form the subepithelial and subendothelial spaces. The foot processes of the epithelial cells (podocytes) are fused together in two glomerular diseases: minimal change disease (MCD) and focal segmental glomerulosclerosis (FSGS). Two diseases that are associated with abnormalities of the basement membrane are diabetes mellitus and Alport's syndrome. Although illustrated in this diagram, Alport's syndrome is usually associated with hematuria (nephritis).

MINIMAL CHANGE DISEASE

- Most common cause of nephrotic syndrome in children
- Selective proteinuria
- Loss of polyanion in basement membrane
- Fusion of foot processes of epithelial cells
- Responsive to steroid therapy

The most common cause of the nephrotic syndrome in children is minimal change disease (MCD). It is called "minimal change disease" because histologic changes are minimal (none, in fact). Electron microscopic examination reveals fusion of the foot processes of the epithelial cells (Fig. 14-2). MCD causes the nephrotic syndrome and never the nephritic syndrome. The proteinuria seen in patients with MCD is a highly selective proteinuria. Selective means that the proteinuria primarily involves proteins of low molecular weight (albumin) rather than high molecular weight (immunoglobulin). MCD is a selective proteinuria because it results from decreased amount of polyanions (mainly heparan sulfate) in the glomerular basement membrane. These polyanions normally block the filtration of the small, but negatively charged albumin molecules. MCD is sometimes called lipoid nephrosis because lipid may be found within tubules and fat bodies in the urine. MCD lacks immunoglobulin or complement deposits (negative immunofluorescence), has no tendency to develop chronic renal failure, and is not associated with hematuria or hypertension. Patients respond quite well to steroid therapy, and the prognosis for this disease is good.

FOCAL SEGMENTAL GLOMERULOSCLEROSIS

- Focal glomerular aggregates of PAS positive material
- Nonselective proteinuria
- Fusion of foot processes of epithelial cells
- May be misdiagnosed as MCD
- Not responsive to steroid therapy

Focal segmental glomerulosclerosis (FSGS) is a rare cause of the nephrotic syndrome. Some cases are associated with intravenous heroin use, while other cases have been associated with HIV infection. FSGS is characterized histologically by aggregates of pink hyaline material within some of the glomeruli. Electron microscopy may reveal fusion of the foot processes of the epithelial cells or thickening of the basement membrane in areas of sclerosis (Fig. 14-2). It is important to realize that not all of the glomeruli are affected, and in fact, some appear normal histologically. The sclerotic areas form first in the deep cortical regions. Therefore a superficial biopsy may not reveal these sclerotic changes, and the normal appearing glomeruli by light microscopy and the fusion of the foot processes by EM can be misdiagnosed as minimal change disease. In contrast to MCD, however, FSGS does not respond to steroid therapy and has a poor prognosis. Other differences between FSGS and MCD include the fact that the proteinuria seen with FSGS is nonselective, and there may be granular deposits of IgM and C3.

Although the names sound similar, it is very important to realize that focal segmental glomerulosclerosis (FSGS) with no cellular proliferation is different from focal segmental glomerulonephritis (FSGN) with cellular proliferation. The main cause of the latter is IgA (Berger) nephropathy.

**CLINICAL EXAMPLES COMPARING
TRANSUDATES AND EXUDATES**

*   Pulmonary edema
*   Pleural effusions
*   Pericardial effusions

PULMONARY EDEMA

Cardiogenic edema

*   Congestive heart failure
*   Renal disease

Noncardiogenic edema

*   Infections
*   Trauma

Now that we have examined in depth the basic mechanisms involved in the production of transudates and exudates, let us look specifically at how these different types of edema can be distinguished clinically at different locations in the body. Pulmonary edema refers to increased fluid within the alveoli (alveolar edema) or the interstitium (interstitial edema) of the lungs. Pulmonary edema results from either abnormalities of the Starling forces acting at the capillary level (cardiogenic edema) or increased capillary permeability due to injury of the blood vessels or alveoli (noncardiogenic edema). Causes of cardiogenic pulmonary edema include increased hydrostatic forces (congestive heart failure and mitral stenosis), decreased oncotic pressure (hypoalbuminemia), and lymphatic obstruction. Noncardiogenic edema may be the result of either endothelial injury (infections and trauma) or alveolar injury (toxins, aspiration, near-drowning). This latter noncardiogenic type of pulmonary edema, if severe and diffuse, may lead to the adult respiratory distress syndrome (ARDS).

The histologic appearance of alveolar edema is pale pink fluid within alveoli. In contrast, pulmonary hemorrhage refers to actual bleeding within the parenchyma of the lung. With the latter numerous erythrocytes are seen histologically within alveoli. Cardiogenic edema may be associated with alveolar hemorrhages and the formation of hemosiderin-laden macrophages (heart failure cells). Pulmonary edema produces restriction of the lung and decreased lung compliance. When a patient with pulmonary edema lies down, the excess pulmonary fluid produces orthopnea and paroxysmal nocturnal dyspnea. Chest X-rays with cardiogenic edema reveal an increase in the caliber of the blood vessels in the upper lobes, perivascular and peribronchial fluid ("cuffing"), and Kerley B lines (fluid in the interlobular septa). Noncardiogenic edema reveals a "white-out" of the lungs.

PLEURAL EFFUSIONS

Noninflammatory edema

- Congestive heart failure
- Renal disease
- Atelectasis
- Tumors

Inflammatory edema

- Infections
- Collagen vascular disease
- Hemorrhagic diathesis
- Tumors

Pleural effusions are caused by the accumulation of fluid within the pleural cavity. Accumulation of this fluid may result in the formation of either a transudate (noninflammatory edema) or an exudate (inflammatory edema). Again the formation of noninflammatory edema is related to abnormalities involving the Starling forces, such as increased hydrostatic pressure (congestive heart failure), decreased oncotic pressure (renal disease), increased intrapleural negative pressure (atelectasis), or decreased lymphatic drainage (tumor). Transudates have a low specific gravity, low protein concentration, and lack inflammatory cells. For the most part the accumulation of transudates in the pleural cavity is called hydrothorax, but other material may accumulate with noninflammatory pleural effusions, such as chylous material or blood. Chylothorax is characterized by milky fluid containing finely emulsified fats. It can result from tumors obstructing the normal lymphatic flow. Accumulation of blood (hemothorax) may be caused by trauma or ruptured aortic aneurysm.

Inflammatory edema results from increased vascular permeability. Inflammatory edema produces exudates that have increased protein, increased cells, and a specific gravity that is >1.020. These pleural exudates can be divided into serofibrinous exudates, suppurative exudates, and hemorrhagic exudates. Serofibrinous exudates may be caused by inflammation in the adjacent lung produced by collagen vascular diseases, while suppurative exudates can be the result of infections. The latter can lead to purulent material (pus) accumulating in the pleural cavity (empyema). Finally, hemorrhagic exudates can result from systemic bleeding disorders or neoplasma.

PERICARDIAL EFFUSIONS

Serous effusions

- Congestive heart failure
- Renal disease (uremia)

Serosanguinous effusions

- Trauma
- CPR

Chylous effusions

- Lymphatic obstruction

Cholesterol effusions

- Myxedema

Bloody effusions

- Rupture of myocardial infarction

Types of pericardial effusions, accumulations of excess fluid within the pericardial cavity, include serous pericardial effusion, serosanguinous effusion (serous effusions mixed with blood), chylous effusion, cholesterol effusion, and hemopericardium. The sudden filling of the pericardial space with fluid is called pericardial tamponade. The three classic signs of pericardial tamponade (Beck's triad) include hypotension, elevated jugular pressure, and muffled heart sounds, the latter because of a dampening effect of the pericardial fluid on the heart sounds. Some patients may also clinically demonstrate a decrease in systemic pressure with inspiration (which is called "paradoxic pulse"). The decrease in cardiac output produces dyspnea (shortness of breath) and hypotension.

HYPEREMIA AND CONGESTION

Hyperemia (active hyperemia)

- Increased arterial blood flow
- Red color
- Blushing, exercise, inflammation

Congestion (passive hyperemia)

- Decreased venous blood flow
- Blue-red color
- Heart-failure cells
- Nutmeg liver

Hyperemia and congestion are two terms that are used to describe increased amounts of blood in organs or tissues. *Hyperemia* (active hyperemia) occurs when arteriolar dilatation produces increased capillary blood flow. Active hyperemia produces a reddish color grossly. Conditions associated with hyperemia include blushing, exercise, and inflammation. In contrast, congestion (passive hyperemia) results from impaired venous drainage. Passive hyperemia produces a blue-red color grossly. Long-term congestion, called chronic passive congestion, most often affects the lungs, liver, and spleen. In the lungs, congested capillaries may rupture and lead to hemorrhage within the alveoli. The red blood cells die within the alveoli and are ingested by macrophages. These hemosiderin-laden macrophages are called heart failure cells because the main cause of pulmonary congestion is heart failure. In the liver, heart failure produces congestion of the central vein and areas of the liver around the central veins (centrilobular regions). This produces a characteristic gross appearance called a nutmeg liver (because it resembles the cut section of a nutmeg).

SHOCK

Definition

- Decreased blood flow to tissue
- Decreased effective cardiac output

Types

- Cardiogenic shock
- Hypovolemic shock
- Septic shock
- Neurogenic shock
- Anaphylaxis

Stages

- Nonprogressive
- Progressive
- Irreversible

There are several types of shock, but the three main types are cardiogenic, hypovolemic, and septic. Cardiogenic shock results obviously from heart disease, while hypovolemic shock can result from hemorrhage or fluid loss, as seen with severe burns, vomiting, or diarrhea. The most common cause of septic shock is infection of the blood (septicemia) with gram-negative endotoxin-producing organisms. The endotoxin lipopolysaccharide (LPS) binds to a receptor on the surface of monocytes and causes them to secrete large amounts of tumor necrosis factor-alpha (TNF-α). Although the actions of TNF-α and IL-1 are useful for acute inflammatory responses, the large amounts of TNF released in septic shock results in cardiovascular collapse.

The three stages of shock are early nonprogressive, and irreversible. In the early nonprogressive stage normal reactive mechanisms can maintain blood flow to vital organs (compensated hypotension). These compensatory mechanisms include baroreceptor reflexes, release of catecholamines, activation of the renin-angiotensin system, release of ADH, and stimulation of the sympathetic system. Symptoms at this stage include increased heart rate (tachycardia) and peripheral vasoconstriction, which causes coolness and pallor of skin. In the progressive stage there is decreased tissue perfusion and reversible tissue damage. The decreased oxygen causes an increase in anaerobic glycolysis. This together with decreased hepatic clearance of lactic acid produces a metabolic lactic acidosis that is characteristic of fully developed shock. In the final irreversible stage the extent of cellular injury is incompatible with survival.

HEMOSTASIS AND INFARCTION

·

HEMORRHAGE

- Hemorrhage → leakage of blood from a blood vessel (bleeding)
- Petechiae → very small, pinpoint hemorrhages
- Purpura → small hemorrhages up to 1 cm in diameter
- Ecchymoses → larger hemorrhages greater than 1 cm in diameter
- Hematoma → localized hemorrhage within tissue

Hemorrhage is a term that describes the process of blood escaping from blood vessels. Several terms describe bleeding based on the size of the hemorrhage. Smaller hemorrhages are called either petechiae or purpura, while larger hemorrhages (bruises) are called *ecchymoses*.

CEREBRAL HEMORRHAGE

Epidural hematoma

- Severe trauma
- Arterial bleeding (middle meningeal artery)
- Symptoms occur rapidly

Subdural hematoma

- Minimal trauma in elderly
- Venous bleeding (bridging veins)
- Symptoms occur slowly

Subarachnoid hemorrhage

- Rupture of berry aneurysm
- "Worst headache ever"
- Bloody or xanthochromic spinal tap

The most common cause of hemorrhage is trauma. Hemorrhage within the central nervous system (CNS) provides a good illustration of hemorrhage and *hematoma* formation. Hemorrhage above the dura and between the dura and the skull (epidural hemorrhage) is most often related to severe trauma that tears a vessel within the dura. This is most often the middle meningeal artery and is associated with fractures of the skull (temporal region). Since the bleeding is of arterial origin, the hematoma expands rapidly and symptoms occur within hours. After the injury the patient may appear normal, but increased intracranial pressure will soon cause headaches, vomiting, papilledema, and changing mental status. Continued bleeding can produce tentorial herniation, oculomotor nerve palsy, and pyramidal tract compression. Compression of the brain stem, if untreated, will lead to coma and death.

Subdural hemorrhage results from bleeding of torn bridging veins (veins that connect the venous system of the brain with the large venous sinuses of the dura). The blood accumulates within the subdural space and is separated from the brain by the arachnoid and subarachnoid space. In contrast to epidural hemorrhage, subdural hemorrhage occurs most often in elderly patients and is associated with minimal trauma. Because the bleeding is of venous origin, the progression is very slow, and symptoms may develop over days to months. Patients present with slowly increasing intracranial pressure, headaches, vomiting, and papilledema. Compression of the underlying brain may cause focal seizures and localizing neurologic symptoms.

Subarachnoid hemorrhages are not usually the result of trauma. Instead, about two-thirds of the cases of subarachnoid hemorrhage are the result of rupture of a preexisting arterial berry aneurysm.

THROMBOSIS

- Formation of a solid mass of blood within the blood vessels or the heart

---

The body reacts to bleeding by trying to stop the bleeding. This process is called hemostasis and involves the formation of a thrombus at the site of vascular injury. Loosely speaking, a thrombus is a blood clot within the blood vessels or heart. Strictly speaking, however, the formation of a "true" blood clot is different from the formation of a thrombus. From a technical standpoint the formation of a blood clot involves the coagulation sequence only. This is really arbitrary and is purely a matter of semantics. "True" blood clots can be formed in tissue, in a test tube in the lab, or inside the blood vessels after death (postmortem clots).

BASIC STEPS OF THROMBOSIS

1. Transient vasoconstriction
2. Platelets form primary plug
   - Platelet adhesion
   - Platelet activation and secretion
   - Platelet aggregation
3. Coagulation cascade forms secondary plug

The process of thrombus formation basically involves three components: the blood vessels, the platelets, and the coagulation system of proteins of the blood. The usual initiating event for the formation of a thrombus is injury to endothelial cells. There may be transient vasoconstriction (due to neurogenic mechanisms), but the most important first step is adhesion of platelets to subendothelial collagen. Usually collagen is hidden from platelets by the endothelial cells that line the blood vessels, but with endothelial injury the collagen is exposed to the platelets. The molecular bridge between platelets and the subendothelial collagen is von Willebrand's factor (vWF). GpIb is the receptor on platelets that binds to vWF.

VON WILLEBRAND'S DISEASE
- Spontaneous bleeding from mucosal membranes
- Excessive bleeding after minor trauma
- Menorrhagia
- Prolonged PTT and bleeding time
- Normal PT and platelet count
- Abnormal platelet aggregation with ristocetin

Abnormal bleeding results from deficiencies of either vWF (von Willebrand's disease) or the GpIb receptor (Bernard-Soulier syndrome). Von Willebrand's disease (vWD) is the most common hereditary coagulation deficiency. It is inherited as an autosomal dominant trait. Patients develop spontaneous bleeding from mucosal membranes, or excessive bleeding after minor trauma. Females may develop excess bleeding during menses (menorrhagia). In contrast to hemophilia, patients with vWD do not develop bleeding into their joints (hemarthrosis). Patients with vWD have a prolonged bleeding time, but a normal platelet count and PT. Because vWF stabilizes factor VIII, patients with vWD also have a secondary deficiency of VIII, which leads to a prolonged PTT. Ristocetin is used to assay the functioning of vWF.

The next step in thrombosis involves the activation of platelets. This process is illustrated in Figure 15-1. This schematic is quite involved, but it illustrates several important second messenger systems. First, notice that platelets can be activated by two separate second messenger systems. On the left side of Figure 15-1 notice that collagen binds to the platelet receptor GpIb, which is linked to phospholipase A2 (PLA2). Through the metabolism of arachidonic acid thromboxane is formed and stimulates other platelets via a different second messenger system (Gq). This system produces both IP3 and DAG. IP3 increases the intracellular concentration of calcium, which causes a change in the shape of the platelets and causes them to move. DAG stimulates protein kinase C (PKC), which causes the release of the contents stored within the platelets. Platelets contain two types of

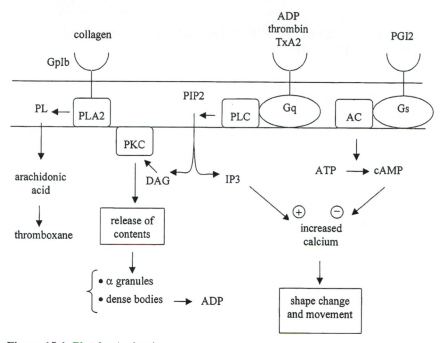

Figure 15-1 Platelet Activation
Activated platelets release the contents of their α granules and dense bodies, change their shape, and move. Binding of platelets to subendothelial collagen via GpIb receptors causes the release of their contents. Binding of ADP, thrombin, or thromboxane (TxA2) to Gq receptors causes shape change and movement. This last process is inhibited by prostacyclin (PGI2), which binds to Gs receptors.

granules. Alpha granules contain fibrinogen, fibronectin, and platelet-derived growth factor (PDGF), while dense bodies contain ADP, ionized calcium, histamine, epinephrine, and serotonin. Note that platelets release ADP, which can also stimulate Gq platelet receptors.

The adherence of platelets to platelets is called platelet aggregation. This is the basis for the formation of the primary plug. Basically platelet aggregation is the result of the stimulation of platelets by three substances: ADP (released from platelet dense bodies), thromboxane (synthesized by activated platelets), and thrombin. Thrombin converts fibrinogen to fibrin, a substance that further stabilizes the platelet plug. This together with platelet contraction converts the primary plug into a much more stable secondary plug. Fibrinogen also forms a molecular bridge between adjacent platelets by linking GpIIb-IIIa receptors on platelets. Patients with thrombasthenia have a deficiency of GpIIb-IIIa.

THE YIN-YANG OF PROSTACYCLIN AND THROMBOXANE

Thromboxane

- Produced by platelets
- Vasoconstriction
- Stimulates platelet aggregation

Prostacyclin

- Produced by endothelial cells
- Vasodilation
- Inhibits platelet aggregation

It is important to compare prostacyclin (PGI2) with thromboxane (TxA2). We covered the yin-yang relationship of these two metabolites of arachidonic acid, namely prostacyclin and thromboxane, in the chapter dealing with cell signaling (Fig. 6-7). To review briefly, thromboxane is produced by platelets and stimulates vasoconstriction and platelet aggregation. In contrast, prostacyclin is produced by the endothelial cells of blood vessels, stimulates vasodilation, and inhibits platelet aggregation. In Figure 15-1 notice that PGI2 functions via Gs receptors, while TxA2 functions via Gq receptors. Gαs activates membrane adenyl cyclase and increases cAMP, while Gαq activates membrane phospholipase C and increases IP3. cAMP inhibits the increase of calcium; IP3 stimulates the increase of calcium.

COAGULATION CASCADE

Intrinsic pathway

- Measured by the PTT (partial thromboplastin time)
- Initiated by contact activation involving factor XII (Hageman factor)

Extrinsic pathway

- Measured by the PT (prothrombin time)
- Initiated by tissue factor activating factor VII

Activation of the coagulation cascade results in the formation of fibrin, which serves to stabilize the initial platelet plug (think of the platelets as being bricks and fibrin as being the mortar). The coagulation cascade consists of two basic pathways, the intrinsic pathway and the extrinsic pathway (Fig. 15-2). Both pathways converge at the point where factor X is activated (after which it's called the common pathway). The intrinsic pathway is activated by surface contact (with collagen), while the extrinsic path is activated by tissue damage (releasing tissue factor). In the intrinsic pathway activated factor XII (Hageman factor) causes the activation in sequence of factors XI, IX, and X. The activation of factor X needs the assistance of factor VIII, calcium, and PF3. Activated factor X forms thrombin from prothrombin (this needs factor V, calcium, and PF3). Thrombin then cleaves fibrinogen to fibrin.

Several laboratory tests can be used to examine the function of the coagulation system. The prothrombin time (PT) measures the extrinsic pathway (V, VII, X, prothrombin, and fibrinogen). The partial thromboplastin time (PTT) measures the intrinsic pathway (XII, XI, IX, VIII, X, V, prothrombin, and fibrinogen).

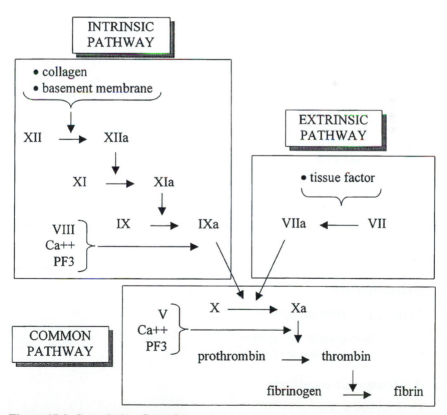

Figure 15-2 Coagulation Cascade

HEMOPHILIA

Factor VIII deficiency (Hemophilia A)

- X-linked disorder
- Massive hemorrhage following trauma or surgery
- Spontaneous hemorrhages
- Hemarthroses
- Prolonged PTT
- Normal PT

Factor IX deficiency (Hemophilia B)

- X-linked disorder
- Clinically similar to factor VIII deficiency
- Prolonged PTT
- Normal PT

Hemophilia A is an X-linked disorder that results from a deficiency of factor VIII. The symptoms produced by this deficiency are variable and depend upon the degree to which factor VII activity is decreased. In symptomatic patients there is massive hemorrhage following trauma or surgery. There are also "spontaneous" hemorrhages in parts of the body that are normally subject to trauma, such as the joints (hemarthroses). Petechiae and ecchymoses are characteristically absent, but large ecchymoses and subcutaneous or intramuscular hematomas are common. Because of the decreased factor VIII activity, patients with hemophilia A have prolonged PTT. Other clinical tests, including bleeding time, tourniquet test, platelet count, and PT, are normal.

Severe factor IX deficiency is clinically indistinguishable from hemophilia A. It is also inherited as an X-linked recessive trait. It is also called Christmas disease, the name of the first patient described with this disorder. The coagulation time is prolonged, and the bleeding time is normal.

THROMBIN

Procoagulation effects

- Stimulates platelet aggregation
- Stimulates conversion of fibrinogen to fibrin

Anticoagulation effects

- Activates protein C

Two facts about the coagulation cascade need special mentioning. First, the vitamin K-dependent factors of coagulation are factors II, VII, IX, X, and proteins C and S. Second, realize that thrombin has both procoagulation and anticoagulation effects. To enhance coagulation, thrombin stimulates platelet aggregation (Fig. 15-1) and in the coagulation cascade stimulates the conversion of fibrinogen to fibrin (Fig. 15-2). The anticoagulation effects of thrombin occur when its function is changed (modulated) by the release of thrombomodulin from endothelial cells. Thrombomodulin is given its name because it modulates the function of thrombin and changes it to the anticoagulation effect. Under the effects of thrombomodulin, thrombin activates protein C. The anticoagulant effects of protein C are discussed in the next section.

ANTICOAGULATION

Plasma protease inhibitors

- Antithrombin III
- Protein C
- Protein S
- Deficiency associated with recurrent thrombosis and spontaneous abortions

Fibrinolysis

- Plasmin
- Produces fibrin split products
- Activated by plasminogen activators (urokinase and streptokinase)

One of the basic concepts of human physiology is that many processes have equal and opposite controlling processes designed to keep them in check. We have seen this yin-yang effect with prostacyclin and thromboxane. It is very important to keep coagulation in check, and this is done by several anticoagulation mechanisms (Fig. 15-3). Examples of these controlling mechanisms include inhibition of the coagulation cascade by certain enzymes (plasma protease inhibitors) and destruction of the blood clot itself (fibrinolysis). The plasma protease inhibitors include antithrombin III and proteins C and S. Antithrombin III (ATIII) inhibits the serine proteases thrombin, XIIa, XIa, Xa, and IXa. It is activated by heparin and heparin-like molecules on endothelial cells. Protein C and protein S are vitamin K-dependent plasma proteins that inactivate factors Va and VIIIa. Protein C is activated by endothelium associated thrombomodulin. Don't confuse protein C with other substances with similar sounding names, such as C-reactive protein (CRP). Clinically a deficiency of these plasma protease in-

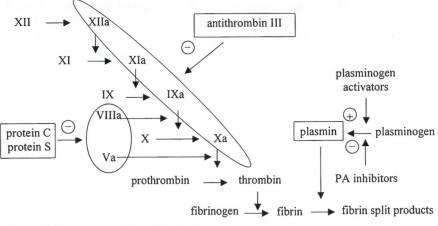

Figure 15-3 Anticoagulation Mechanisms

hibitors (especially proteins C and S) is associated with recurrent thrombus formation and recurrent spontaneous abortions in females.

The main component of the fibrinolytic system is plasmin. Don't confuse plasmin and thrombin. Their names sound similar, but their functions are quite different. Plasmin functions by splitting fibrin into fibrin split products (FSP), which are also known as fibrin degradation products (FDP). How is plasmin formed? It is formed from plasminogen by substances called plasminogen activators (PA). Substances that can activate plasmin include urokinase-like PA (u-PA), tissue-type PA (t-PA), and streptokinase. Myocardial infarction (MI) results from occlusion of a coronary artery by a thrombus. Streptokinase can be used in the treatment of MI to dissolve this thrombus by activating plasmin.

ENDOTHELIAL CELLS

Procoagulation effects

- Tissue factor (thromboplastin)
- Platelet activating factor
- von Willebrand factor
- t-PA inhibitor

Anticoagulation effects

- Heparin-like molecule
- Protein C

- Protein S
- Thrombomodulin
- Prostacyclin
- Nitric oxide
- t-PA

In the yin-yang world of clotting and bleeding, endothelial cells are big-time players, so much so that they participate in both clotting and bleeding (truly a schizophrenic situation). The normal endothelial cells may promote hemostasis, or they may inhibit hemostasis (Fig. 15-4). As unusual as this might seem at first glance, it does make sense. If the endothelium of the blood vessels is intact, then endothelial cells inhibit hemostasis and keep the blood flowing. When there is trauma to the blood vessel, the injured endothelial cells stimulate hemostasis to stop the bleeding.

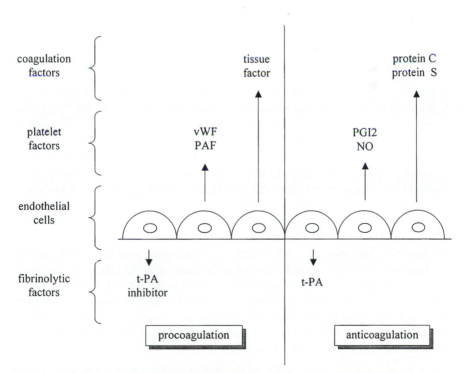

Figure 15-4 Procoagulation and Anticoagulation Effects of Endothelial Cells

How do endothelial cells participate in procoagulation activities? They can influence all areas of hemostasis, including coagulation factors, platelets, and fibrinolytic system. Endothelial cells can secrete many different substances that affect all of these areas (left side of Fig. 15-4). Likewise, endothelial cells can secrete many different substances that can inhibit these three areas (right side of Fig. 15-4).

MORPHOLOGY OF THROMBI

Premortem thrombi

- Arterial thrombi may have lines of Zahn
- May attach to the blood vessel wall
- May show evidence of reorganization

Postmortem blood clots

- "Chicken fat" appearance overlying dark "currant jelly" base

---

Thrombi may form within the heart, the arteries, or the veins. When they are formed in areas where the blood is flowing (no stasis), such as the arteries, thrombi may have laminations called the lines of Zahn. These laminations are formed by layers with abundant platelets separated by layers with abundant white cells. These lines are not found in thrombi formed in areas of stasis, such as thrombi formed in the veins. Both arterial and venous thrombi are formed during life (premortem). It is important to be able to tell these premortem thrombi from blood clots formed after death (postmortem clots). The latter is obviously of no clinical significance, but thrombi formed during life can certainly be significant. Consider the case of a thrombus that forms in a leg vein, breaks off, and travels to the lungs. How could you tell this premortem thrombus from a postmortem blood clot? Grossly postmortem clots are usually rubbery and gelatinous. Large postmortem clots may have a "chicken fat" appearance (due to plasma without erythrocytes) overlying a dark "currant jelly" base (plasma with many erythrocytes). Also, postmortem clots are never attached to the wall of the blood vessel (although this can be difficult to determine grossly). Histologically postmortem clots lack the fibrin strands that attach premortem thrombi to the vessel wall. If the premortem thrombus had been formed several days prior to death, there may be evidence of reorganization of the clot.

THROMBOTIC STATES

Endothelial injury

* Atherosclerosis

Abnormal blood flow

* Myocardial infarction
* Aortic aneurysm
* Venous stasis

Hypercoagulable states

* Familial deficiencies of plasma protease inhibitors
* Secondary hypercoagulable states

Thrombosis is a very good thing to prevent excessive bleeding, but too much of a good thing can be bad. Abnormal formation of thrombi generally results from injury to endothelial cells, abnormal blood flow, and excess activity of the coagulation system. Endothelial injury is important in the formation of thrombi in the arterial system, such as atherosclerosis. We will discuss the pathology of atherosclerosis in detail below.

Abnormalities of blood flow include turbulence and stasis. Turbulent blood flow can result from myocardial infarction or abnormal dilations of arteries (aneurysms). Because of the turbulence, thrombi can form inside the heart after an MI or within an aneurysm of the aorta. Blood stasis is important in the formation of thrombi in the venous system, such as in dilated veins (varicose veins). Other clinical situations associated with an increased risk for venous thrombosis (phlebothrombosis) include bed rest, pregnancy, oral contraceptives, and cancer. Trousseau's sign, migratory thrombophlebitis, is associated with visceral cancer.

Excess activity of the coagulation system (hypercoagulability of the blood) may be caused by primary (familial) deficiencies of substances that control coagulation (antithrombin III, protein C, or protein S), or it may be secondary to other diseases or conditions, such as severe trauma, burns, cancer, or pregnancy. Other risk factors for developing secondary hypercoagulable states include smoking and obesity.

Some patients who develop antibodies against certain phospholipids (cardiolipin) have a high frequency of arterial and venous thrombosis. This antibody binds to phospholipids on platelets, makes them "sticky," and promotes thrombosis. This unusual antibody is called the lupus anticoagulant because some of these patients have symptoms of systemic lupus erythematosus. This name is a misnomer, though, for two reasons. First, most patients with the lupus anticoagulant don't have lupus (a disease we will cover in the chapter on immunology). Second, the antibody is not an anticoagulant; it promotes coagulation. (The reason it's called an anticoagulant is because of its actions in the laboratory.)

ARTERIOSCLEROSIS

- Atherosclerosis
- Arteriosclerosis
- Mönckeberg's arteriosclerosis

Arteriosclerosis is a general term that refers to sclerosis (rigidity) of arteries. Three vascular diseases are characterized by arteriosclerosis: atherosclerosis, arteriolosclerosis, and Mönckeberg's arteriosclerosis. The latter disease is also called medial calcific sclerosis and is characterized, as the name suggests, by calcification in the media of medium-sized muscular arteries. It is a disease of older individuals that produces stiff "pipestem" arteries. There is no loss of function, however, because the lumens of the affected vessels are not decreased in size, and there is no decrease in blood flow. We will discuss the changes of arteriolosclerosis after we discuss the pathology of atherosclerosis.

ATHEROSCLEROSIS

- Formation of fibrous plaques (atheromas)
- Medium to large sized arteries
- Fatty streaks may be precursor lesion
- Infarcts and gangrene

Atherosclerosis is the major cause of morbidity and mortality in the United States. Atherosclerosis is characterized by the formation of *atheromas* (fibrous plaques) in medium to large sized arteries. Atheromas have a cholesterol-laden core with an overlying fibrous cap. In addition, routine atheromas are composed of cells, extracellular matrix material, and lipid. The cells within an atheroma include smooth muscle cells, macrophages, and leukocytes. (Both smooth muscle cells and macrophages can ingest lipid to form foam cells.) The extracellular matrix material within atheromas (secreted by smooth muscle cells) includes collagen, elastic fibers, and proteoglycans. Intracellular and extracellular lipid (derived from the cholesterol of abnormal LDL) is also present. In contrast to routine atheromas, complicated atheromas may develop calcification, rupture, ulceration, or overlying thrombosis. Fatty streaks are thought to be precursors of atheromatous plaques (however, this is controversial). They form multiple yellow, flat lesions that are composed of lipid-filled foam cells. Fatty streaks can be found early in life in children.

Atheromas most frequently affect the proximal portions of the coronary arteries, the branches of the carotid arteries, the circle of Willis, the large vessels of the lower extremities, and the renal and mesenteric arteries. Atherosclerosis blocks the flow of blood and can cause strokes, heart attacks, and gangrene of the legs. Mild obstruction of the iliac vessels can cause pain in the legs when walking (claudication), while more severe occlusions can produce gangrene. Obstruction of the carotid vessels can cause strokes, and rupture of atheromatous plaques produces cholesterol emboli. In the smaller vessels, such as the carotids or the coronary arteries, ulceration of the fibrous caps can cause thrombosis. Atherosclerosis involving the coronary arteries can lead to ischemic heart disease and myocardial infarctions.

RISK FACTORS FOR ATHEROSCLEROSIS

Major risk factors

- Hypertension
- Hyperlipidemia
- Cigarette smoking
- Diabetes mellitus

Minor risk factors

- Lack of physical exercise
- Obesity
- Male gender
- Stress
- Increased serum homocysteine

Multiple risk factors are related to the development of atherosclerosis. Some factors are associated with a greater risk of developing atherosclerosis than are other factors. For example, after the age of 45, hypertension is a stronger risk factor than increased cholesterol. Serum lipid levels, however, are a very important risk factor. Types of fats include fatty acids, triglycerides, phospholipids, glycolipids, and cholesterol. Fatty acids contain a long alkyl (not acetyl) chain and a terminal carboxyl group. Saturated fats contain no double bonds and are bad. Unsaturated fatty acids have double bonds and are good (in an atherosclerosis-producing sense). Triglycerides contain glycerol (3 carbons and 3 hydroxyl groups) and 3 fatty acids.

LIPOPROTEINS

Chylomicrons

- Exogenous triglyceride
- Apoprotein B-48
- Apoproteins C and E

Very low density lipoprotein (VLDL)

- Endogenous triglyceride
- Apoproteins C and E

Intermediate density lipoprotein (IDL)

- Cholesterol and triglyceride

Low density lipoprotein (LDL)

- Cholesterol ("bad")
- Apoprotein B-100

High density lipoprotein (HDL)

- Cholesterol ("good")
- Apoprotein A
- Apoproteins C & E

Lipids are transported in the blood within lipoproteins, which are named according to their density. The lipoproteins are composed of lipid and protein, and it is their protein content that determines their density and their name. The main lipids within lipoproteins are triglycerides and cholesterol. Triglycerides are obtained either from the diet (exogenous triglycerides) or the liver (endogenous triglycerides). Exogenous triglycerides are the main component of chylomicrons, while endogenous triglycerides are the main component of very low density lipoprotein (VLDL). Cholesterol is the main component of low density lipoprotein (LDL) and high density lipoprotein (HDL). Within intermediate density lipoprotein (IDL) the triglyceride and cholesterol levels are approximately the same.

Lipoproteins are also composed of one or more apoproteins. The major apoprotein of HDL (alpha-lipoprotein) is apoprotein A, while LDL (beta-lipoprotein) is composed of apoprotein B. (Note that there are two forms of apoprotein B, namely, B-48 found in chylomicrons and chylomicron remnants, and B-100 found in LDL, VLDL, and IDL.) Apoproteins C and E are also found in VLDL, HDL, and chylomicrons.

Atherosclerosis results from the infiltration of an artery by cholesterol from low density lipoproteins (LDL). The severity of atherosclerosis is directly related to the level of cholesterol in the blood in the form of LDL. In contrast, levels of high density lipoproteins (HDL) are inversely proportional to the risk of atherosclerosis. Therefore the cholesterol in LDL is the "bad" cholesterol, while the cholesterol in HDL is the "good" cholesterol. Increased serum levels of triglycerides also increase the risk of developing atherosclerosis. High dietary levels of cholesterol and saturated fats raise the serum cholesterol levels. A diet low in cholesterol and with a low ratio of saturated to polyunsaturated fats lowers the cholesterol levels.

Why do these different forms of cholesterol (LDL versus HDL) have different risks for developing atherosclerosis? To understand the pathology involved we first need to review the normal metabolism of lipids (Fig. 15-5). Cholesterol comes from two sources, the dietary ingestion of cholesterol and the synthesis of cholesterol in the liver from saturated fats in the diet. Dietary lipids composed of triglycerides (TG) and cholesterol are adsorbed in the gut and conjugated to proteins to form chylomicrons. These lipid carriers contain on their surface the apoproteins A, B48, CII, and E. The chylomicrons (carrying dietary TG and cholesterol) are converted into the chylomicron remnants by the endothelial enzyme lipoprotein lipase. This reaction releases free fatty acids to the tissue, which can be used for oxidation (muscle) or storage (adipose tissue). The remnants of the chylomicrons, which contain mainly cholesterol, are then transported to the liver where they are taken up by receptors to the apoprotein E.

In the liver the cholesterol is combined with TG to form very low density lipoprotein, VLDL (Fig. 4-1). VLDL, which has the apoproteins CII, E and B100, is released into the blood where it transports endogenous triglycerides to the adipose tissue. In the capillaries VLDL is hydrolyzed by lipoprotein lipase to release the triglycerides and this leaves behind an intermediate fragment called intermediate density lipoprotein (IDL). The IDL (the VLDL remnant) contains TG and cholesterol and the apoproteins B100 and E. It is converted to LDL after removal of the apoprotein E (leaving apoB100). This is accomplished by the enzyme hepatic lipase.

LDL has a high cholesterol content and is the principal transport form of cholesterol. LDL is normally taken up and cleared by the liver, which has LDL receptors (for apoB100 and apoE). The LDL is broken down in lysosomes to free the cholesterol, which then can be utilized for steroid or membrane synthesis, or it can be excreted in the bile. Additionally LDL can be taken up by monocytes

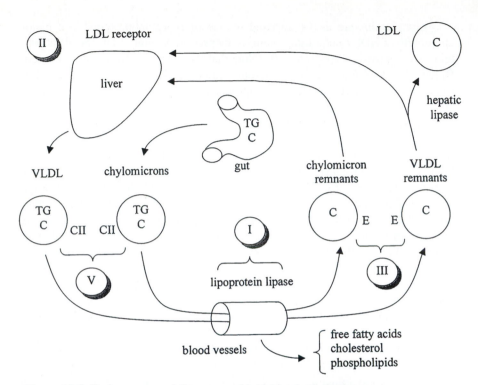

Figure 15-5 Endogenous and Exogenous Lipid Metabolic Pathways
Note the similarity of the exogenous chylomicron pathway with the endogenous VLDL
pathway. Both types of lipoproteins transport mainly triglycerides with some cholesterol.
Both are broken down by the enzyme lipoprotein lipase into remnants while giving lipids
(free fatty acids) to the tissues. Both contain the apoproteins CII and E, but chylomicrons
also have apoA and B48, while VLDL has apoB100. (The Roman numerals in the shad-
owed circles represent the familial types of hyperlipidemias.)

and fibroblasts. In high concentrations LDL can pass through the normal
endothelium, and this permeability is increased if the endothelium is damaged. In
the vessel wall LDL is not taken up directly by macrophages, because they have
few LDL receptors. Instead free LDL is oxidized by free radicals in the blood
vessel wall. (Oxidation does not occur in the bloodstream because of the high
concentration of antioxidants, such as vitamin E.) The oxidation of LDL is important in the pathogenesis of atherosclerosis (see below).

High density lipoproteins (HDL) contain mainly phospholipids and have
low cholesterol. HDL serves two main functions. One is to transport free cholesterol from cells and peripheral tissues back to the liver for excretion. HDL is
thought to be capable of removing cholesterol from arterial walls, and possibly

this can be protective against atherosclerosis. The other main function of HDL is to give the apoproteins C and E to chylomicrons and VLDL.

HYPERLIPIDEMIA
Primary hyperlipidemia

1. Increased cholesterol
   - Type II familial hyperlipidemia
2. Increased triglyceride
   - Type I familial hyperlipidemia
   - Type IV familial hyperlipidemia
   - Type V familial hyperlipidemia
3. Increased cholesterol and triglyceride
   - Type III familial hyperlipidemia

Secondary hyperlipidemia

1. Increased cholesterol
   - Diet
   - Nephrotic syndrome
2. Increased triglyceride
   - Diet
   - Diabetes mellitus
3. Increased cholesterol and triglyceride
   - Alcohol
   - Pregnancy

To reiterate, increased serum lipid levels (hyperlipidemia) is a major risk factor for the development of atherosclerosis. Hyperlipidemia may be either a primary genetic defect, or it may be secondary to another disorder. Clinically hyperlipidemias can be classified as being either primary or secondary hyperlipidemias. Secondary hyperlipidemias can result in the elevation of serum cholesterol levels, triglyceride levels, or both cholesterol and triglyceride levels. The hypertriglyceridemia in patients with diabetes mellitus occurs secondary to increased blood levels of VLDL (Fig. 4-1). This increased level is due to increased secretion of VLDL by the liver (due to increased mobilization of free fatty acids from adipose tissue) and decreased removal of VLDL by lipoprotein lipase (the activity of which diminishes secondary to the prolonged elevated levels of VLDL).

FAMILIAL HYPERLIPIDEMIA

Type I hyperlipoproteinemia (familial hyperchylomicronemia)

- Mutation in lipoprotein lipase gene
- Increased serum chylomicrons

Type II hyperlipoproteinemia (familial hypercholesterolemia)

- Mutation involving LDL receptor
- Increased serum LDL
- Increased serum cholesterol

Type III hyperlipidemia (floating or broad β disease)

- Mutation in apolipoprotein E
- Increased chylomicron remnants and IDL
- Increased serum triglyceride and cholesterol

Type IV hyperlipidemia (familial hypertriglyceridemia)

- Unknown mutation
- Increased serum VLDL
- Increased serum triglyceride and cholesterol

Type V hyperlipidemia

- Mutation in apolipoprotein CII
- Increased serum chylomicrons and VLDL
- Increased serum triglyceride and cholesterol

Familial defects in the enzymes or receptors involved in the normal lipid pathway can lead to an increased risk of atherosclerosis by increasing serum lipid levels (Fig. 15-4). Type I hyperlipidemia is a rare disorder. Patients tend not to develop atherosclerosis, but they do develop fatty tumors (xanthomas) of the skin over elbows and buttocks. Type II hyperlipidemia is a more common disorder. Patients who are homozygous for the defect develop tendinous xanthomas, *xanthelasmas* (yellow fatty deposits around the eyelids), and early severe atherosclerosis. Type III hyperlipidemia is also a rare disorder that is caused by a mutation in the apolipoprotein E gene. Patients develop palmar and tuberous xanthomas and are predisposed to atherosclerosis. Type IV hyperlipidemia is a common disorder, the cause of which is unknown. (Note that excess VLDL can also be seen secondary to several disorders such as obesity, alcohol ingestion, and excessive carbohydrate ingestion.) Type V hyperlipidemia is a rare disorder that is due to defective tissue lipase activity. Patients are prone to abdominal pain and pancreatitis.

Each of the five types of primary (familial) hyperlipoproteinemias produces a characteristic pattern with electrophoresis of the serum (Fig. 15-6). The normal pattern seen in fasting blood reveals an alpha band (HDL), a prebeta band (VLDL), and a beta band (LDL). Chylomicrons are not normally found in fasting

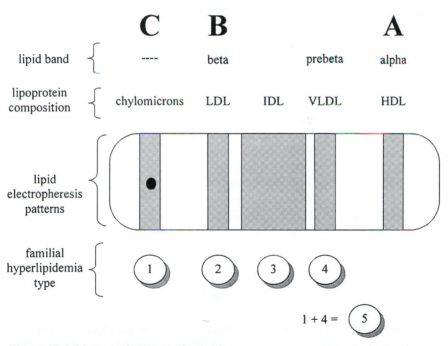

Figure 15-6 Lipoprotein Electrophoresis
Lipoproteins can be separated by electrophoresis into different bands. Chylomicrons do not migrate and stay at the origin, HDL migrates the farthest, and the band that they form is called the alpha band. LDL migrates the least, and its band is called the beta band. Between HDL and LDL is the prebeta band with VLDL, while IDL forms a broad band between VLDL and LDL.

blood, while IDL are found in the area between the beta and prebeta bands. Type 1 hyperlipidemia has increased chylomicrons and produces a large band at the origin. Type 2 hyperlipoproteinemia has increased LDL and produces a large beta band. Type 3 has increased chylomicron remnants and IDL and produces a large broad band (broad beta) between the beta and the prebeta areas. Type 4 produces a large prebeta band, while type 5 produces a large prebeta band and a large band at the origin.

PATHOGENESIS OF ATHEROSCLEROSIS

- Endothelial damage
- Influx of macrophages
- Smooth muscle proliferation and migration
- Formation of foam cells
- Deposition of extracellular matrix material

There are two major theories concerning the pathogenesis of atherosclerosis, namely, the lipid infiltration theory and the reaction to injury theory. In the former the initial event that produces atherosclerosis is lipid accumulation within blood vessels; in the latter the initial event is endothelial damage. It is important to realize that many of the risk factors for atherosclerosis (such as hypertension and cigarette smoking) are associated with endothelial damage. This endothelial injury causes increased permeability of the blood vessel to various components of the blood. Monocytes adhere to endothelial cells, enter the intima, transform into macrophages, and accumulate lipid (forming foam cells). Macrophages express receptors for LDL and can phagocytize LDL, but their uptake of normal LDL is too slow to produce foam cells. Instead macrophages have receptors for the uptake of oxidized LDL. These receptors for oxidized LDL are called scavenger receptors.

In addition to the influx of macrophages, atherosclerosis is associated with the proliferation of smooth muscle cells. Factors released from activated platelets or monocytes can cause migration of smooth muscle cells from the media to the intima. Once within the intima the smooth muscle cells proliferate and then begin to synthesize substances of the extracellular matrix. The pathogenesis of atherosclerosis depends upon the transformation of smooth muscle cells from normal resting cells (spindle-shaped cells that have a contractile function) into proliferating and migrating smooth muscle cells. This change in smooth muscle is the result of interactions between smooth muscle cell growth promoters and growth inhibitors. Growth promoters of smooth muscle cells include platelet-derived growth factor (secreted by platelets, endothelial cells, and macrophages), basic fibroblast growth factor, and IL-1. Growth inhibitors of smooth muscle cells include heparan sulfate, nitric oxide, gamma-interferon, beta-transforming growth factor, and heparin-like molecules. Smooth muscle cells can also accumulate cholesterol like macrophages and form foam cells within the atheromatous plaque.

ANEURYSMS

Atherosclerotic aneurysms

- Located in the abdominal aorta (between the renal arteries and the bifurcation of the aorta)
- Pulsatile mass
- May rupture

Luetic aneurysms

- Due to syphilis infection
- Obliterative endarteritis
- May produce aortic regurgitation or rupture

Dissecting aneurysms

1. Result of cystic medial necrosis of aorta
   - Hypertension
   - Marfan syndrome
2. "Double-barrel" aorta

Berry aneurysms

- Located at bifurcation of arteries in circle of Willis
- Most commonly bifurcation of anterior communicating artery
- Subarachnoid hemorrhage
- Associated with polycystic renal disease

An *aneurysm* is an abnormal dilatation of any vessel. Aneurysms can be classified based on their cause, their shape, or their location. There are many causes of aneurysms, but one of the most important is atherosclerosis. Atherosclerotic aneurysms usually form in the abdominal aorta distal to the renal arteries and proximal to the bifurcation of the aorta. Many atherosclerotic aneurysms are asymptomatic, but if they rupture they produce sudden, severe abdominal pain. Prior to rupture, physical examination reveals a pulsatile mass in the abdomen.

Don't confuse atherosclerotic aneurysms with other types of aneurysms. Syphilitic (luetic) aneurysms are caused by obliterative endarteritis of the vasa vasorum of the aorta, which leads to fibrous scars and a "tree-bark" appearance of the aorta. Luetic aneurysms occur in the thoracic aorta and may lead to luetic heart disease by producing insufficiency of the aortic valve. Dissecting aneurysms (also found in the aorta) are seen in patients with hypertension or Marfan syndrome and are the result of cystic medial necrosis of the aorta. Berry aneurysms are found at the bifurcation of arteries in the circle of Willis and are due to congenital defects in the vascular wall.

INFARCTION

White infarcts

- Arterial occlusion
- Solid organs (heart, spleen, kidneys)

Red infarcts

- Venous occlusion
- Congested tissue
- Dual circulation (liver and lungs)
- Collateral circulation (small intestines and brain)

An infarction is an area of ischemic necrosis that results from decreased arterial or venous blood flow. Infarcts can be classified on the basis of their color (white or red) or by the presence of bacteria (septic or bland). Infarcts may be anemic (white) or hemorrhagic (red). White infarcts occur with arterial occlusion in solid tissues. Red infarcts occur with venous occlusion, congested tissues, or organs with a double or collateral blood supply. Infarcts are usually wedge-shaped, with the apex of the wedge pointing to the occlusion. Histologically most infarcts reveal coagulative necrosis, the classic example being a myocardial infarction. The exception to this histologic appearance is infarction of the brain, which typically reveals liquefactive necrosis. We will examine both these important infarctions separately.

MYOCARDIAL INFARCTION

Distribution of infarcts

- Right coronary artery → 30%
- Left circumflex artery → 20%
- Left anterior descending (LAD) artery → 50%

Types of infarcts

- Transmural
- Subendocardial

Sequence of events

- Coronary atherosclerosis
- Fissures in coronary plaque
- Formation of overlying thrombus

Diagnosis of infarction

- Symptoms
- EKG changes
- Serum enzyme changes

Acute myocardial infarction ("heart attack") refers to acute necrosis of myocardial cells that is due to decreased blood flow (ischemia). The most common cause of myocardial ischemia is atherosclerosis of the coronary arteries, and the most common cause of myocardial infarction is the complete occlusion of coronary vessels by the formation of an occluding thrombus on top of an atherosclerotic plaque. Other rarer causes of ischemic heart disease include inflammation of the coronary arteries (Kawsaki disease), coronary artery vasospasm (Prinzmetal angina and cocaine use), and coronary artery embolism. Don't confuse thrombosis of the coronary arteries (common) with embolism of the coronary arteries (very rare).

There are two basic types of myocardial infarctions, namely, transmural infarction and subendocardial (nontransmural) infarction. In transmural infarction, the more common type, the ischemic necrosis involves the full thickness of the ventricular wall in the distribution of a single coronary artery. In contrast, subendocardial infarction is limited to the inner one-third of the ventricular wall and often extends beyond the distribution area of a single coronary artery.

The area of the heart that becomes necrotic depends upon the site of the occlusion and the anatomic distribution of the occluded coronary vessel. The LAD supplies the anterior left ventricle, the apex, and the anterior two-thirds of the interventricular septum. The left circumflex artery supplies the lateral and posterior wall of the left ventricle. The right coronary artery supplies the right ventricle and the posterior one-third of the interventricular septum (right dominant distribution). In general, posterior (inferior or diaphragmatic) infarcts result from occlusion of the right coronary artery; anterior infarcts (anterior left ventricle) from occlusion of the LAD; and posterolateral infarcts from occlusion of the left circumflex artery.

The necrotic myocardium undergoes a series of changes that consists of typical ischemic coagulative necrosis followed by inflammation and repair. We have previously examined these changes in depth, but to review briefly coagulative necrosis characteristically retains the outline of the necrotic cells. At first there will be an acute inflammatory response that is composed of neutrophils. This is followed by an influx of macrophages and proliferation of blood vessels to form granulation tissue. Finally deposition of collagen will produce a fibrous scar.

The clinical diagnosis of myocardial infarction depends upon correlating clinical symptoms, EKG findings, and serum cardiac enzyme changes. The classic description of the pain produced by an MI is crushing, substernal pain that may radiate down the left arm of the patient. The pain may be associated with sweating, nausea, and vomiting. EKG findings associated with MI include ST segment elevation (which may return to normal), inverted T waves, and abnormal Q waves. Serum enzymes that can be elevated following an MI include CPK, SGOT (AST), and LDH (which are increased sequentially in that order). CPK exists in 3 isoenzymes (MM, MB, and BB, where M stands for muscle and B stands for brain). Elevation of the CPK MB isoenzyme is seen following an MI. LDH exists in 5 isoenzyme forms. Normally serum LDH2 is greater than LDH1, but following an MI this ratio is "flipped" (that is, LDH1 is greater than LDH2).

COMPLICATIONS OF MYOCARDIAL INFARCTION

1. Sudden death
   - Usually due to an arrhythmia
2. Left ventricular failure
3. Dressler syndrome
   - Pericarditis
   - 1–3 weeks following MI

4. Mural thrombosis
    • May embolize
5. Ventricular aneurysms
6. Rupture
    • Hemopericardium

Sudden death occurs within two hours of a myocardial infarction in about 20% of patients. Of the remaining 80% of patients that survive, approximately 80% will develop complications that include arrhythmias, left ventricular failure, extension or expansion of the infarcts, pericarditis, mural thrombosis, ventricular aneurysmal formation, rupture of intraventricular septum, rupture of ventricular free wall, and rupture of a papillary muscle. The latter can lead to acute mitral regurgitation, which produces a pansystolic and diastolic flow murmur and increased left atrial pressure during systole.

CEREBRAL INFARCTION

Diffuse ischemia

• Watershed (border-zone) infarcts
• Laminar necrosis

Localized ischemia

• Thrombosis
• Emboli
• Hypertension

Decreased brain perfusion (ischemia) may be a diffuse (global) or localized process. Global ischemia results from generalized decreased blood flow, such as with shock, cardiac arrest, and systemic hypoxia. Global hypoxia produces watershed (border-zone) infarcts and laminar necrosis. Border-zone infarcts typically occur at the border of area supplied by the anterior and middle cerebral arteries. In contrast, laminar necrosis produces small linear infarcts at the ends of the short penetrating vessels that originate from pial arteries. (Areas that are particularly sensitive to hypoxia are the Purkinje cells of the cerebellum and the pyramidal neurons of Sommers sector in the hippocampus.)

Localized (focal) infarction of the brain results from the local absence of blood flow to the brain. Occlusion of blood vessels can result from thrombosis, emboli, or arteritis. In general thrombosis is more common in the extracerebral carotid system, while embolism is more common in the intracranial arterial system. The majority of thrombi are the result of atherosclerosis and typically produce nonhemorrhagic (pale) infarcts. Common sites for atherosclerotic occlusions include the bifurcation of the carotid artery, the origin of the middle cerebral artery, and at either end of the basilar artery. In contrast, emboli are often associated with cardiac mural thrombi, which can be produced in the heart due to several cardial diseases, such as myocardial infarction, valvular heart disease, atrial fibrillation, or infective endocarditis. Emboli typically produce hemorrhagic (red) infarcts within the brain. The hemorrhage is the result of collateral blood flow or reperfusion that follows the dissolution of the embolus.

The microscopic changes of a cerebral infarction are first seen at about 24 hours and are characterized by ischemic neuronal change (red neurons). After several days there is the influx of inflammatory cells, mainly neutrophils and macrophages. It is important to remember that ischemic necrosis of the brain produces liquefactive necrosis. After several weeks to months a cavity forms that is surrounded by numerous glial cells (gliosis).

Finally, an important type of small ischemic infarcts located deep within the substance of the brain are called lacunar infarcts. They are the result of hypertension (not thrombi or emboli). Hypertensive hemorrhages have a predilection for the distribution of the lenticulostriate arteries and produce small (lacunar) hemorrhages or large hemorrhages that can destroy the corpus striatum. Hypertension results in the deposition of lipid and hyaline material in the walls of cerebral arterioles (lipohyalinosis). This weakens the wall and forms small Charcot-Bouchard aneurysms that can rupture.

ARTERIOLOSCLEROSIS

Hyaline arteriolosclerosis

- Benign hypertension
- Benign nephrosclerosis

Hyperplastic arteriolosclerosis

- Malignant hypertension
- Malignant nephrosclerosis

We mentioned above that there are abnormalities other than atherosclerosis that are associated with scarring of the walls of the smaller muscular arteries. These abnormalities include arteriolosclerosis and medial calcification. Arteriolosclerosis is a disease of small muscular arteries that is related to hypertension. It is divided into a hyaline form and a hyperplastic form. The hyaline form is seen commonly in diabetics, but also occurs in individuals with benign hypertension. Histologically the artery of the affected blood vessel is narrowed by an infiltration of proteins that come from the blood into the intima of the vessel. This infiltration produces a hyaline thickening of the intima. This form of arteriolosclerosis is also associated with changes in the small arteries of the kidneys and results in diffuse ischemia, atrophy, and scarring of the kidney called benign nephrosclerosis. Characteristically the surface of the affected kidneys have a finely granular appearance.

The hyperplastic form of arteriolosclerosis is seen mainly with severe (malignant) hypertension. Malignant hypertension refers to diastolic pressures greater than 130 mm Hg. Malignant hypertension is associated with retinal changes and papilledema. Intimal and medial cells proliferate within affected small blood vessels to produce a characteristic "onion-skinning" thickening of the vessel. In the kidney these changes are called malignant nephrosclerosis. Characteristically the surface of the affected kidneys has multiple small hemorrhages (petechiae) and has been described as a "flea-bitten" kidney.

It is important to compare the above two forms of arteriolosclerosis with a rarer cause of hypertension that is associated with stenosis of the renal artery. The stenosis may occur secondary to either an atheromatous plaque at the orifice of the renal artery or fibromuscular dysplasia of the renal artery. The former is more common in elderly men, while the latter is more common in young women. The decrease in blood flow to the kidney with the renal artery obstruction causes hyperplasia of the juxtaglomerular apparatus and increased renin production. This kidney grossly becomes small and shrunken due to the chronic ischemia (Goldblatt kidney). This small kidney, however, is protected from hypertensive damage by the stenosis. The other kidney is not protected from the increased blood pressure and may develop microscopic changes of benign nephrosclerosis (hyaline arteriolosclerosis).

EMBOLI

Venous emboli

- Originate in veins
- Terminate in veins

Arterial emboli

- Originate in arterial system
- Terminate in arteries

Paradoxical emboli

- Originate in veins
- Terminate in arteries

An *embolus* is a mass that is formed within the vascular system and then is carried by the flow of blood to another site in the vascular system. There are several types of emboli depending upon what the mass is composed of and where the mass is formed. Most emboli are formed from thrombi, and most originate in veins (venous emboli). Most venous emboli end up in the vessels of the lungs, and conversely most emboli within the lungs (pulmonary embolus) originate as thrombi in the large veins of the lower legs.

In contrast to venous emboli, systemic emboli end up within systemic arteries (arterial emboli). Most systemic emboli originate from thrombi formed within the heart, and are frequently the result of a previous myocardial infarction. In contrast to venous emboli (which usually end up within the lungs), arterial emboli have a more varied pathway and may embolize to the lower extremities, the brain, the viscera, or the upper extremities.

A strange and rare type of embolus originates in veins (such as the deep veins of the legs) and terminates in systemic arteries. This type of embolus is called a paradoxical embolus. In order for this to occur there must be a connection between the venous system and arterial system that bypasses the lungs, such as a hole in the septum of the heart.

NONTHROMBOTIC EMBOLI

- Amniotic fluid emboli
- Air emboli
- Fat emboli (associated with fractures)
- Bone marrow emboli (associated with CPR)

For the most part you can assume that an embolus is formed from a thrombus, but this isn't always the case. Types of nonthrombotic emboli include amniotic fluid emboli, air emboli, and fat emboli. Amniotic fluid emboli are complications of pregnancy usually seen around the time of labor and delivery. They are caused by a tear in the placental membranes and rupture of uterine veins. Postmortem examination of the lungs can reveal squamous epithelial cells from fetal skin within pulmonary vessels. Air emboli can also be formed as a complication of delivery, or they can be formed because of too rapid decompression of divers (decompression sickness). The quantity of air needed to produce an air embolus is probably around 100 cc (which makes this complication quite unlikely if you accidentally introduce air into a vessel while drawing blood). Decompression sickness, due to nitrogen and helium bubbles, may be an acute disease ("the bends") or a chronic disease (Caisson disease). Fat emboli are associated with trauma and fractures to long bones. This type of embolus can be particularly serious because free fatty acids released from the fat globules can damage endothelial cells and lead to respiratory failure. Bone marrow emboli are usually the result of rib fractures caused by CPR. They are usually incidental findings.

IMMUNOLOGY—PART ONE: CELLS OF THE IMMUNE SYSTEM

·

· · · · · · · · · · · ·

CELLS OF THE IMMUNE SYSTEM

- Lymphocytes
- Natural killer cells
- Macrophages
- Dendritic cells
- Langerhans cells

LYMPHOCYTES

B lymphocytes

- Form plasma cells that secrete immunoglobulin
- Surface antigen receptor composed of immunoglobulin
- Rearrange immunoglobulin genes

T lymphocytes

- Secrete lymphokines
- Surface antigen receptor is attached to CD3
- Rearrange genes for T cell receptor

Natural killer cells

- Large granular lymphocytes
- Do not need previous sensitization

The immune system is composed of many different types of cells working together to protect the body from infectious organisms. Lymphocytes are a special type of white blood cell (leukocyte) that actively participate in immune reactions. There are two basic types of lymphocytes: B lymphocytes (B cells) and T lymphocytes (T cells). B lymphocytes form plasma cells and secrete immunoglobulins; T lymphocytes secrete lymphokines.

Both B lymphocytes and T lymphocytes originate from the same stem cell, but the developmental sequence for each is different. The maturation of B lymphocytes and T lymphocytes is characterized by gene rearrangement and the acquisition of surface markers. B lymphocytes recognize antigens by their unique surface receptor, which is composed of immunoglobulin. There are literally millions of different types of B cell immunoglobulin surface receptors, each of which binds a particular antigen. This vast diversity of B cell surface receptors is the result of rearrangement of the immunoglobulin genes. In every other cell in the body, the immunoglobulin genes are in the native (germline) configuration. That is, they are not rearranged. The rearrangement of immunoglobulin genes occurs only in B lymphocytes. Therefore, the presence of rearranged immunoglobulin genes in a lymphoid cell indicates that that cell is a B lymphocyte.

In an analogous fashion, T lymphocytes have a surface antigen-binding receptor that consists of CD3 proteins attached to a heterodimer. This heterodimer is composed of alpha, beta, gamma, or delta polypeptide chains and is formed by a process similar to the formation of immunoglobulin. Rearrangement of the genes for the T cell receptor (TCR) serves as a molecular marker for T lymphocytes (just as rearrangement of the immunoglobulin genes is a marker for B lymphocytes).

A third type of lymphocyte in the peripheral blood does not have either a T cell receptor or surface immunoglobulin. In the past these cells were called "null cells" because they lacked these surface receptors, but now they are called natural killer (NK) cells. NK cells comprise about 15% of the peripheral blood lymphocytes. These cells are larger than B or T lymphocytes and have azurophilic cytoplasmic granules. Because of this morphologic appearance they are called large granular lymphocytes (LGL). NK cells transform into lymphokine-activated killer (LAK) cells. These special cells are being evaluated for possible use in the treatment of some types of malignancies.

CLUSTER DOMAINS

T lymphocytes

- CD2 → receptor for sheep erythrocyte
- CD3 → attached to T cell receptor
- CD4 → helper T cells, binds with MHC class II antigens
- CD5 → pan-T cell marker
- CD7 → pan-T cell marker
- CD8 → cytotoxic T cells, binds with MHC class I antigens

B lymphocytes

- CD19 → pan-B cell marker
- CD20 → pan-B cell marker, also called L26
- CD21 → pan-B cell marker, receptor for EBV
- CD22 → pan-B cell marker

NK cells

- CD16 → receptor for Fc portion of IgG

Antibodies can be formed that specifically react to antigens located on the surface membranes of leukocytes. Antibodies that have similar membrane target regions are given cluster designation (*CD*) numbers. Different leukocytes are characterized by different surface antigens, and therefore have different CDs on their surface. For example, peripheral blood T lymphocytes have the surface markers CD2, CD3, CD5, and CD7. T lymphocytes can be divided into two subtypes based on their surface CD markers. Helper T lymphocytes are CD4 positive, while cytotoxic T lymphocytes are CD8 positive.

Similarly there are certain CD markers that are fairly specific for B lymphocytes. Examples of these markers seen in most types of B cells (pan-B cell markers) include CD19, CD20, CD21, and CD22. NK cells can also be identified by two cell surface molecules, CD16 and CD56. CD16 is the receptor for the Fc portion of immunoglobulin G (IgG). It enables NK cells to destroy cells that have been coated with IgG.

Not only can CDs be used to tell B cells from T cells, but they can also be used to help diagnose certain types of leukemias and lymphomas. For example, CD10 is present in certain types of acute lymphocytic leukemias, while both CD15 and CD30 are markers that are useful in the diagnosis of Hodgkin disease.

CDs have many diverse functions, such as serving as adhesion molecules or receptors for certain substances. For example, CD18 forms a portion of the integrin adhesion molecules, while CD21 is the receptor for the Epstein-Barr virus (EBV). Deficiencies of particular CDs may be associated with some diseases. For example, CD55 is decay accelerating factor (DAF), a factor that is important in limiting the activation of complement. A deficiency of CD55 in a cell (such as an erythrocyte) leads to excess complement destruction of that type of cell.

B LYMPHOCYTE DEVELOPMENT

- Pre-pre B cells → rearrangement of heavy chain genes
- Pre-B cells → cytoplasmic mu heavy chains
- Immature B cells → surface IgM
- Mature B cells → surface IgM and IgD
- Plasma cell → cytoplasmic immunoglobulin

B lymphocytes develop from precursors found in the bone marrow. (The letter "B" comes from the fact that in fowl these cells develop in the bursa of Fabricius.) Mature B cells are found in the peripheral blood (10–20% of small lymphocytes), lymph nodes (follicles, germinal centers), and spleen (white pulp).

B cell maturation is defined by the production of immunoglobulin (Ig), which consists of heavy chains and light chains (Fig. 16-2, on p. 308). In order to form immunoglobulin molecules the genes for the heavy chains and the genes for the light chains of immunoglobulin must be rearranged and activated. The genes that code for the heavy chains are rearranged first, but until the light chain genes are rearranged no immunoglobulin can be formed. The heavy chain of immunoglobulin consists of constant regions and variable regions. There are several loci for the genes that code for the variable regions (called V, D, and J), and there are different genes that code for the constant regions. The great diversity of antibodies comes from the fact that there are many different genes in each of the V, D, and J areas, and these genes are selectively rearranged during B cell maturation.

The first step in immunoglobulin gene rearrangement involves one D gene combining with one J gene (all the rest of the D and J genes are deleted). This step defines the pre-pre-B cell (Fig. 16-1). Next one V gene is combined with the DJ combination, and the resulting new gene combination is transcribed with the adjacent Cμ heavy chain locus to produce μ-heavy chain. After this rearrangement, μ-heavy chain is expressed within the cytoplasm, and the cells are called pre-B cells. These pre-B cells also demonstrate surface CD10 and the pan-B cell markers CD19, CD20, and CD22.

Next the developing B cells begin to synthesize light chains. The light chain genes must be rearranged in a process similar to the rearrangement of the heavy

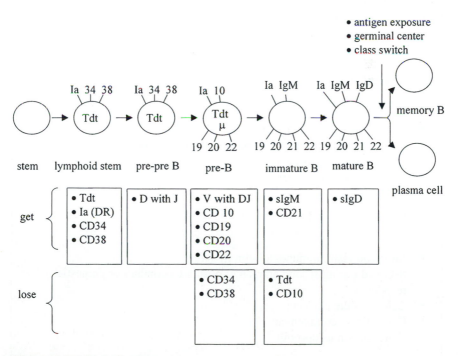

Figure 16-1 B Cell Development

chain genes (except that there are no D light chain genes). The light chain genes are either kappa or lambda. Kappa genes are found on chromosome 2 and are rearranged first. If something goes wrong in this process, then the lambda genes on chromosome 22 are rearranged (otherwise they stay in their germline configuration). The synthesized light chains combine with the intracytoplasmic mu heavy chains to form IgM, which is then transported to the surface where it forms surface IgM (sIgM). These cells, which have also acquired CD21 but have lost TdT and CD10, are called immature B cells. Next the developing B cells produce IgD, which is also expressed on the cell surface (sIgD). These cells are mature B cells. They are also called "virgin" B cells because they have not encountered any foreign antigen. (All of the preceding steps occur in the developing fetus in the bone marrow.)

Subsequent binding of antigen to membrane bound surface Ig results in activation of the B cell. Activate B lymphocytes form either memory cells or plasma cells. Before becoming plasma cells there may be a class switch (isotype switch) to a particular surface Ig that the plasma cell will then secrete. This activation occurs within germinal centers where morphologically the proliferating B cells are classified as being either small cleaved lymphocytes, large cleaved lymphocytes, small noncleaved lymphocytes (with prominent nucleoli), and large noncleaved lymphocytes (with prominent nucleoli). Prior to forming plasma cells these activated B lymphocytes are called B immunoblasts. Plasma cells are characterized by the presence of cytoplasmic immunoglobulin.

IMMUNOGLOBULINS

IgM

- Large molecule (pentamer)
- Secreted early in immune response (primary response)
- Cannot cross the placenta
- Can activate complement
- Contains a J chain

IgG

- Most abundant immunoglobulin in serum
- Secreted during second antigen exposure (secondary or amnestic response)
- Can cross the placenta
- Can activate complement
- Can function as opsonin

IgE

- Allergies, asthma, parasitic infection
- Found on the surface of basophils and mast cells
- Not found on eosinophils
- Participates in type I hypersensitivity reactions

IgA

- Usually a dimer with a J chain and a secretory component
- Found along GI tract
- Secretory immunoglobulin
- Can activate alternate complement pathway

IgD

- Receptor for B cells
- Found on the surface of mature B cells

Immunoglobulins (Ig) are the product of plasma cells. They are composed of light chains and heavy chains, each of which is composed of a variable region and a constant region (Fig. 16-2). The variable regions of both of these chains combine to form the antigen-binding region of Ig (the Fab portion). The portion of immunoglobulin that binds complement is called the Fc portion. Not only can the Fc portion of Ig bind to complement, but it can bind to cells that have Fc receptors, such as monocytes, macrophages, NK cells, mast cells and basophils.

There are two types of light chains (kappa and lambda), and five types of heavy chains (M, D, A, E, and G). The combination of one type of light chain with a particular heavy chain will form each of the five types of immunoglobulin. IgM is a large molecule (pentamer) that is formed and secreted early in the immune response (first exposure to antigen). The monomeric form of IgM is found on the surface of some B cells, while the pentameric form is found in the serum. The fact that IgM is a large pentamer is very important. Because it is so large it cannot cross the placenta, but because it is so large it is very effective at activating complement. Just one molecule of IgM can fix and activate complement.

The most abundant immunoglobulin in the serum is IgG. It is secreted during the second response to certain antigens, not the first response. In contrast to IgM, IgG is a small molecule that usually exists as a monomer. Because it is small

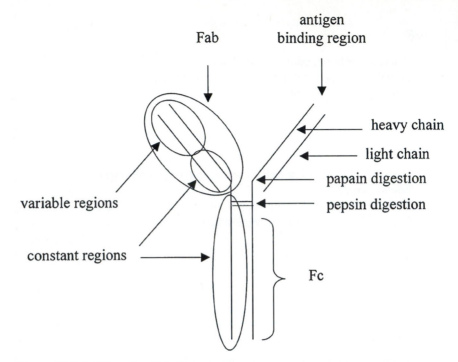

Figure 16-2 IgG Immunoglobulin
IgG is a monomer composed of a light chain and a gamma heavy chain. The light chains, either kappa or lambda, and the heavy chain both have a variable and a constant region. The portion of the immunoglobulin molecule that binds antigen is called Fab, while the portion that binds complement is called Fc. Papain cleaves IgG at the hinge region and produces 1 Fc fragment and 2 Fab fragments. In contrast, pepsin produces 1 Fc fragment and 1 F(ab)$'_2$, fragment; the latter consists of the 2 Fab portions still bound together.

it can cross the placenta, but because it is small it takes several IgG molecules to activate complement.

IgE is found attached to the plasma membrane of mast cells and basophils and participates in type I hypersensitivity reactions, such as allergies, asthma, and *anaphylaxis*. IgE is used to fight parasitic infections. IgA is found on mucosal surfaces (especially the GI tract) and can activate complement through the alternate pathway. IgA exists as a monomer in the serum and a dimer in glandular secretions. It is the most common type of immunoglobulin found in secretions. IgD, which forms less than 1% of serum Ig, is found on the cell surface of some B cells and functions as a receptor for the activation of these B cells.

MULTIPLE MYELOMA

- Monoclonal proliferation of plasma cells in bone marrow
- M spike in peripheral blood (due to monoclonal production of immunoglobulin)
- Multiple lytic bone lesions
- Increased calcium in blood
- Increased protein in blood (due to immunoglobulin)
- Renal disease, anemia, and increased risk of infection

Multiple myeloma, a clonal proliferation of neoplastic plasma cells, is the most common primary hematologic malignancy of bone. In most cases a monoclonal (M) spike is found in the peripheral blood as the result of the monoclonal production of immunoglobulin, most commonly IgG or IgA. (Production of IgM, IgD, or IgE in patients with multiple myeloma is rare.) Monoclonal plasma cells can sometimes produce only light chains (Bence-Jones proteins). These small proteins may be filtered from the blood into the urine. In this case there will be no M spike in the blood, because all of the light chains are in the urine. These Bence-Jones proteins can precipitate within the glomeruli or the tubules as deposits of amyloid.

The diagnosis of multiple myeloma is made by clinical-pathologic correlation. Multiple myeloma is associated with the presence of more than 20% plasma cells in the bone marrow. Clinically, the patient will have multiple lytic bone lesions and increased serum calcium (hypercalcemia). The bone lesions are due to production of osteoclast activating factors (OAF) by the myeloma cells, while the hypercalcemia is due to reabsorption of bone by OAF. Patients with myeloma are at an increased risk of infection, which is the most common cause of death in these patients. These infections are usually due to encapsulated bacteria, because patients with myeloma have abnormal humoral immunity. In contrast, these individuals have no increase in viral infections because their cell-mediated immunity is normal.

WALDENSTRÖM'S MACROGLOBULINEMIA

- Monoclonal production of IgM
- Hyperviscosity syndrome
- No lytic bone lesions or hypercalcemia

Waldenström's macroglobulinemia (WM) is associated with the monoclonal production of IgM, but is clinically distinct from multiple myeloma. Similar to patients with myeloma, patients with macroglobulinemia have a monoclonal production of immunoglobulin (IgM) that produces an M spike in the blood. Unlike myeloma, there are no lytic bone lesions, no hypercalcemia, and the bone marrow shows the proliferation of both plasma cells, lymphocytes, and plasmacytoid lymphocytes. WM is associated with infiltration by neoplastic cells of organs outside of the bone marrow, such as lymph nodes and the spleen. Involvement of these organs is unusual in patients with multiple myeloma. Because IgM is a large molecule (a pentamer), patients with WM are prone to developing the hyperviscosity syndrome, which consists of visual abnormalities, neurologic signs (headaches and confusion), bleeding, and cryoglobulinemia.

T LYMPHOCYTE DEVELOPMENT
Prethymus stage
- Surface markers → TdT, CD34, CD38

Thymus stage
- Stage I surface markers → CD2, CD5, CD7
- Stage II surface markers → CD3, CD4, CD8, TCR
- Stage III surface markers → CD4 or CD8

Postthymus stage
- CD4-positive → helper T cells
- CD8-positive → cytotoxic T cells

T cells arise from precursors in the bone marrow that migrate to the thymus and mature (hence the "T" in their name). As they mature these developing T cells express different cell surface molecules, some of which are given CD numbers (Fig. 16-3). The sequence of events in T cell development is the initial expression of nuclear terminal deoxynucleotide transferase (TdT) in the nucleus and surface CD34 and CD38. This stage is called the lymphoid stem cell and it occurs prior to the cells reaching the thymus (prethymus stage). It is the same cell that gives rise to B lymphocytes.

The next three developmental stages occur within the thymus. Stage I occurs in the outer cortex of the thymus, where the developing T lymphocytes (thymocytes) obtain the surface antigen CD7 followed by CD2 and CD5. The stage I

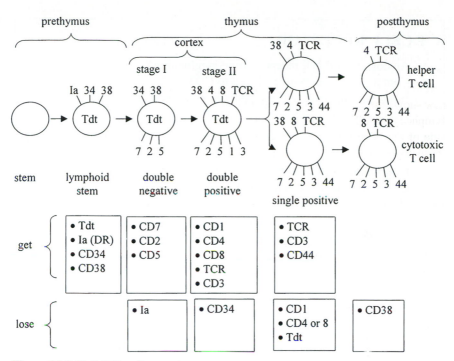

Figure 16-3 T Cell Development

(early) thymocytes lack both CD4 or CD8 and are called "double negative" cells. They comprise about 10% of the thymocytes in the thymus.

The next stage, which starts in the cortex and continues into the medulla, involves generation of an intact T cell receptor (TCR) on the cell surface. Early in the formation of TCR, called stage II, the intermediate (or common) thymocytes acquire both CD4 and CD8 molecules. These cells are called "double positive" T cells and are the majority thymocyte in the thymus (80%). As they leave the thymus, T cells lose either the CD4 or the CD8 antigen. This stage III occurs in the medulla where the T cells also lose TdT. These mature thymocytes comprise about 15% of the thymus thymocytes.

The end result is that postthymus T cells have CD2, CD3, CD5, TCR, and either CD4 or CD8. The CD4-positive cells function as helper cells, and CD8-positive T cells function as cytotoxic cells. In normal healthy individuals, the helper/suppressor ratio (CD4/CD8 ratio) in the peripheral blood is about 2. That is, about 40% of peripheral lymphocytes are helper cells and 20% of peripheral lymphocytes are cytotoxic T cells. These postthymus T cells are found in the peripheral blood (60–70% of small lymphocytes), lymph nodes (paracortical area), and spleen (periarteriolar sheaths, most of white pulp).

T CELL RECEPTOR

- Analogous to B cell receptor (immunoglobulins)
- Composed of heterodimer linked to CD3
- Binds to antigens attached to antigen-presenting cells
- Genes are rearranged only in T lymphocytes

The structure of the T cell receptor (TCR) is very similar to the structure of immunoglobulins. Whereas immunoglobulins are composed of light chains and heavy chains with constant and variable regions, the TCR is composed of either an alpha and a beta chain or a gamma and a delta chain. Each of these chains has a variable (antigen binding) region and a constant region. The TCR is noncovalently linked to the CD3 molecule complex and functions through the second messenger system that increases intracellular IP3 and calcium (Fig. 16-4, opposite).

The genetic organization of the TCR is remarkably similar to that of immunoglobulins. The beta chain is assembled from the genes of four regions, namely V, D, J, and C (variable, diversity, joining, and constant). Every somatic cell contains the TCR genes in the germline configuration, but they are expressed (rearranged) only in T lymphocytes. During processing of the mRNA, the intervening sequences between the genes are spliced off, so that the products of VDJC regions come together. First D joins to J, then they bind to V, and finally they bind to C.

T CELL RECEPTOR SUBTYPES

TCR-2

1. Composed of alpha and beta chains
2. Majority of T lymphocytes
3. Associated with major histocompatibility complex
4. Subpopulations of lymphocytes
   a. CD4+ lymphocytes
      - Helper T lymphocytes
      - Respond to MHC class II antigens
   b. CD8+ lymphocytes
      - Cytotoxic T lymphocytes
      - Respond to MHC class I antigens

TCR-1

- Composed of gamma and delta chains
- Minority of T lymphocytes
- Found in mucosal epithelium
- Not associated with major histocompatibility complex

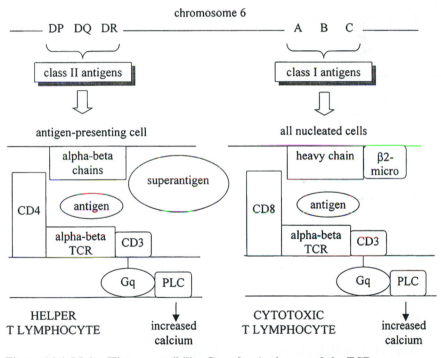

Figure 16-4 Major Histocompatibility Complex Antigens and the TCR
Genes that code for class I and class II antigens are found in the major histocompatibility complex on chromosome 6. Class I antigens are found on the membranes of all nucleated cells in the body and are complexed with beta-2 microglobulin. Antigens that are attached to class I antigens are recognized by the TCR of CD8-positive cytotoxic T lymphocytes. In contrast, class II antigens are found on the membranes of antigen-presenting cells. Antigens that are attached to class II antigens are recognized by the TCR of CD4-positive helper T lymphocytes. In either case, the TCR is attached to CD3 and functions by increasing intracellular concentrations of IP3 and calcium.

About 95% of T cells have a TCR that is composed of an alpha chain and a beta chain. These cells (TCR-2 cells) are subdivided into subpopulations consisting of CD4+ cells and CD8+ cells. These TCR-2 cells need to be exposed to major histocompatibility complex class I or II antigens on antigen-presenting cells (APC) to function (see below). CD4-positive cells react to class II antigens, while CD8-positive cells react to class I antigens (Fig. 16-4). About 5% of T cells have a TCR composed of a gamma chain and a delta chain. These cells (TCR-1 cells) home to mucosal epithelia and do not need MHC class I or II antigens to function.

CD4-POSITIVE T CELL SUBTYPES
T-helper-1 cells (T$_H$1)

- Secrete → IL-2, IL-3, GM-CSF, γ-interferon, and lymphotoxin (β TNF)
- Stimulate cell-mediate immune reactions → fight intracellular organisms

T-helper-2-cells (T$_H$2)

- Secrete → IL-3, IL-4, IL-5, IL-6, IL-10, and GM-CSF
- Stimulate antibody production by plasma cells to fight extracellular organisms

---

CD4-positive T lymphocytes (helper cells) are further divided into two subtypes based on the substances that they secrete and the immune mechanisms with which they participate.

ANTIGEN-PRESENTING CELLS
Macrophages

- Derived from peripheral blood monocytes
- Phagocytic cells
- Release monokines

Dendritic cells of lymph nodes

- Express surface HLA class II antigens
- Poorly phagocytic

Langerhans cells

- Found in epidermis
- Express surface HLA class II antigens
- Contain Birbeck granules

Macrophages originate from monocytes in the peripheral blood and are members of the mononuclear phagocytic system. Macrophages have many functions. They are required to process antigen to T cells. They are phagocytic cells that have receptors for the Fc portion of IgG and C3a. Macrophages are the dominant type of inflammatory cell in chronic inflammation. If macrophages cannot digest the antigen they phagocytized, they may become epithelioid cells or giant cells and a granulomatous reaction can develop. Macrophages produce and secrete many substances including complement components, prostaglandins, interferons, monokines and hemopoietic growth factors.

Dendritic cells are found in lymphoid tissue, while Langerhans cells are found in the epidermis. They both have large amounts of class II antigens on their cell surfaces and are extremely efficient in antigen presentation, but they are both poorly phagocytic. Langerhans cells are also characterized by cytoplasmic Birbeck granules, which by EM examination appear shaped like tennis rackets.

LANGERHANS CELL HISTIOCYTOSIS (LCH)
Acute disseminated LCH

- Letterer-Siwe disease
- Young children
- Systemic disease
- Fatal without therapy

Multifocal LCH

- Hand-Schuller-Christian disease
- Children
- Lytic bone lesions in the skull
- Diabetes insipidus
- Exophthalmus

Unifocal LCH

- Eosinophilic granuloma
- Adults
- Single bone lesions

Langerhans cell histiocytosis (histiocytosis X) refers to a spectrum of clinical diseases that are associated with the proliferation of Langerhans cells. There are three general clinical forms of Langerhans histiocytosis. Acute disseminated Langerhans cell histiocytosis (Letterer-Siwe disease) affects children before the age of three. These children have prominent cutaneous lesions (that resemble seborrhea), hepatosplenomegaly, and lymphadenopathy. The clinical course is usually rapidly fatal without chemotherapy.

Multifocal Langerhans cell histiocytosis (Hand-Schuller-Christian disease) usually begins between the second and sixth years of life. The characteristic triad consists of lytic bone lesions (particularly in the calvarium and the base of the skull), diabetes insipidus, and exophthalmus (bulging outward of the eyes). The diabetes insipidus results from aggregates of Langerhans cells within the hypothalamus or posterior pituitary, while the exophthalmus results from aggregates located behind the eye.

Unifocal Langerhans cell histiocytosis (eosinophilic granuloma), seen in older patients, is usually a unifocal disease (hence the name), most often affecting the skeletal system. The lesions are granulomatous and are made up of a mixture of lipid-laden Langerhans cells, macrophages, lipid-laden lymphocytes, and sheets of eosinophils.

CYTOKINES

IL-1

- Secreted by macrophages, antigen-presenting cells (APC), and other somatic cells
- Activates antigen-presenting cells and helper T cells
- Stimulates neutrophils and B cells
- Induces fever ("endogenous pyrogen")
- Increases acute phase reactants

IL-2

- Secreted by helper T cells
- Stimulates T cell growth (helper T cells and cytotoxic T cells)

IL-3

- Secreted by activated T cells
- Stimulates growth and differentiation of cells of bone marrow

IL-4

- Secreted by helper T cells
- Stimulates B cell growth
- Regulates heavy chain class switch to IgE

IL-5

- Secreted by helper T cells
- Stimulates and activates eosinophils
- Stimulates B cell differentiation
- Increases production of IgA (class switch)

IFN-gamma

- Secreted by helper T cells and cytotoxic T cells
- Potent activator of macrophages (granulomas)
- Stimulates neutrophils and NK cells

The cytokines are chemical mediators of immune reactions that are released from several different immune cells. For example, products of lymphocytes are called lymphokines, and products of monocytes are called monokines. Two of the most important categories of cytokines are the interleukins and the interferons. There are numerous interleukins, all of which have different (and sometimes overlapping) functions. There are two classes of interferons (IFN), namely, anti-viral IFNs (α IFN, β IFN, and omega IFN) and immune IFN (γ IFN). γ IFN is the most potent activator of macrophages. As such it produces epithelioid cells (granulomas). It also stimulates neutrophils and NK cells.

MAJOR HISTOCOMPATIBILITY COMPLEX

- Human leukocyte antigen (HLA) complex
- Products classified into three classes
- Bind foreign proteins during presentation to antigen-specific T cells

CLASS I ANTIGENS

- Found on all nucleated cells
- Transmembrane alpha glycoprotein chain with beta-2 microglobulin
- React with antibodies and CD8-positive lymphocytes
- Fight virus infected cells and transplants

Some foreign antigens are rejected by host tissue when they are transplanted. The genes that code for these foreign transplant antigens are called histocompatibility genes. The genes that code for the strongest transplantation antigens are grouped together on chromosome 6 and are called the major histocompatibility complex (MHC). This complex is also known as the human leukocyte antigen (HLA) complex.

The products of the MHC gene complex are classified into three classes. Class I and class II genes encode for cell surface glycoproteins, while class III genes encode for components of the complement system. Class I antigens are coded by three closely linked loci called HLA-A, HLA-B, and HLA-C. The three class I loci on each chromosome form a single series that is inherited unbroken from each parent. Therefore an individual will have 6 class I HLA antigens, three of maternal origin and three of paternal origin. The products of these genes are glycoproteins that are present on virtually all nucleated cells and platelets (Fig. 16-4). These surface molecules are closely associated with a beta-2 microglobulin. All class I surface antigens result in the formation of humoral antibodies in nonidentical individuals; that is, they can be serologically defined. In general these class I molecules bind to proteins that are synthesized within the cell, such as viral antigens.

CLASS II ANTIGENS

- Found on antigen-presenting cells, B cells, and T cells
- Transmembrane alpha chain and beta chain
- React with CD4-positive lymphocytes
- Fight exogenous antigens that have been processed by antigen-presenting cells

In contrast to class I antigens, class II antigens exist as bimolecular complexes that are composed of an alpha chain and a beta chain. Unlike class I antigens, class II antigens are found on only certain cells (mainly antigen-presenting cells, B cells, and some activated T cells). Similar to class I antigens, most class

II antigens result in antibody production and can be serologically defined. There are, however, some class II antigens that cannot be defined serologically. Instead they are detected by tests that utilize the proliferation of incompatible lymphocytes. Class II molecules bind foreign peptides that are different from the intracellular products bound by class I molecules. In general, class II antigens are associated with exogenous antigens that are processed in endosomes or lysosomes, such as bacteria.

The importance of MHC lies in the way the body controls and regulates the immune cell-to-cell interactions. T cell subtypes can recognize foreign antigen only if the antigen is complexed with a specific type of MHC class antigens. For example, T-helper cells (CD4-positive) can recognize antigen only in association with class II antigens on the surface of the presenting cell, while cytotoxic T cells (CD8-positive) can recognize viral antigens only if they are associated with self class I molecules. This is called HLA-restricted killing.

It is important to make note of a special type of antigen that is capable of binding to both class II MHC and the TCR outside of the normal antigen binding area. These antigens are called *superantigens* and are capable of causing massive activation of T cells in the peripheral blood. An example of this is the TSST-1 toxin, which is associated with the toxic shock syndrome (TSS) and is secreted by some strains of *staph aureus*. Most patients with TSS are females between 15 and 25 years of age who use tampons. Patients present with acute onset of high fever, hypotension, nausea, vomiting, and diarrhea. Patients also characteristically develop a diffuse skin rash that leads to desquamation of the skin.

DISEASES ASSOCIATED WITH HLA TYPES

Inflammatory disease

* Ankylosing spondylitis → HLA-B27

Inborn errors of metabolism

* Hemochromatosis → HLA-A3
* 21-Hydroxylase deficiency → HLA-BW47

Autoimmune disease

* Rheumatoid arthritis → HLA-DR4
* Insulin-dependent diabetes mellitus → HLA-DR3/DR4
* Systemic lupus erythematosus → HLA-DR2/DR3

It is interesting to note that some types of HLA are associated with certain diseases. That is, certain HLA types are found with an increased frequency in patients with certain disease. The reason why is not known, but there are many, many examples of these associations.

Ankylosing spondylitis is a chronic inflammatory disorder that primarily affects the sacroiliac joints and produces bony fusion (ankylosis) of the joints. Patients (usually young adult men) develop low back pain and stiffness. Calcification of the vertebral joints and paravertebral ligaments produces a characteristic "bamboo spine" X-ray appearance. Ankylosing spondylitis is also classified as one of the spondyloarthropathies, others of which include Reiter's syndrome (urethritis, conjunctivitis, and arthritis), psoriatic arthritis, and arthritis associated with inflammatory bowel disease.

IMMUNOLOGY—PART TWO: HYPERSENSITIVITY REACTIONS

HYPERSENSITIVITY REACTIONS
Antibody-dependent reactions

1. IgE
   • Type I
2. IgG or IgM
   • Type II
   • Type III

Antibody-independent reactions (T lymphocytes)

• Type IV

Immunologic responses to antigens, either antibody-mediated (humoral) or cell-mediated, are called hypersensitivity reactions. The antigens can be exogenous, homologous, or autologous. Exogenous antigens are from the environment, such as plant pollens or poison ivy. Homologous antigens are antigenic differences between individuals, such as transfusions or transplants. Autologous antigens are an individual's own antigens and are associated with autoimmune disorders.

Hypersensitivity reactions are classified into four types based on the immune mechanisms that they involve. Antibodies are involved in type I, II, and III hypersensitivity reactions, but they are not involved in type IV reactions (antibody-independent cell-mediated reactions). In contrast, type IV reactions involve T lymphocytes. Type I hypersensitivity reactions involve IgE, while type II and III reactions primarily involve IgG and IgM and the activation of complement.

TYPE I HYPERSENSITIVITY REACTIONS
First exposure

• Antigen binds to antigen-presenting cell
• TH2 cell secretes IL-4, IL-5, IL-6
• B lymphocytes form plasma cells which secrete IgE
• IgE binds to receptors on mast cells and basophils

Reexposure

• Antigen binds to IgE bound to mast cells and basophils
• Mast cells and basophils release intracytoplasmic granules
• Mast cells and basophils synthesize new substances

The basic concept about type I hypersensitivity reactions is that they involve IgE antibodies that are bound to the surface of mast cells and basophils. Type I reactions occur rapidly after an antigen binds to these surface-bound IgE antibodies. How are these IgE antibodies formed, and how do they end up bound to mast cells and basophils? An antigen initially binds to an antigen-presenting cell and causes it to activate TH2 cells. These activated cells then secrete IL-4, IL-5, and IL-6, substances that stimulate B cells to transform into plasma cells and secrete IgE. Mast cells and basophils have cell surface receptors for the Fc portion of IgE and bind the secreted IgE. At this point the mast cells and basophils are "armed and dangerous." All of these events have taken place during the first exposure to the antigen (Fig. 17-1). When the "armed" mast cell or basophil reen-

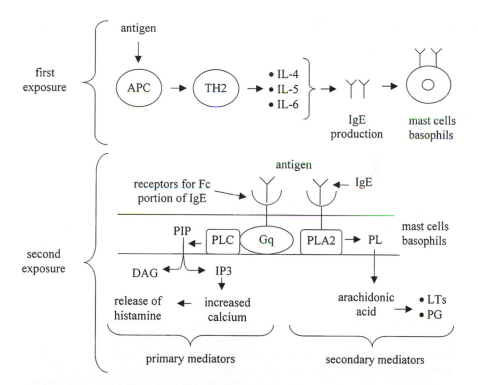

Figure 17-1 Type I Hypersensitivity Reaction
Type I hypersensitivity reactions involve IgE antibodies bound to mast cells and basophils. During the first exposure to an appropriate antigen, antigen-presenting cells (APC) stimulate TH2 lymphocytes to secrete factors that stimulate plasma cells to secrete IgE antibodies. These antibodies become bound to receptors on mast cells and basophils and during reexposure to the same antigen cause these cells to release primary vasoactive mediators and synthesize other secondary mediators of type I reactions.

counters that antigen, it binds to and forms a bridge between two IgE molecules. This causes mast cells to release preformed (primary) mediators and also causes them to synthesize secondary mediators. This primary reaction involves IgE bound to surface receptors that are connected to Gq surface receptors. The degranulation of the mast cells is the result of increased intracellular IP3 and DAG.

MEDIATORS OF TYPE I HYPERSENSITIVITY REACTIONS

Primary mediators

1. Histamine
   - Vasodilation
   - Increased vascular permeability
   - Contraction of bronchial smooth muscle

Secondary mediators

- Arachidonic acid metabolites
- Platelet-activating factor
- IL-4, IL-5, α-tumor necrosis factor

The primary mediators of type I hypersensitivity reactions produce rapidly occurring symptoms because the granules have already been made and are stored within the granules of mast cells. These substances include biogenic amines such as histamine, which cause increased vascular permeability, vasodilation, and bronchial smooth muscle contraction.

Mast cells also produce new products (secondary mediators) by a series of reactions within their cell membrane. These reactions lead to the production of lipid mediators and cytokines. The lipid mediators are generated from arachidonic acid. Membrane receptors bound to IgE activate phospholipase A2, which then cleaves membrane phospholipids into arachidonic acid. The enzyme lipoxygenase produces leukotrienes, including LtB4 (chemotactic) and the leukotrienes C4, D4, and E4, which are the most potent vasoactive and spasmogenic agents known. They used to be called SRS-A (slow reactive substance of anaphylaxis). Prostaglandin D2, which is produced via the enzyme cyclooxygenase, is abundant in lung mast cells. It causes bronchospasm and increased mucus production.

CLINICAL EXAMPLES OF TYPE I HYPERSENSITIVITY REACTIONS

Localized

- Urticaria
- Angioedema
- Asthma
- Allergies
- Allergic rhinitis
- Conjunctivitis

Systemic

- Anaphylaxis

Clinically, type I reactions may be either local or systemic. Local reactions include urticaria ("hives"), angioedema, allergic rhinitis ("hay fever"), conjunctivitis, food allergies, and allergic bronchial asthma. Systemic reactions usually follow parenteral administration of the antigen, such as drug reactions (penicillin) or insect stings. (It is important to realize that the dose of the antigen may be very small.) Systemic symptoms include vomiting, cramps, diarrhea, itching, wheezing, and shortness of breath. Severe systemic symptoms produced with type I reactions are called systemic anaphylaxis. These reactions occur within minutes because the antigen reacts with preformed antibodies already on the surface on mast cells. Death may occur within minutes.

TYPE II HYPERSENSITIVITY REACTIONS

- Antibodies bind to antigens in situ
- Complement-mediated destruction
- Antibody-dependent cell-mediated cytotoxicity (ADCC)
- Cell dysfunction

Type II reactions involve antibodies combining with antigens that are located at the site where they should be located. The antibodies attach to the antigens and then something happens. If the antigen is on a particular cell that cell may be destroyed, or it may malfunction. Type II reactions destroy cells in two basic ways. One way involves complement and the other does not. In complement-mediated reactions antibodies react with a cell surface antigen, and then they activate complement. The cell may then be either lysed by the MAC (C5-9), or it may be phagocytized after being coated with the opsonin C3b.

Cells may be destroyed by type II hypersensitivity reactions that do not involve the activation of complement. These reactions still involve antibodies and are called antibody-dependent cell-mediated cytotoxicity (ADCC) reactions. They are called cell-mediated because the antigens bound to antibodies are attacked by nonsensitized cells having Fc receptors, such as neutrophils, eosinophils, macrophages, and NK cells.

CLINICAL EXAMPLES OF TYPE II HYPERSENSITIVITY REACTIONS

Blood cells

- Transfusion reactions
- Autoimmune hemolytic anemia
- Erythroblastosis fetalis

Connective tissue

- Skin → pemphigus and pemphigoid
- Basement membrane of lungs and kidneys → Goodpasture's disease

Hyperfunction

- Graves' disease

Hypofunction

- Myasthenia gravis
- Pernicious anemia

Many times the antibodies involved in type II hypersensitivity reactions are against blood cells, but the antibodies can be directed against other structures, such as the glomerular basement membrane (Goodpasture's disease) or against parts of the skin (bullous skin diseases). Immunofluorescence staining in type II reactions reveals a linear pattern of antibody and complement deposition. Clinical situations involving antibodies that are directed against blood cells include transfusion reactions, erythroblastosis fetalis, and autoimmune hemolytic anemia.

HEMOLYTIC ANEMIA

Autoimmune hemolytic anemia (AIHA)

* Warm AIHA
* Cold AIHA

Isoimmune hemolytic anemia

* Transfusion reactions
* Hemolytic disease of the newborn

Antibody-mediated destruction of red blood cells is a very good example of a type II hypersensitivity reaction. The antibodies can be directed against antigens of the individual's own red blood cells (autoimmune hemolytic anemia), or they can be directed against antigens on another person's red blood cells (isoimmune hemolytic anemia). This is a very important basic concept to understand. Destruction of cells within the blood (red cells, white cells, or platelets) by antibodies can be an autoimmune or isoimmune reaction.

Autoimmune hemolytic anemia (AIHA) is caused by antibodies that react against normal or altered red cell membranes. The diagnosis depends on the demonstration of these anti-red cell antibodies. The laboratory method used to detect anti-red cell antibodies is called the Coombs antiglobulin test (direct antiglobulin test, DAT). Antihuman globulins (prepared in animals) agglutinate red cells that are coated with antibody. The indirect Coombs test is used to detect antibodies that are free in the patient's serum. Normal red cells are incubated with the patient's serum, and then a DAT is performed. Other signs of AIHA include microspherocytes in the peripheral smear (the result of progressive phagocytosis of red cell membrane material by macrophages within the spleen or the liver), increased serum levels of LDH (released from destroyed red cells), and decreased serum levels of haptoglobin (a protein that tries to bind free hemoglobin in the blood).

The autoimmune hemolytic anemias are divided into two main types: those secondary to "warm" antibodies and those secondary to "cold" antibodies. Cases of warm AIHA are associated with the formation of IgG (rarely IgA) antibodies (not monoclonal) that are active at 37 degrees C. These antibodies are usually directed against Rh antigens. The antibody-coated red cells are sequestered and destroyed in the spleen, which leads to splenomegaly. Most of the cases of warm AIHA are idiopathic. The remainder of the cases are secondary to an underlying disease, such as autoimmune diseases (SLE), leukemias, lymphomas, or drugs.

MECHANISMS OF DRUG-INDUCED HEMOLYTIC ANEMIA

Hapten model

- Penicillin
- Cephalosporins

Immune complex model

- Quinidine
- Phenacetin

Autoantibody model

- Alpha-methyldopa

Many of the cases of warm AIHA are secondary to the use of drugs. Three mechanisms have been developed to describe drug-induced warm AIHA. The hapten model refers to drugs combining with red cell membranes to induce antibody production. In the immune complex model, the drugs combine with plasma proteins to induce the production of antibodies, which then attach to the "innocent bystander" red blood cells. This is an example of a type III hypersensitivity reaction, which we will discuss below. Finally, with the autoantibody model, illustrated by alpha-methyldopa, antibodies are directed against intrinsic red cell antigens, in particular the Rh antigens.

COLD AUTOIMMUNE HEMOLYTIC ANEMIA

Cold agglutinins

- IgM autoantibodies
- Anti-I → mycoplasma pneumonia
- Anti-i → infectious mononucleosis

Cold hemolysins

- Paroxysmal cold hemoglobinuria
- Biphasic Donath-Landsteiner antibody

Cold autoimmune hemolytic anemia can be due to antibodies that either cause red blood cells to clump together (agglutinins) or destroy red blood cells (hemolysins). Cold agglutinins are monoclonal IgM antibodies that react at 4 to 6 degrees C. They are called agglutinins because IgM can agglutinate red cells because of its large size (pentamer). Additionally, IgM can activate complement and cause intravascular (IV) hemolysis. Two diseases are classically associated with cold agglutinin formation. They are mycoplasma pneumonitis (associated with anti-I autoantibodies) and infectious mononucleosis (associated with anti-i autoantibodies).

In contrast to cold agglutinins, cold hemolysins are seen in patients with PCH (paroxysmal cold hemoglobinuria). These antibodies are IgG antibodies that are directed against the P blood group antigen. These cold hemolysins are unique: they are biphasic antierythrocyte autoantibodies. They are called biphasic because they attach to red cells and bind complement at low temperatures, but they don't activate complement until the temperature is increased. This antibody, called the Donath-Landsteiner antibody, was previously associated with syphilis, but may follow various infections, such as mycoplasmal pneumonia.

TRANSFUSION REACTIONS

ABO incompatibility

- Severe reactions (risk of death)
- Intravascular hemolysis

Rh incompatibility

- Less severe reactions
- Extravascular hemolysis (spleen)

Isoimmune hemolytic anemias result from the destruction of the red cells of one individual by antibodies from another individual. This can occur with incompatible blood transfusions or during pregnancies in which there is a blood type incompatibility between the mother and the fetus. Transfusion reactions can produce intravascular or extravascular hemolysis. Both of these reactions produce hypotension, fever, chills, headache, and pain. Intravascular hemolysis, however, is the more serious type of reaction and is often the result of ABO incompatibility. The majority of these mismatches are due to human error. Massive intravascular hemolysis can produce hypovolemic shock, disseminated intravascular coagulation (DIC), and renal failure.

In contrast to intravascular hemolysis, extravascular hemolysis is usually due to an undetected antibody in the patient's serum that is directed against an antigen that is found on the red cells in the donor blood. An example is an antibody to Rh antigens. There are five major Rh antigens, which are called CDEce. Note that there is no d antigen (called "small d"). In common terms, Rh-positive means the person is D-antigen positive, and Rh-negative means that no D-antigen is present (which is usually indicated by two "d"). About 85% of the population is Rh-positive. Antibodies to Rh antigens are IgG antibodies that do not fix complement. Instead the antibody-coated red cells are removed in the spleen, because the macrophages in the spleen have receptors to the Fc portion of IgG. Patients typically develop chills and fever about one hour after the incompatible transfusion.

HEMOLYTIC DISEASE OF THE NEWBORN

Rh incompatibility

- Depends upon presence of D antigen on fetal erythrocytes
- Initial response is production of IgM antibodies → disease unlikely with first pregnancy
- Subsequent responses → IgG
- Prevention → anti-D immunoglobulin

ABO incompatibility

- Depends upon presence of A, B, or AB antigens on fetal erythrocytes
- IgG antibodies may be present → disease is possible with first pregnancy
- No known prevention
- Disease tends to be less severe

Hemolytic disease of the newborn (HDN) is a type of isoimmune hemolytic anemia that is caused by maternal antibodies that react against fetal red blood cells. Once the maternal antibodies cross the placenta, the fetal red cells are destroyed (hemolytic anemia). The breakdown of hemoglobin leads to hyper-bilirubinemia (jaundice), which is a severe unconjugated hyperbilirubinemia. The released heme is not easily conjugated by the immature newborn liver because it is deficient in the enzyme glucuronyl transferase. The unconjugated bilirubin is water insoluble and has an affinity for lipids. In an infant with a poorly developed blood-brain barrier, the bilirubin may bind to the lipids in the brain and produce kernicterus (yellow brain). The severe anemia may produce congestive heart failure, which together with hypoproteinemia (reduced hepatic synthesis) can lead to generalized edema (anasarca). In its most severe form this disorder is called hydrops fetalis. In the peripheral blood of affected newborns, many immature red blood cells can be found (nucleated RBCs or normoblasts). This finding is called erythroblastosis, which is why another name for HDN is erythroblastosis fetalis.

HDN is caused by the transplacental passage of maternal antibodies that are directed against fetal erythrocyte antigens. The mother's red blood cells must lack the sensitizing erythrocyte antigens, while the child erythrocytes must have these antigens (inherited from the father). The most important erythrocyte antigens are the Rh antigens and the ABO antigens. The most important Rh antigen is the D antigen. Therefore for Rh incompatibility, the mother must be Rh-negative (d), while the child is Rh-positive (D). The antibody response depends on the dose of the immunizing agent, so that the Rh-negative mother needs to be exposed to a significant amount of Rh-positive cells (more than 1 ml). This amount of red cells can be seen by the mother during the bleeding of childbirth. The initial response to this incompatibility is the production of IgM antibodies, but these antibodies cannot cross the placenta because they are large pentamers. Rh disease is therefore uncommon with the first pregnancy, but subsequent incompatible pregnancies can lead to the production of IgG antibodies, and these smaller antibodies can cross the placenta. Rh-negative mothers are given anti-D globulin soon after the delivery of an Rh-positive infant. The anti-D antibodies bind to the fetal red cells and hide the antigenic sites from the mother. ABO incompatibility in an Rh-negative mother normally helps to protect the mother against immunization by Rh antigens (the D antigen) because any fetal cells with the Rh antigen that enter her circulation would be destroyed before the mother's immune system could react to them.

ABO incompatibility is the most common cause of hemolytic disease of the newborn. ABO incompatibility usually involves a group O mother with a group A or B fetus. Most antibodies against A and B red cell antigens are IgM antibodies that cannot cross the placenta. However, some group O individuals without prior sensitization by previous pregnancy or blood transfusion have anti-A or anti-B antibodies that are IgG antibodies. Therefore, group O mothers may have infants with HDN in their first pregnancy due to ABO incompatibility. Usually the disease is less severe than HDN caused by Rh incompatibility because there is poor expression of blood group antigens A and B on neonatal red cells. Since these IgG antibodies can be formed naturally, there is no way to protect against ABO reactions.

GOODPASTURE'S DISEASE

- Autoantibodies against basement membranes of lungs and kidneys
- Linear IF staining patterns
- Hemoptysis
- Hematuria

Goodpasture's disease is the result of antibodies being formed that are directed against the noncollagenous domain of the $\alpha 3$ chain of collagen type IV.

The main type of collagen in basement membranes is type IV collagen. Therefore, the antibodies in patients with Goodpasture's disease react against basement membranes, in particular, the basement membranes of the lungs and kidneys. This results in hemorrhage within the lungs (intra-alveolar hemorrhage) and the kidneys (glomerular and tubular hemorrhage). Clinically this hemorrhage results in patients coughing up blood (hemoptysis), and there may be blood in the urine (hematuria). Patients are typically young males, who may develop signs of anemia due to the prolonged bleeding. Diagnostic immunofluorescent (IF) studies reveal linear deposits of IgG (classic type II immunofluorescence pattern) in both the lungs and the kidneys. The prognosis for individuals with this disease has been improved by intensive plasma exchange, which attempts to filter the autoantibodies from the blood.

VESICULOBULLOUS DISEASES OF THE SKIN

Pemphigus vulgaris

- IgG autoantibodies against intraepidermal intercellular antigens
- Linear IF ("chicken-wire" appearance)
- Acantholysis
- Intraepidermal bullae
- Severe disease

Bullous pemphigoid

- IgG autoantibodies against lamina lucida of basement membrane zone
- Linear IF at epidermal-dermal junction
- Acantholysis is absent
- Subepidermal bullae
- Less severe disease

Dermatitis herpetiformis

- IgA antibody-antigen immune complexes at tips of dermal papillae
- Type III hypersensitivity reaction
- Subepidermal bullae
- Associated with gluten-sensitive enteropathy

Several important skin diseases result in the formation of vesicles and bullae (blisters). These vesiculobullous diseases include pemphigus vulgaris, bullous pemphigoid, and dermatitis herpetiformis. Pemphigus vulgaris is a severe (possibly fatal) chronic skin disease that is characterized by the formation of large bullae in the skin and oral mucosa. It is an autoimmune disease (type II hypersensitivity reaction) that is caused by IgG antibodies that are directed against keratinocyte antigens involved in intercellular attachment. Pemphigus vulgaris is characterized by separation of the keratinocytes (*acantholysis*) which results in intraepidermal (suprabasal) bullae. Clinically the bullae are large, flaccid, and easily ruptured because of the roof of the bullae is thin. This can produce large denuded areas of skin. Physical examination reveals that pressure extends the bullae (Nikolsky sign). Immunofluorescence reveals a uniform, "chicken-wire" appearance to the skin.

Bullous pemphigoid is also an autoimmune disease (type II hypersensitivity reaction) that is caused by IgG antibodies, but these antibodies are directed against a glycoprotein that is located in the lamina lucida of the basement membrane zone. Therefore, bullous pemphigoid is characterized by subepidermal blisters and linear deposits of IgG and C3 in the lamina lucida. The vesicles contain predominantly eosinophils. In contrast to pemphigus vulgaris, acantholysis is absent, and mucosal lesions are rare. Because the roof of the bulla is much thicker than that of pemphigus vulgaris, the bullae rarely rupture, and the Nikolsky sign is negative.

Dermatitis herpetiformis (DH) is a bullous disease of the skin that is related to gluten sensitivity (celiac disease). In contrast to the linear deposits of pemphigus and pemphigoid, DH is characterized by granular deposits (type III hypersensitivity) of IgA, fibrin, and neutrophils at the dermal-epidermal junction in the tips of papillae (necrotizing papillitis). These changes result in subepidermal vesicles. Clinical examination reveals symmetrical groups of small papules and erythematous vesicles that are associated with severe itching. The clinical course is self-limited.

GRAVES' DISEASE

- Hyperthyroidism (thyroid-stimulating antibodies)
- Exophthalmus
- Pretibial myxedema

Sometimes instead of destroying cells, the antibodies cause the cells to malfunction. The dysfunction may result in hyperfunction or hypofunction. Graves' disease is an autoimmune disease caused by thyroid-stimulating immunoglobulins (TSI) or thyroid-growth immunoglobulins (TGI). These antibodies, originally called long-acting thyroid stimulators (LATS), activate receptors for thyroid-stimulating hormone (TSH) and produce hyperfunctioning of the thyroid gland. In addition to hyperthyroidism, Graves' disease is associated with characteristic changes of the eyes (ophthalmopathy) and the skin (dermatopathy). The eye changes consist of lid retraction, stare, and *exophthalmus* (protrusion of the eyes). These changes are the result of lymphocytic infiltration of the adipose tissue behind the eye and the muscle of the eye (antibodies to thyroid microsomes cross-react with eye muscles). The skin changes (pretibial myxedema) consist of localized edematous skin in the pretibial area, the result of localized accumulation of mucopolysaccharide. Although it sounds similar to myxedema, pretibial myxedema is associated with Graves' disease, while generalized myxedema is associated with hypothyroidism.

Histologic examination of the thyroid gland in patients with Graves' disease reveals characteristic changes of hyperfunctioning of the thyroid. These changes include increased numbers of follicular cells and scalloping of the colloid. The latter change refers to finding multiple clear areas within the follicles that are adjacent to the follicle cells. These clear cells are the result of the follicle cells taking up colloid material from the lumen of the follicle to obtain thyroid hormones. Additionally, there may be a lymphocytic infiltrate within the interstitium. Grossly the thyroid gland is likely to be diffusely enlarged. This type of enlarged thyroid is called a diffuse toxic goiter. (Toxic means hyperfunctioning, and goiter refers to any enlargement of the thyroid gland.)

HYPOFUNCTIONING AUTOIMMUNE DISEASES
Hashimoto's thyroiditis

- Multiple autoantibodies
- Hypothyroidism
- Lymphocytic infiltrate with Hürthle cell formation

Pernicious anemia

- Autoantibodies to parietal cells or intrinsic factor
- Chronic atrophic gastritis
- Vitamin B12 deficiency
- Megaloblastic anemia
- Subacute combined degeneration of the spinal cord

Myasthenia gravis

- Autoantibodies to acetylcholine receptors at myoneural junction
- Increased muscle fatigability
- Ptosis and diplopia
- Associated with thymic abnormalities

Eaton-Lambert syndrome

- Autoantibodies to calcium channels on the motor nerve terminals
- Clinically similar to myasthenia gravis
- Not aggravated by repeated effort

Autoantibodies may also cause hypofunctioning of organs. Hypofunctioning of the thyroid gland (hypothyroidism) can be the result of the autoimmune disease Hashimoto's thyroiditis. Hashimoto's thyroiditis is associated with high titers of circulating autoantibodies, such as antimicrosomal antibodies, antithyroglobulin, and anti-TSH receptor antibodies. Histologic examination of the thyroid gland reveals infiltration of the thyroid stroma by numerous lymphocytes, which may form lymphoid follicles and germinal centers. This lymphocytic infiltrate destroys the thyroid follicles and transforms the follicular cells into acidophilic cells (oxyphilic cells, oncocytes, or Hürthle cells). Hashimoto's thyroiditis may be associated with other autoimmune diseases. The combination of Hashimoto's disease, pernicious anemia, and type 1 diabetes mellitus is called Schmidt's syndrome. This is one type of the multiglandular syndromes.

Pernicious anemia is associated with chronic atrophic (type A) gastritis and is characterized by the presence of antibodies to parietal cells or intrinsic factor. These autoantibodies decrease the functioning of intrinsic factor and produce a deficiency of vitamin B12 and megaloblastic anemia. A deficiency of vitamin B12 (or folate) is characterized by impaired DNA synthesis, which delays mitotic division and causes cells and their nuclei to be enlarged. The synthesis of RNA and the cytoplasm are not affected. This combination of effects is called nuclear-cytoplasmic asynchrony and affects all rapidly proliferating cells in the body. In the bone marrow this defective DNA synthesis produces enlarged erythroid precursors (megaloblasts) and enlarged red cells (macro-ovalocytes). These megaloblasts undergo autohemolysis within the bone marrow, which is called ineffective erythropoiesis. Granulocyte precursors are also enlarged (giant metamyelocytes) and produce enlarged hypersegmented neutrophils. The megakaryocytes are large and have nuclear abnormalities. Although the platelet count is decreased, the platelets are not enlarged (no macrothrombocytes).

Neurologic changes are frequent in patients with pernicious anemia and are related to degeneration of the posterior and lateral spinal tracts. These degenerations produce symptoms of sensory ataxia and severe paresthesias in the lower limbs. Loss of vibratory sensation in the lower extremities is the first neurologic finding in this disease. These neurologic abnormalities of B12 deficiency (subacute combined degeneration of the spinal cord) do not occur with folate deficiency. They are thought to be the result of abnormal myelin production, due to either excess methionine or abnormal fatty acid production (fatty acids with an odd number of carbons, such as propionate).

Myasthenia gravis is an acquired autoimmune disease that is characterized by circulating antibodies to the acetylcholine receptors at the myoneural junction. These autoantibodies causes abnormal muscle fatigability and typically involve the smallest motor units first, such as the extraocular muscles. This will produce the clinical findings of ptosis and diplopia. Other muscles may also be involved and cause additional symptoms, such as problems with swallowing (dysphagia). Characteristically, repeated contraction of the affected muscles makes the symptoms worse. The symptoms, however, are promptly reversed with Tensilon, a short-acting anticholinesterase. Two-thirds of patients with myasthenia gravis have thymic abnormalities, the most common being thymic hyperplasia. A minority of patients have a tumor of the thyroid gland, called a thymoma.

The Eaton-Lambert (myasthenic) syndrome is a paraneoplastic syndrome that is associated with small-cell carcinoma of the lung. Patients develop autoantibodies that are directed against the calcium channels of the motor nerve terminals. Clinically patients develop muscular weakness that is similar to that of myasthenia gravis (with involvement of the ocular muscles). In contrast to myasthenia gravis, the weakness is not aggravated by repeated effort.

TYPE III HYPERSENSITIVITY REACTIONS
Pathogenesis

- Formation of immune complexes
- Deposition of immune complexes
- Complement activation and inflammation

Forms

- Systemic → serum sickness
- Local → Arthus reaction

Signs and symptoms

- Blood vessels → vasculitis
- Kidneys → glomerulonephritis
- Joints → arthritis
- Serosa → serositis

The pathogenesis of type III hypersensitivity reactions involves the formation of immune complexes by the reaction of antibodies with antigens. It is the formation and deposition of immune complexes that is the basic abnormality of type III reactions. The immune complexes are formed either within the circulation and then deposited outside of blood vessels, or they are formed at extravascular sites where the antigen has been deposited (in situ immune complex formation). These two possibilities define the two major types of immune complex injury, namely, systemic reactions and local reactions. Serum sickness is a systemic type III reaction that results from a single large exposure to antigen. This disease is seldom seen today, but previously it was related to treatments that used horse antisera. Symptoms typically occur 5 to 7 days following exposure to the antigen (the antisera). The immune complexes can precipitate in multiple sites, such as the blood vessels (vasculitis), kidneys (glomerulonephritis), joints (arthritis), and serosal surfaces (serositis). Once deposited they initiate an acute inflammatory reaction. Local damage is done through complement activation, and therefore only complement-fixing antibodies are involved in type III reactions, namely, IgG and IgM (and IgA by the alternate pathway). One of the histologic hallmarks of this complement activation in type III hypersensitivity reactions is fibrinoid necrosis of blood vessels (fibrin from microthrombi and necrosis from the neutrophils).

In contrast to serum sickness, the Arthus reaction is an example of a localized type III hypersensitivity reaction. There is a focal area of tissue necrosis that results from acute immune complex vasculitis. The Arthus reaction develops over a few hours and peaks at 4 to 10 hours. Microscopically there is fibrinoid necrosis of vessel walls. Farmer's lung is an example of a local hypersensitivity reaction in the lung that is the result of molds that grow on hay.

Now is a good time to compare type II and type III reactions. Complement is activated by immune complexes in both type II and type III reactions, but in type II reactions the immune complexes are formed where the antigens should be located, while in type III reactions the immune complexes are formed where the antigens aren't normally found (such as circulating in the blood or deposited in the skin). Don't make the mistake of assuming that because the immune complexes are formed within the blood it must be a type III reaction. (Recall that transfusion reactions are type II reactions.) Another major difference involves immunofluorescence examination (IF). Type II reactions characteristically reveal a linear IF staining pattern, while type III reactions have a granular (lumpy) IF pattern. This is especially important with the immune glomerular diseases (see below).

CLINICAL EXAMPLES OF TYPE III HYPERSENSITIVITY REACTIONS

Drugs

- Foreign serum → serum sickness
- Heroin → glomerulonephritis
- Quinidine → hemolytic anemia

Infections

- Bacteria → poststreptococcal glomerulonephritis
- Virus (hepatitis B) → polyarteritis nodosa
- Fungi (actinomyces) → farmer's lung

Endogenous antigens

- Nuclear antigens → systemic lupus erythematosus
- Immunoglobulin → rheumatoid arthritis

Many different clinical abnormalities involve the formation and deposition of immune complexes. These abnormalities differ in the antigens that are involved in the immune reactions, either exogenous antigens or endogenous antigens. Exogenous antigens include foreign protein, bacteria, or viruses; endogenous antigens include nuclear antigens and immunoglobulins themselves. We will discuss two important examples of diseases associated with endogenous antigens (SLE and rheumatoid arthritis) later, but for now we will concentrate on the glomerular diseases involved with immune complex deposition.

GLOMERULAR ELECTRON-DENSE DEPOSITS
Subepithelial deposits

- Diffuse proliferative glomerulonephritis (DPGN)
- Membranous glomerulonephropathy (MGN)

Intramembranous deposits

- Membranoproliferative glomerulonephritis (MPGN), type II

Subendothelial deposits

- Membranoproliferative glomerulonephritis, type I
- SLE

Mesangial deposits

- Focal segmental glomerulonephritis (FSGN)
- Henoch-Schönlein purpura

Most diseases associated with inflammation of the glomeruli (glomerulonephritis) produce the nephritic syndrome. In contrast to the nephrotic syndrome, the nephritic syndrome is associated with hematuria (blood in the urine). The major causes of the nephritic syndrome involve immune-related processes and the production of electron-dense deposits. Electron-dense deposits composed of immunoglobulin and complement can be deposited in multiple locations within the glomerulus. The location of the deposit indicates the type of glomerular disease that is present (Fig. 17-2).

Deposits located between the epithelial cells and the basement membrane (subepithelial deposits) are characteristic of either diffuse proliferative glomerulonephritis (DPGN), such as poststreptococcal glomerulonephritis, or membranous glomerulonephritis (MGN). The size and distribution of the deposits can differentiate these two. The deposits of MGN are small, uniform in size, and evenly distributed. In contrast, the deposits of DPGN are large, single, and unevenly deposited.

Deposits within the basement membrane are seen in type II membranoproliferative glomerulonephritis (MPGN). These deposits are very long and ribbonlike. They are also very dark, which is why the other name for type II MPGN is "dense deposit disease." Subendothelial deposits are seen in type I MPGN and

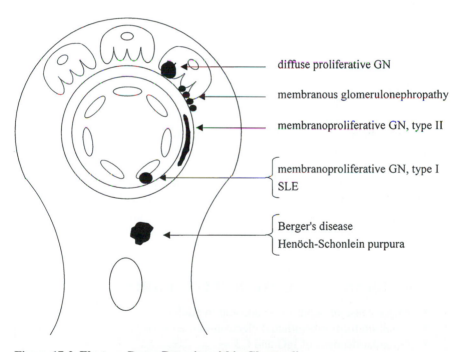

diffuse proliferative GN

membranous glomerulonephropathy

membranoproliferative GN, type II

membranoproliferative GN, type I
SLE

Berger's disease
Henöch-Schonlein purpura

Figure 17-2 Electron-Dense Deposits within Glomeruli
Electron-dense deposits are characteristically located in four locations within the glomerulus: between the epithelial cell and the basement membrane (subepithelial deposits), within the basement membrane (intramembranous deposits), between the endothelial cell and the basement membrane (subendothelial deposits), and within the mesangium (mesangial deposits). For an explanation of the structures seen in this schematic see Figure 14-2.

systemic lupus erythematosus. Deposits within the mesangial matrix are found in IgA nephropathy (Berger's disease) and Henoch-Schönlein purpura.

Electron-dense deposits are not usually found within the Bowman space, nor are they usually found in patients with Goodpasture's disease or lipoid nephrosis.

DIFFUSE PROLIFERATIVE GLOMERULONEPHRITIS

- Poststreptococcal glomerulonephritis
- Granular deposits of IgG and C3
- Single large subepithelial electron-dense deposits

Diffuse proliferative glomerulonephritis most commonly follows a streptococcal infection of the pharynx or skin (poststreptococcal glomerulonephritis). The streptococcal infection is usually caused by a group A beta hemolytic streptococcus (*streptococcus pyogenes*), and it usually occurs in children. Acute poststreptococcal glomerulonephritis has a classic clinical presentation, typically beginning 1–3 weeks following the streptococcal infection. Patients present with hematuria, mild periorbital edema, increased blood pressure, and red cell casts in the urine. Throat cultures taken at the time of the renal disease will fail to grow the organism, but serum ASO titers (antistreptococcal antibodies) will be elevated, and serum C3 levels will be decreased. Most children with acute poststreptococcal glomerulonephritis recover, but the prognosis is much worse in adults, where therapy is supportive care only.

Microscopic examination of the kidneys reveals a proliferation of the endothelial cells and mesangial cells within the glomerulus. There may also be an infiltrate of neutrophils within the glomeruli. IF reveals granular deposits of IgG and C3, while EM reveals large single subepithelial deposits.

MEMBRANOUS GLOMERULONEPHROPATHY

- Major cause of nephrotic syndrome in adults
- Small uniform subepithelial electron-dense deposits
- Granular deposits of IgG and C3
- Formation of basement membrane "spikes and domes"

Membranous glomerulonephropathy (MGN) is a major cause of the nephrotic syndrome (nonselective proteinuria) in adults. It is important to realize the MGN is associated with the nephrotic syndrome and not the nephritic syndrome. That is, MGN is not an inflammatory glomerular disease, and the more accurate name is membranous glomerulonephropathy and not membranous glomerulonephritis.

Most cases are idiopathic, but some cases of MGN are secondary to other diseases, such as some types of cancer, some infections (typically hepatitis B), toxic metals (gold), and some drugs (penicillamine). MGN is associated with small uniform subepithelial electron-dense deposits of IgG and C3. These immune complex deposits activate complement and damage the basement membrane (leading to proteinuria), but there is no influx of inflammatory cells (no proliferative disease).

The subepithelial deposits stimulate the production of new basement membrane material (hence the name "membranous"). MGN is subdivided into 3 stages based on the changes seen in the basement membrane (Fig. 17-3). In stage I, there are uniform subepithelial deposits, but the basement membrane is within normal limits. In stage II MGN, new basement membrane material forms between these uniform subepithelial deposits. This produces characteristic abnormalities called *spikes*. In stage III MGN, new basement membrane is found between and overlying the uniform subepithelial deposits. This latter abnormality is called *domes*.

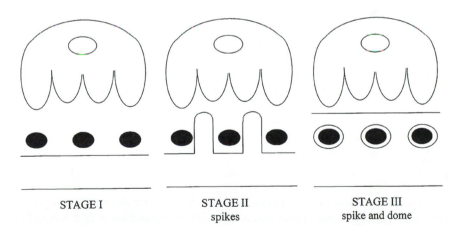

| STAGE I | STAGE II | STAGE III |
| | spikes | spike and dome |

Figure 17-3 Formation of "Spikes and Domes" in Membranous Glomerulonephropathy

---

MEMBRANOPROLIFERATIVE GLOMERULONEPHRITIS

Type I

*   Subendothelial deposits of IgG, IgM, and complement

Type II

*   Associated with C3 nephritic factor in serum
*   Dense ribbonlike deposits of C3 and properdin within the basement membrane

---

Membranoproliferative glomerulonephritis (MPGN) is characterized by a thickened basement membrane ("membrano") and an increase in the number of mesangial cells ("proliferative"). There are two basic types of MPGN. Type I MPGN is more common and is characterized by subendothelial deposits of IgG, IgM, and complement. Type II MPGN is much rarer, but is much more interesting from a pathologic standpoint. It is characterized by very dense, ribbonlike, electron-dense deposits within the basement membrane. In both types of MPGN (but especially type I), proliferation of mesangial cells and mesangium into the basement membrane cause it to split apart and produce a characteristic *tram-track* appearance.

Clinically MPGN is quite variable in its presentation. Patients may present with the nephrotic syndrome, the nephritic syndrome, or combinations of both. Type I MPGN is seen primarily in children and young adults.

FOCAL SEGMENTAL GLOMERULONEPHRITIS

*   Mesangial deposition of IgA
*   Berger's disease
*   Henoch-Schönlein purpura

Focal segmental glomerulonephritis (FSGN) is the result of the focal proliferation of mesangial cells and is associated with the deposition of IgA within the mesangium. The two main diseases associated with the deposition of IgA within the mesangium are Berger's disease (IgA nephropathy) and Henoch-Schönlein purpura). Berger's disease is the most common cause of the nephritic syndrome worldwide. Hematuria usually follows an upper respiratory infection, but IgA nephropathy may also be associated with certain GI diseases (celiac disease) or skin diseases (dermatitis herpetiformis). Henoch-Schönlein purpura is a disease of children that is characterized by systemic vasculitis, involving especially the skin, joints, and kidneys. Patients develop purpuric lesions of the arms, legs, and buttocks and nonmigratory arthralgia.

RAPIDLY PROGRESSIVE GLOMERULONEPHRITIS

Linear immunofluorescence → antimembrane antibody

- Goodpasture's disease

Granular immunofluorescense → immune complexes

- Other glomerular or systemic disease

Minimal or negative immunofluorescence → pauci-immune disease

- Wegener's granulomatosis
- Microscopic polyarteritis nodosa

The finding of crescents within the Bowman space in a patient with rapidly progressing renal failure is diagnostic of rapidly progressive (crescentic) glomerulonephritis (RPGN). *Crescents* are formed by proliferation of epithelial cells within the Bowman space of the glomerulus. RPGN may be subdivided into 3 types based on the IF staining pattern. Type I RPGN reveals linear staining of IgG and C3. The majority of these patients have Goodpasture's disease (anti-GBM disease). Type II RPGN reveals immune complex deposition (granular staining). These patients may have other glomerular or systemic diseases, which include poststreptococcal GN, membranoproliferative GN, IgA nephropathy (Berger's disease), and SLE. (Membranous GN is not a cause of RPGN.)

Finally, type III RPGN reveals minimal immune changes and is referred to as pauci-immune crescentic GN. Antineutrophil cytoplasmic antibodies (ANCA), which are found in some patients with vasculitis, are found in many of these patients with pauci-immune GN. ANCAs are either perinuclear (P-ANCA, against myeloperoxidase) or cytoplasmic (C-ANCA, against proteinase 3). P-ANCA is found in patients with microscopic polyarteritis and idiopathic crescentic GN, while C-ANCA is found in patients with Wegener's granulomatosis.

Microscopic polyarteritis nodosa (hypersensitivity angiitis) refers to a group of immune complex-mediated vascular diseases (vasculitis). Particularly common in these patients are necrotizing lesions that involve the glomeruli and pulmonary capillaries. Major symptoms of microscopic polyarteritis include hemoptysis and hematuria. Skin involvement may produce a palpable purpura. Many times the disease is triggered by an antigen such as a drug (penicillin), a microorganism, a virus, or a tumor antigen. Neutrophils accumulate in small vessels and may become fragmented, hence the alternate name leukocytoclastic angiitis. Henoch-Schönlein purpura with renal involvement is included in this group and is characterized by hemorrhagic urticaria and upper respiratory infections.

Wegener's granulomatosis is characterized by acute necrotizing granulomas that affect the upper and lower respiratory tract; focal necrotizing vasculitis that affects small to medium-sized vessels; and renal disease. Histologically Wegener's disease demonstrates granuloma formation with giant cells, while small arteries may develop fibrinoid necrosis. This disease, which has a peak incidence in the fifth decade, is highly fatal within one year, unless it is treated with immunosuppressive agents.

TYPE IV HYPERSENSITIVITY REACTIONS
Delayed-type hypersensitivity

- Gamma-interferon → activates macrophages and forms epithelioid cells (granulomas)
- IL-2 → activates other CD4 cells
- TNF-alpha → activates endothelial cells

Cell-mediated cytotoxicity

- Cytotoxic T lymphocytes

Type IV hypersensitivity reactions are hypersensitivity reactions that are mediated by cells (T cells) rather than by antibodies. There are two subtypes of cell-mediated hypersensitivity. One involves lymphocytes and other cells, mainly macrophages, and is called delayed-type hypersensitivity. The other involves only T cells and is called cell-mediated cytotoxicity. Delayed-type hypersensitivity reactions primarily involve CD4-positive lymphocytes. Upon first exposure to an antigen, macrophages ingest and process the antigen to helper cells. This process is dependent upon class II antigens (HLA-D). The end result is formation of "memory" T cells. Upon reexposure, these memory cells are activated and secrete biologically active factors, the lymphokines. Specifically, CD4 TH1 cells are activated and secrete gamma-interferon, IL-2, and TNF-alpha.

In contrast to delayed-type hypersensitivity, cell-mediated cytotoxicity involves sensitized T cells (CD8-positive) that can by themselves kill antigen-bearing target cells. These cells are called cytotoxic T lymphocytes (CTLs).

CLINICAL EXAMPLES OF TYPE IV HYPERSENSITIVITY REACTIONS

Delayed-type hypersensitivity

- Contact dermatitis
- Poison ivy and poison oak
- Tuberculin skin test (Mantoux)
- Lepromatin test (leprosy)
- Granulomatous inflammation

Cell-mediated cytotoxicity

- Fight viral infections
- Transplant rejections

Delayed-type hypersensitivity is involved in reactions against a variety of intracellular pathogens, including mycobacteria and fungi. The classic reaction is the tuberculin skin test (Mantoux reaction). A local area of erythema and induration peaks at about 48 hours following intradermal injection of tuberculin. Granulomatous inflammation (aggregates of epithelioid cells), poison ivy reactions, and contact dermatitis are other types of delayed-type hypersensitivity. In contrast, cell-mediated cytotoxic hypersensitivity reactions are important in viral infections, tumors, and graft rejection.

TRANSPLANT PATHOLOGY

Terminology

- Autograft (autologous) → self to self (always accepted)
- Isograft → between identical twins (always accepted)
- Allograft → person to person (variable acceptance)
- Xenografts (heterologous) → between species (strong rejection)

Host-versus-graft disease

- Hyperacute rejection
- Acute rejection
- Chronic rejection

Graft-versus-host disease

- Bone marrow transplants

The rejection of organ transplants is called host-versus-graft disease. It involves both humoral and cell-mediated immunologic reactions. There are basically three types of rejections of grafts: hyperacute rejection, acute rejection, and chronic rejection. Hyperacute rejection occurs within minutes after transplantation and is due to preformed antibodies against antigens on the graft. Histologic examination of a transplanted kidney that develops hyperacute rejection would reveal neutrophils within the glomerulus and peritubular capillaries. These changes illustrate an antigen-antibody reaction at the vascular endothelium, similar to the Arthus reaction.

Acute rejection may occur within days or much longer after transplantation. It is called acute because once it begins, the changes progress rapidly. Acute rejection can result from vasculitis or lymphocytic infiltration of the interstitium. Vasculitis is the result of humoral rejection (acute rejection vasculitis), while the interstitial mononuclear infiltrate is the result of cellular rejection (acute cellular rejection). Acute rejection is the result of CD8 lymphocytes responding to class I HLA antigens and causing CD4 helper cells to proliferate. Acute cellular rejection is responsive to immunosuppressive therapy, but acute rejection vasculitis is not.

In chronic rejection of a transplanted kidney, tubular atrophy, mononuclear interstitial infiltration, and vascular changes are found. The vascular changes are probably the result of the proliferative arteritis seen in acute and subacute stages. Vascular obliteration, primarily the result of antibodies, leads to interstitial fibrosis, tubular atrophy, and loss of renal function.

Graft-versus-host (GVH) disease occurs with the transplantation of bone marrow or liver. Immunocompetent lymphocytes from the donor marrow attack the recipient's tissue. GVH may be acute or chronic. Acute GVH is manifested by changes in the skin (dermatitis), the intestines (diarrhea, malabsorption), and the liver (jaundice). Chronic GVH produces changes in the skin (fibrosis) that are similar to the skin changes seen in patients with progressive systemic sclerosis.

IMMUNOLOGY—PART THREE: AUTOIMMUNE AND IMMUNODEFICIENCY DISEASE

- Autoimmune Diseases
- Types of Autoantibodies
- Antinuclear Antibodies (ANAs)
- Antineutrophil Cytoplasmic Antibodies (ANCAs)
- Systemic Lupus Erythematosus
- WHO Classification of Renal Disease in Patients with SLE
- Sjögren's Syndrome
- Progressive Systemic Sclerosis
- CREST Syndrome
- Inflammatory Myopathies

- Rheumatoid Arthritis
- Polyarteritis Nodosa
- Immunodeficiency Diseases
- Severe Combined Immunodeficiency Disease
- X-Linked Agammaglobulinemia of Bruton
- Common Variable Immunodeficiency
- Isolated Deficiency of IgA
- DiGeorge's Syndrome
- AIDS

AUTOIMMUNE DISEASES

- Loss of self-tolerance
- Immune reactions against self-antigens

TYPES OF AUTOANTIBODIES

1. nuclear: several → see ANA chart
2. cytoplasmic: mitochondria → primary biliary cirrhosis
3. cells: smooth muscle → lupoid hepatitis (autoimmune chronic active hepatitis)
                      neutrophils → Wegener's granulomatosis and microscopic polyarteritis
                      parietal cell and intrinsic factor → pernicious anemia
                      microvasculature of muscle → dermatomyositis
4. proteins: immunoglobulin → rheumatoid arthritis
                      thyroglobulin → Hashimoto's thyroiditis
5. structural antigens: lung and glomerular basement membranes → Goodpasture's disease
                      intercellular space of epidermis → pemphigus vulgaris
                      epidermal basement membrane → bullous pemphigoid
6. receptors: acetylcholine receptor → myasthenia gravis
                      thyroid hormone receptor → Graves' disease
                      insulin receptor → diabetes mellitus

ANTINUCLEAR ANTIBODIES (ANAs)

1. diffuse (homogenous) DNA → many
                         histone → drug-induced SLE
2. rim (peripheral);   double-stranded DNA → SLE
3. speckled: non-DNA extractable nuclear proteins → many including:
                              Smith → SLE
                              SS-A and SS-B → Sjögren's syndrome
                              Scl-70 → progressive systemic sclerosis (PSS)
4. nucleolar: RNA → many (think PSS)
5. centromere: CREST syndrome

ANTINUETROPHIL CYTOPLASMIC ANTIBODIES (ANCAs)

1. c-ANCA (cytoplasmic):   proteinase 3 → Wegener's granulomatosis
2. p-ANCA (perinuclear):   myeloperoxidase → microscopic polyarteritis

Autoimmune reactions may involve humoral or cell-mediated hypersensitivity reactions. Humoral mechanisms involve antibodies against self-antigens (autoantibodies). There is a tremendous number of autoantibodies; some are directed against nuclear antigens, some are directed against cytoplasmic antigens, and others are directed against proteins or cells themselves.

One of the most important type of autoantibodies is antinuclear antibodies (ANA). The most commonly used clinical test to detect these antibodies examines the indirect immunofluorescence pattern that they produce. The pattern of nuclear staining suggests the type of antibody that is present in the patient's serum. This can help to identify the type of autoimmune disease an individual has. Four basic patterns are found: diffuse (homogenous) pattern, which reflects staining to DNA and histone; rim (peripheral) pattern, which indicates antibodies to double-stranded DNA (native DNA); speckled pattern, which reflects antibodies to non-DNA nuclear components; and a nucleolar pattern, which represents antibodies to RNA.

It is important to realize that autoantibodies are not always specific indicators of disease. That is, sometimes autoantibodies are associated with certain diseases (high specificity), and at other times they can be found in many different diseases (low specificity). This is particularly true for antinuclear antibodies (ANA), which seem to be present in almost any type of autoimmune disease. For example, positive tests for antinuclear antibody (ANA) occur in greater than 95% of patients with systemic lupus erythematosus (high diagnostic sensitivity), but the test is not specific because positive results are also frequently found in other autoimmune diseases. Antibodies to double-stranded DNA (anti-ds DNA) are clinically useful, however, since these antibodies are found in about 50 percent of patients with SLE (sensitive) and are rare in other autoimmune diseases (specific).

SYSTEMIC LUPUS ERYTHEMATOSUS

Type III reactions

- Vasculitis → fibrinoid necrosis
- Arthritis → most common symptom
- Synovitis
- Serositis → pleural effusions
- Glomerulonephritis
- Skin rash

Type II reactions

- Thrombocytopenia
- Hemolysis

Systemic lupus erythematosus (SLE) is the prototypic autoimmune disorder. Clinically SLE is a chronic, remitting and relapsing, multisystem disease. Basically patients with SLE have a marked B-cell hyperactivity that leads to a polyclonal production of antibodies to self and nonself antigens. It is the numerous antibodies to self-antigens (autoantibodies) that produce the pathology of SLE. These autoantibodies are directed against nuclear and cytoplasmic cell components, but the antinuclear antibodies (ANA) are the laboratory hallmark of SLE (especially anti-double-stranded DNA antibodies). There is no evidence, however, that these antinuclear antibodies can penetrate intact cells. Instead damaged cells lose their nuclei, which then react with the autoantibodies and can form LE bodies (hematoxylin bodies). These bodies are pathognomonic for lupus. In vivo, phagocytic cells (such as a neutrophil or macrophage) can ingest these LE bodies and form LE cells. This same process is the basis of an in vitro test that tries to produce LE cells by taking blood and agitating it to damage cells. This test is positive in most patients with SLE.

These autoantibodies react with antigens via type II or type III hypersensitivity reactions. The majority of the signs and symptoms seen in patients with SLE are due to type III reactions where antibodies react with antigens and form immune complexes. Subsequently these complexes are deposited in many sites, such as blood vessels (vasculitis), joints (arthritis), the synovium (synovitis), and the kidneys (glomerulonephritis). A common histologic finding that demonstrates this immune complex deposition is acute necrotizing vasculitis affecting small arteries and arterioles. Histologically there is necrosis and fibrinoid deposits (accumulations of pink-staining homogeneous masses of fibrin, immunoglobulins, and other plasma proteins) within the walls of the vessels (fibrinoid necrosis). In patients with SLE chronic inflammation may induce perivascular fibrosis (onionskin lesions).

Type II reactions are rarer in patients with SLE. These reactions may destroy red cells (hemolysis) or platelets. These antibodies may cause a false positive laboratory test, the classic example being a false positive test for syphilis.

Clinically most patients with SLE are female, and the disease usually becomes symptomatic in the second and third decades. The classic lesion in SLE is an erythematous (red) rash that is located over the bridge of the nose, a characteristic "butterfly" rash. Sunlight makes this rash worse. Histologically there is liquefactive degeneration of the basal layer of the epidermis and lymphoid infiltrates around blood vessels. Deposits of immunoglobulin and complement can be demonstrated at the epidermal-dermal junction. Finding immunoglobulin deposits in uninvolved adjacent skin is considered highly specific for SLE. This is called the "lupus band test." The most common symptom is caused by immune involvement of the joints (arthritis), which produces a nonerosive synovitis. The heart may also be involved in patients with SLE. Small growths (vegetations) may develop on the heart valves and are called Libman-Sacks endocarditis. The vegetations are from 1 to 3 mm and are found on either side of the leaflet of the valve (this is an important gross diagnostic feature).

There are several variant forms of SLE, including chronic discoid lupus and drug-induced lupus. Chronic discoid lupus affects only the skin, while drug-induced SLE, associated with antihistone antibodies, is a multisystem disease. The only exceptions to the latter are lack of involvement of the kidneys and central nervous system. Drugs associated with drug-induced lupus include procainamide (an antiarrhythmic drug), hydralazine (a hypertensive drug), and isoniazid (used to treat TB).

WHO CLASSIFICATION OF RENAL DISEASE IN PATIENTS WITH SLE

Type I

- No changes

Type II

- Mesangial glomerulonephritis
- Mild disease, slow progression
- Most common type

Type III

- Focal proliferative glomerulonephritis

Type IV

- Diffuse proliferative glomerulonephritis (proliferation of endothelial cells)
- "Wire-loop" lesions
- Severe, rapidly progressive disease

Type V

- Diffuse membranous glomerulonephritis
- Nephrotic syndrome
- Slow progression

Renal disease is the presenting sign in only about 5% of patients with SLE, but it is the major cause of death. All of the glomerular diseases in patients with SLE are the result of the deposition of immune complexes (DNA-anti-DNA complexes) in mesangial, intramembranous (inside the basement membrane), subepithelial, or subendothelial locations within the glomeruli. WHO (the World Health Organization) classifies the glomerular disease of patients with SLE into five distinct patterns. In membranous glomerulonephritis the deposits are in a subepithelial location; in diffuse proliferative lupus GN, the deposits are mainly in a subendothelial location. Subendothelial deposits produce a characteristic "wire loop" histologic appearance due to thickening of the capillary wall. The immunofluorescence findings may be variable in patients with SLE, but finding a little bit of everything ("full house" pattern) is fairly characteristic.

SJÖGREN'S SYNDROME

* Keratoconjunctivitis sicca (dry eyes) due to destruction of lacrimal glands
* Xerostomia (dry mouth) due to destruction of salivary glands
* Arthritis

Sjögren's syndrome results from autoimmune destruction of the lacrimal and salivary glands. This destruction produces dry eyes and a dry mouth. Like most autoimmune diseases, Sjögren's syndrome affects females more often than males. Patients are usually over the age of 40. Sjögren's syndrome can be an isolated disorder (primary form or sicca syndrome), or it can be associated with other autoimmune diseases (secondary form), rheumatoid arthritis being the most common.

As with SLE, patients with Sjögren's syndrome have a polyclonal hypergammaglobulinemia and numerous autoantibodies. Most patients have rheumatoid factor (even without arthritis) and antinuclear antibodies. About 70% of patients have autoantibodies to two nuclear nonhistone proteins, SS-A and SS-B. Anti-SS-B antibodies are considered specific for Sjögren's syndrome.

Histologic examination of affected organs reveals a periductal and perivascular lymphocytic infiltrate. Most of the cells are T cells of the helper phenotype (CD4+). B cells may be present and may form germinal centers. Some patients have such a marked lymphocytic infiltrate that can simulate a malignant process. This can be a challenging diagnostic problem, especially considering that patients with Sjögren's syndrome have a markedly increased risk of developing B-cell lymphomas.

PROGRESSIVE SYSTEMIC SCLEROSIS

Skin

- Sclerotic atrophy
- Loss of adnexal structures

GI

- Dysphagia

Kidneys

- Occlusion of small blood vessels ("onion-skinning")
- Hypertension

Lungs

- Interstitial fibrosis

Progressive systemic sclerosis (PSS) is characterized by inflammatory and fibrotic changes throughout the body. The fibrosis is due to the increased production of collagen by fibroblasts secondary to the release of fibroblast growth factors. As with many other autoimmune diseases, patients with PSS have hypergammaglobulinemia and antinuclear antibodies. Some patients even have rheumatoid factor. One antinuclear antibody that is particularly unique to systemic sclerosis is Scl-70 (an antibody to a nonhistone nuclear protein). Histologic examination of affected organs reveals abnormal blood vessels having intimal fibrosis ("onion-skinning") and fibrinoid necrosis.

The vast majority of patients with systemic sclerosis have involvement of the skin (hence another name for this disease is scleroderma). In the skin the changes begin in the fingers and hands and produce sclerotic atrophy. There is increased dermal collagen, epidermal atrophy, and loss of skin adnexal structures. The loss of adnexal structures is the best histologic diagnostic sign of PSS. When the disease affects the face, patients may first notice a loss of wrinkles. This pleasant change is rapidly replaced by severe symptoms, because PSS is a severe progressive disease.

The gastrointestinal tract is affected in over half of the cases. The esophagus is commonly involved, but the colon is rarely affected. Sclerosis of the esophagus leads to problems swallowing food (dysphagia). In the kidneys changes of the small arteries ("onion-skinning") can lead to hypertension. Patients also develop diffuse interstitial fibrosis of the lung, which can lead to problems with breathing (restrictive pulmonary disease) and right-sided heart failure.

CREST SYNDROME

- Calcinosis
- Raynaud phenomenon
- Esophageal dysmotility
- Sclerodactyly
- Telangiectasia

A variant of PSS is called the CREST syndrome. The name of this disease is an acronym that stands for the combination of calcinosis, Raynaud syndrome (episodic ischemia of digits), esophageal dysmotility, sclerodactyly, and telangiectasia (dilated blood vessels). Pulmonary hypertension and primary biliary cirrhosis are common in the CREST syndrome, but the kidneys are usually spared. An autoantibody that is specific for this syndrome is the anticentromere antibody.

INFLAMMATORY MYOPATHIES

Polymyositis

- Proximal muscle weakness
- Increased incidence of visceral malignancies

Dermatomyositis

- Proximal muscle weakness
- Bimodal age distribution (children and adults)
- Heliotrope rash of upper eyelids with periorbital edema
- Red rash over knuckles

Inclusion-body myositis

- Most frequent form of myositis in the elderly
- Histology reveals numerous rimmed vacuoles within muscle

The inflammatory myopathies are characterized by immune mediated inflammation and injury of skeletal muscle. The inflammatory myopathies include polymyositis, dermatomyositis, and inclusion-body myositis. Polymyositis is a diffuse inflammatory disorder of skeletal muscles that can occur at any age. It is about twice as common in females as in males. Proximal muscle weakness is the usual presenting symptom. Skin lesions are present in almost half of the patients and when present, the diagnosis of dermatomyositis is made. In contrast to polymyositis, dermatomyositis is more common in children. Patients typically have a purple discoloration on their eyelids (heliotrope rash) and an erythematous rash on their knuckles (Gorton sign). Malignant neoplasms may be found in some adults with dermatomyositis. The most commonly associated neoplasms are carcinomas of the lung, breast, colon and stomach.

The inflammatory myopathies are associated with numerous types of autoantibodies, one of which is the anti-Jo-1 antibody. In children with dermatomyositis, antibodies to small blood vessels within the muscle produce a characteristic atrophy of the muscle fibers located at the periphery of the muscle fiber fascicle (perifascicular atrophy).

RHEUMATOID ARTHRITIS

- Rheumatoid factor (antibody against antibody)
- Pannus formation in synovium
- Ulnar deviation of fingers
- Subcutaneous rheumatoid nodules (at pressure points)
- Pain worse in morning

Rheumatoid arthritis is a systemic disease that frequently affects the small joints of the hands and feet. It is characterized by a nonsuppurative (no neutrophils) proliferative synovitis. Rheumatoid arthritis is associated with the formation of rheumatoid factor, autoantibodies to immunoglobulin. These antibodies, usually IgM, are directed against the Fc fragment of IgG. In the joints, the synovial membrane is thickened by granulation tissue (pannus) that is infiltrated by many inflammatory cells (lymphocytes and plasma cells, not neutrophils). Involvement of the hands and feet typically affects the proximal interphalangeal joints. Involvement of the metacarpophalangeal (MCP) joint results in the classic sign of ulnar deviation. Patients present with swollen, painful, stiff joints (the symptoms are worse in the morning). Also associated with rheumatoid arthritis is the formation of subcutaneous rheumatoid nodules, which are characterized histologically by central fibrinoid necrosis and peripheral palisading epithelial histiocytes.

POLYARTERITIS NODOSA

- Focal fibrinous necrosis of small blood vessels
- Type III hypersensitivity reaction
- More common in males

Polyarteritis nodosa (PAN) is characterized by necrotizing inflammation of medium- to small-sized arteries. This inflammation (arteritis) is focal and causes destruction of the collagen and elastin in the vessel wall. This destruction produces a small outpouching (microaneurysm), which has been described as a focal "ballooning" of the vessel (nodose means "ballooning"). Polyarteritis is one of the very few autoimmune diseases that affects males more often than females. It is a disease of young adults, but can occur at any age.

Hepatitis B virus is thought to be the cause of PAN in about one-third of the cases. Two findings support this theory. First, there is a high incidence of hepatitis B surface antigen (HBsAg) in the blood of patients with PAN. Second, circulating HBsAg-anti-HBs immune complexes are found in the serum. These immune complexes may be responsible for the histologic finding of fibrinoid necrosis of small blood vessels (a type III hypersensitivity reaction).

IMMUNODEFICIENCY DISEASES
Both B cell and T cell defects

- Severe combined immunodeficiency

B cell defects

- X-linked agammaglobulinemia of Bruton
- Common variable immunodeficiency
- Isolated deficiency of IgA

T cell defects

- DiGeorge's syndrome
- Acquired immunodeficiency syndrome

Immunodeficiency diseases result from defects in the normal maturation of lymphocytes. These diseases can affect B cells, T cells, or both B cells and T cells. The peripheral blood in patients with immune deficiencies may reveal either decreased numbers of T lymphocytes, decreased numbers of B lymphocytes, or decreased numbers of T lymphocytes and B lymphocytes. Therefore, the total lymphocyte count in the peripheral blood may or may not indicate that a deficiency is present. Normally about 60% of the lymphocytes in the peripheral blood are T lymphocytes (40% helper cells and 20% cytotoxic cells), 20% are B lymphocytes, and 20% are null cells (large granular lymphocytes). Since T lymphocytes comprise the largest number of lymphocytes in the peripheral blood, a deficiency of T lymphocytes will most likely produce a decrease in the total lymphocyte count in the peripheral blood. In contrast, since B lymphocytes are a minority of the normal population of peripheral lymphocytes, a deficiency of B lymphocytes may not decrease the peripheral lymphocyte count below normal levels.

All of the immune diseases are associated with recurrent infections. The type of infection depends on whether humoral immunity or cellular immunity is abnormal. In general, defects of cellular immunity, which primarily involve T lymphocytes, lead to recurrent infections with mycobacteria, fungi, and viruses. In contrast, defects of humoral immunity, which primarily involve B lymphocytes and the production of antibodies, lead to recurrent infections with bacteria. Patients with defects in both cellular and humoral immunity, such as patients with severe combined immunodeficiency (SCID), have problems with recurrent infections involving bacteria, mycobacteria, fungi, viruses, and some parasites.

SEVERE COMBINED IMMUNODEFICIENCY DISEASE

X-linked form

- Defect in IL-2 receptor

Autosomal recessive form (Swiss type)

- Lack of adenosine deaminase
- Prenatal diagnosis and gene therapy possible

Patients with severe combined immunodeficiency disease (SCID) have defects that involve lymphoid stem cells, and therefore both T cells (cellular immunity) and B cells (humoral immunity) are affected. Patients are at risk for infection with all types of organisms (bacteria, mycobacteria, fungi, viruses, and parasites). There are two forms of SCIDs. One form has an X-linked pattern of inheritance and is due to a defect in the IL-2 receptor. The other form (the Swiss type of SCID) has an autosomal recessive pattern of inheritance and is due to a lack of the enzyme adenosine deaminase (ADA) in red cells and leukocytes. This enzyme deficiency leads to the accumulation of adenosine triphosphate and deoxyadenosine triphosphate, both of which are toxic to lymphocytes.

X-LINKED AGAMMAGLOBULINEMIA OF BRUTON

- Defective maturation of B lymphocytes past the pre-B stage
- Absence of germinal centers and plasma cells
- Bacterial infections begin at the age of 6 months
- Therapy with immunoglobulin injections

X-linked agammaglobulinemia is one of the most common forms of primary immunodeficiency. This disease, which is found in male infants, is caused by a defect in the differentiation of pre-B cells to B cells (Fig. 16-1). This leads to markedly decreased levels of all immunoglobulins and of mature B lymphocytes (seen histologically as absence of germinal centers and plasma cells in lymph nodes). In contrast to the B cell abnormalities, T lymphocytes are normal in function and number. Therefore, patients develop recurrent pyogenic infections, but they have no problems with fungal and viral infections since cell-mediated immunity is unaffected. These infections begin in affected infants at about 6 months of age when maternal immunoglobulin levels have decreased.

COMMON VARIABLE IMMUNODEFICIENCY

- Variable clinical presentation
- Recurrent infections → especially bacteria and *Giardia lamblia*
- Hyperplastic B cell areas
- Therapy with immunoglobulin injections

As its name implies, common variable immunodeficiency is a disorder that has a variable clinical presentation. It may be congenital or acquired, sporadic or familial. The feature common to all patients with this disorder is hypogamma-globulinemia. Typical B cell areas of lymphoid tissue are hyperplastic, but plasma cells are absent because of a failure of the end-stages of B cell differentiation. Clinically patients have recurrent bacterial infections and an increased incidence of both autoimmune diseases and lymphoid malignancies.

ISOLATED DEFICIENCY OF IgA

- Most patients are asymptomatic
- May develop anti-IgA antibodies
- Risk of anaphylaxis with transfusion

Isolated deficiency of IgA is probably the most common form of immuno-deficiency. It results from a block in the terminal differentiation of B lymphocytes. Most patients are asymptomatic, but some patients may develop chronic sinopulmonary infections. Patients also have an increased incidence of autoimmune disease (Hashimoto's thyroiditis). Laboratory findings seen in patients with this disorder include decreased serum and salivary IgA levels, but levels of IgG and IgM are normal. Clinically it is important to recognize this disease because these individuals can develop anti-IgA antibodies and are at risk of developing anaphylaxis with transfusions or immunoglobulin therapy.

DiGEORGE'S SYNDROME

1. Development failure of pharyngeal pouches 3 and 4
2. Abnormal development of thymus
   - T cell defect
   - Abnormal cell-mediated immunity
3. Abnormal development of parathyroids
   - Hypocalcemia
   - Tetany
4. Typical facial appearance
   - Wide-set eyes (hypertelorism)
   - Low-set ears
5. Congenital defects of heart and great vessels

DiGeorge's syndrome is a T-cell deficiency that results from hypoplasia of the thymus. The basic defect in patients with DiGeorge's syndrome is abnormal development of the third and fourth pharyngeal pouches. Normally the thymus develops from pharyngeal pouch 3, but abnormal embryonic development of this pouch leads to hypoplasia of the thymus. The resultant T-cell defect causes defective cellular immunity and problems with recurrent viral and fungal infections. Since the inferior parathyroid glands develop from pouch 3 and the superior parathyroid glands develop from pouch 4, defective development of both of these pouches results in hypoplasia of the parathyroid glands. This causes decreased concentrations of calcium in the peripheral blood (hypocalcemia), which can lead to sustained muscle contraction (tetany).

AIDS

Pathogenesis

- Cause → HIV
- Infection of CD4+ T lymphocytes
- Inversion of CD4:CD8 ratio
- Decreased humoral and cell-mediated immunity

Clinical phases

- Acute phase → early
- Chronic phase → middle
- Crisis phase → AIDS

Acquired immune deficiency syndrome (AIDS) is an immunodeficiency disease that is caused by an RNA retrovirus called HIV (human immunodeficiency virus). HIV binds to the CD4 surface protein of helper T lymphocytes, infects these cells, and kills them. This causes decreased humoral and cell-mediated reactions. Laboratory examination reveals a characteristic decrease in the peripheral CD4:DC8 cell ratio, which is normally about 2 to 1. It is important to note that CD4 is also present on other types of cells including monocytes/macrophages (which may be reservoirs or vehicles for viral entry into the CNS), microglial cells, and endothelial cells of the brain. High-risk populations for AIDS include homosexual or bisexual men, IV drug abusers, heterosexual partners of high-risk groups, recipients of multiple blood transfusions (hemophiliacs), and infants of high-risk mothers.

The natural history and progression of HIV infection is divided into several phases. The early (acute) phase is the initial response and is characterized by viral production and infection of lymphoid tissue. About 2 to 4 weeks following infection, the majority of individuals develop a self-limited acute illness (acute seroconversion illness) that is characterized by sore throat, rash, and myalgia. This usually resolves in 2 to 3 weeks.

In the middle (chronic) phase, which lasts 7 to 10 years, there is clinical latency, but viruses are still being formed within lymphoid tissue. Patients may be asymptomatic, or they may develop persistent generalized lymphadenopathy (PGL). Patients may eventually develop fever, rash, fatigue, or other symptoms that reflect the declining function of the immune system. In the past, the combination of these symptoms was called ARC (AIDS-related complex), but that term is no longer in use.

With the final (crisis) phase, patients may develop chronic fever, fatigue, weight loss, and diarrhea. In this phase patients develop full-blown AIDS. Without therapy the mean life expectancy is then less than 3 years. AIDS is defined by a helper T cell count that is less than $200/mm^3$. Patients with full-blown AIDS develop many different diseases related to their severe immunodeficiency. Patients are at a high risk of developing opportunistic infections with many different organisms, including *Pneumocystis carinii* (pneumonia), CMV, mucor, typical and atypical mycobacteria (MAC), *Candida, cryptosporidia, coccidioides, cryptococcus* (especially CNS), Toxoplasma (especially CNS), *Giardia*, etc. Patients are also at an increased risk of developing certain types of malignancies, including Kaposi's sarcoma, and lymphoma (typically B-cell immunoblastic non-Hodgkin lymphomas).

NEOPLASIA—PART ONE: BENIGN AND MALIGNANT TUMORS

·

· · · · · · · · · · · · ·

NEOPLASIA

- Irreversible process of uncontrolled cell growth
- May produce tumor masses

Uncontrolled growth of cells produces abnormal masses of tissue commonly called tumors. Although the word "tumor" literally refers to *any* swelling (recall the 4 cardinal signs of acute inflammation), commonly the word refers to neoplastic growths only. Neoplastic tumors are composed of the neoplastic cells themselves, the surrounding connective tissue, and blood vessels. Sometimes tumors promote fibrosis of the surrounding stroma, this process being called desmoplasia.

BENIGN TUMORS VERSUS MALIGNANT TUMORS

BENIGN TUMORS	MALIGNANT TUMORS
• Slow growth	• Rapid growth
• Remain localized	• Locally invasive
• May have well-developed fibrous capsule	• Irregular growth with no capsule
• Do not metastasize	• Capable of metastasis
• Well-differentiated histologically	• Variable degrees of differentation

Tumors exhibit many different growth characteristics. They may remain localized, they may infiltrate into adjacent tissue, or they may metastasize to other parts of the body. Localized tumors are called benign tumors, while infiltrating and metastasizing tumors are called malignant tumors. Most benign tumors grow slowly, so slowly in fact that they may be surrounded by a fibrous capsule. In contrast, malignant tumors grow into surrounding tissue (infiltration) in a crablike fashion. This feature led Hippocrates to call these tumors karkinoma after *karkinos*, the Greek word for "crab." (*Cancer* is Latin for "crab.")

Metastasis is the hallmark characteristic for the diagnosis of malignancy. There are, however, a few tumors that rarely metastasize. (The main exceptions are some malignant tumors of the central nervous system and the most common types of skin malignancies.) Malignant tumors metastasize through either the vascular system or the lymphatic system.

There are many other differences between benign and malignant neoplasms, such as their histologic characteristics. In addition to their infiltrative growth pattern, malignant cells have hyperchromatic nuclei, a high nuclear to cytoplasmic ratio (due to the large nuclei), and large nucleoli. Mitoses are also present within malignant tumors. The presence of nucleoli and mitoses are not diagnostic of malignant cells, because non-neoplastic reactive and proliferating cells can have nucleoli and mitoses. Malignant tumors, however, are characterized by bizarre (atypical) mitoses (such as tripolar mitoses).

Another important basic histologic characteristic of neoplastic cells is their differentiation, which refers to the extent that the neoplastic cells resemble normal cells, both morphologically and functionally. Tumors that resemble normal cells are called well differentiated, while tumors that have very little resemblance to normal cells are called poorly differentiated (and those tumors somewhere in between are called moderately differentiated). In general, benign tumors resemble the cells of origin, while malignant tumors do not. Some malignant tumors do not resemble any cell of origin, and these tumors are said to be undifferentiated (anaplastic).

GRADE VERSUS STAGE

- Grade = histologic estimate of the degree of differentiation of a tumor
- State = clinical extent of the size and the spread of a tumor

---

Once the diagnosis of a malignancy is made, it is important to determine the prognosis for the patient. The prognosis depends not only on the type of malignancy (some tumors are more aggressive than others), but also on the grade and the stage of the tumor. The grade is determined by a pathologist who examines the tumor histologically; the stage is determined clinically.

The *grade* of a malignant tumor is based on the histologic degree of differentiation of the tumor cells. Many times the number of mitoses is a good predictor of the aggressiveness of the tumor. In contrast, the *stage* of cancers is based on the size of the primary lesion and the presence or absence of metastases. The system generally used to stage malignant tumors is the TNM classification. ("T" stands for tumor, "N" stands for lymph node metastases, and "M" stands for blood-born metastases.) Staging has proved to be of greater clinical value than grading.

DYSPLASIA

- Mild dysplasia → dysplasia involving basal one-third of epithelium
- Moderate dysplasia → dysplasia involving basal two-thirds of epithelium
- Severe dysplasia → dysplasia extending into upper one-third of epithelium
- Carcinoma in situ (CIS) → full-thickness dysplasia (no maturation)

INTRAEPITHELIAL NEOPLASIA

- Cervix → cervical intraepithelial neoplasia (CIN)
- Vulva → vulvar intraepithelial neoplasia (VIN)
- Prostate → prostatic intraepithelial neoplasia (PIN)

Many neoplastic growths are preceded by a non-neoplastic proliferation of cells within the epithelium from which they arise. These proliferations are non-neoplastic because they are potentially reversible. Something caused the cells to start proliferating in an abnormal fashion, and if this initiating stimulus is removed the cells may revert to normal (although it may not be possible to remove this stimulus). If the cells in these non-neoplastic growths have a disorganized pattern, the growth process is called dysplasia.

Dysplastic cells are abnormal histologically. Characteristics of dysplastic epithelium include disorganization of the cells, abnormal location of mitoses, and nuclei that are darker than normal (hyperchromatic). The cells themselves look dissimilar from each other as they vary in size and shape (pleomorphism). The degree of dysplasia is usually determined by the thickness of the epithelium having these abnormal changes. The degrees of dysplasia include mild dysplasia, moderate dysplasia, and severe dysplasia. This basic concept of intraepithelial neoplasia is very important to dysplastic processes involving the cervix, vulva, and prostate.

CARCINOMA IN SITU

- Nonreversible dysplastic change
- Involvement of the entire epithelial thickness
- No invasion into the underlying tissue
- No risk of metastasis

The concept of carcinoma in situ and its relationship to invasion carcinoma can be illustrated by examining breast cancer. Malignant carcinomas of the breast may be either noninvasive or invasive. Noninvasive carcinomas (carcinoma in situ) may be within the ducts (intraductal carcinoma) or within the lobules (lobular carcinoma in situ). There are several variants of intraductal carcinoma including comedocarcinoma, cribriform carcinoma, or intraductal papillary carcinoma, but they all lack infiltration into underlying tissue. Comedocarcinoma grows as a solid intraductal sheet of cells with a central area of necrosis. Cribriform carcinoma is characterized by round ductlike structures within solid intraductal sheets of epithelial cells. Intraductal papillary carcinoma has a predominant papillary pattern.

Invasive malignancies are characterized by infiltration of the stroma, which may produce a desmoplastic response within the stroma. In the breast this reaction produces a firm mass and is sometimes called a schirrous carcinoma. Infiltrating ductal carcinomas also produce yellow-white chalky streaks that are the result of deposition of elastic tissue around ducts (elastosis).

TERMINOLOGY OF TUMORS

CELL OF ORIGIN	BENIGN TUMOR	MALIGNANT TUMOR
Glandular	Adenoma	Adenocarcinoma
Fibrous tissue	Fibroma	Fibrosarcoma
Smooth muscle	Leiomyoma	Leiomyosarcoma
Skeletal muscle	Rhabdomyoma	Rhabdomyosarcoma
Adipose tissue	Lipoma	Liposarcoma
Cartilage	Chondroma	Chondrosarcoma
Bone	Osteoma	Osteosarcoma
More than one germ cell layer	Benign teratoma	Malignant teratoma

Tumors are named according to the type of neoplastic cell that is proliferating. Benign tumors are usually named by attaching the suffix "oma" to the cell of origin. "Adeno" is a prefix meaning glandular, so an adenoma is a benign glandular neoplasm. A *papilloma* refers to a benign glandular neoplasm that has papillary (fingerlike) projections and a fibrovascular core. In contrast, malignant tumors are named by adding the suffix "carcinoma" or "sarcoma" to the cell of origin depending on whether the tumor arises from epithelial structures or mesenchymal structures (see below).

MISNAMED TUMORS
Non-neoplastic lesions

- Hamartoma
- Choristoma

Malignant lesions

- Melanoma
- Hepatoma
- Seminoma
- Lymphoma
- Myeloma

Unfortunately the terminology of tumors is not as consistent or simple as it should be. Some terms are in common usage but are inappropriate and misleading. For example, the names of some malignant tumors end in "oma" and sound benign, such as melanoma (a malignant tumor derived from melanocytes), hepatoma (a malignant tumor of the liver), seminoma (a malignant testicular tumor), and lymphoma (a malignant tumor derived from lymphocytes). Some tumors have names that sound like bad-acting tumors, but they aren't; and some lesions have names that sound like neoplasms, but they aren't. For example, hamartoma is a term that is used to describe tissue in the right place, but with the wrong architecture (bronchial hamartoma). In contrast, choristoma is a term used to describe tissue in the wrong place, such as ectopic gastric epithelium in an out-pouching of the small intestines.

EXAMPLES OF BENIGN TUMORS

- Uterus → leiomyoma
- Breast → fibroadenoma
- Meninges → meningioma

A few examples can illustrate the basic concepts and features of benign neoplasms. Leiomyomas ("fibroids") are benign smooth muscle tumors that are found in the wall of the uterus. They are the most common tumor in women and are usually symptomatic. Because of their size, however, they can produce abnormal uterine bleeding, urinary frequency, abdominal pain, or infertility. Grossly these tumors are well circumscribed and on cut section have a characteristic whorled tan appearance. Histologically they are composed of interlacing bundles of smooth muscle. Mitoses are absent, and there is no invasion or metastases present.

The most common benign neoplasm of the breast is the fibroadenoma. It typically occurs in the upper outer quadrant of the breast in women between the ages of 20 and 35. These tumors originate from the terminal duct lobular unit and histologically reveal a mixture of fibrous connective tissue and ducts. Clinically fibroadenomas are rubbery, freely movable, oval nodules that usually measure 2 to 4 cm in diameter. They are estrogen-sensitive and frequently enlarge during pregnancy or during the normal monthly cycle.

Meningiomas are benign tumors of adults that arise from the meningothelial cells of the arachnoid. They are external to the brain and can be removed surgically. They are slow growing tumors, but because they may have progesterone receptors, they can exhibit rapid growth during pregnancy. Histologically these tumors may display several patterns, such as a whorled pattern that is associated with the formation of psammoma bodies.

MALIGNANT TUMORS

Arise from totipotential or multipotential cells

- Germ cell tumors
- Leukemias and lymphomas

Arise from differentiated cells

- Carcinomas
- Sarcomas

In general, malignant tumors are named and subdivided based on their cell or origin. Basically malignancies can arise from either totipotential cells or differentiated cells. Totipotential cells are cells that are capable of differentiating into other types of cells. The basic type of malignant tumors that arise from these types of cells are called germ cell tumors. These tumors are further divided into different types based on their differentiation.

GERM CELL TUMORS

Minimal differentation

- Seminoma (testis)
- Dysgerminoma (ovary)
- Germinoma (pineal)

Ectodermal differentiation

- Embryonal carcinoma (testis)

Endodermal differentiation

- Yolk sac carcinoma (testis and ovary)

Multiple embryonic layer differentiation

- Teratoma (testis and ovary)

Trophoblastic differentiation

- Choriocarcinoma

Seminomas are germ cell tumors of the testis that have minimal differentiation from the totipotential germ cells. They are the most common germ cell tumor (about one-third of testicular neoplasms). Grossly they grow as large, gray-white, lobulated fleshy masses. Microscopically seminomas are composed of a uniform population of large polygonal cells that have distinct cell membranes and clear cytoplasm. Their nucleus is centrally located, hyperchromatic, and has one or two prominent nucleoli. Mitotic figures are infrequent, and there is usually a prominent lymphocytic infiltrate. About 10% of the tumors have syncytial giant cells that contain or secrete human chorionic gonadotropin (HCG). The tumors are extremely radiosensitive (important), metastasize late in the course of the disease, and have a relatively good prognosis. Seminomas can occur in sites outside of the testes, such as the retroperitoneum, mediastinum, ovary (dysgerminoma), and pineal (germinoma). An important, distinct variant of seminoma is the spermatocytic seminoma. It is characterized by two unique features: It is found in older individuals and it does not metastasize. Histologically, a spermatocytic seminoma has maturation of the tumor cells, some of which histologically resemble secondary spermatocytes.

Embryonal carcinomas are generally more aggressive than seminomas. Grossly they are gray-white masses with areas of hemorrhage and necrosis. Histologically these tumors are poorly differentiated malignancies and have varying histologic patterns including glandular and tubular formation. Giant cells may be present and may produce HCG, alpha fetoprotein (AFP), or both.

Yolk sac tumors are rare tumors in adults, but are the most common tumor of the testes in children under the age of three. Other names for a yolk sac tumor include infantile embryonal carcinoma and endodermal sinus tumor. The histology of these malignancies is quite varied and occasionally they are found admixed with embryonal carcinoma in adults. Sometimes endodermal sinuses are seen within these tumors. These are structures that appear to be somewhat like glomerular structures with a central blood vessel. They are characteristic of yolk sac tumors and are called Schiller-Duval bodies. The tumor cells of yolk sac tumors characteristically produce alpha-fetoprotein (AFP).

Teratomas are tumors that are derived from all three embryonic germ layers (endoderm, ectoderm, and mesoderm). Teratomas may be benign or malignant. Benign teratomas are composed of mature elements and are rare in the testis. In contrast, malignant teratomas are characterized histologically by immature neural elements or undifferentiated mesenchymal cells. It is important to realize that the biological behavior of teratomas in males is quite different from that in females. In females, most teratomas are benign, mature, and cystic (dermoid cysts). In contrast, all teratomas in adult males should be considered malignant (even if immature elements are not found), while in children under the age of 12 years, they act in a benign fashion.

Choriocarcinomas are highly malignant tumors that metastasize early via the bloodstream. Grossly, a tumor with a necrotic, hemorrhagic appearance is characteristic. Two malignant components are seen histologically: cytotrophoblasts (masses of cuboidal cells) and syncytiotrophoblasts (sheets of syncytial epithelium with abundant cytoplasm). The syncytiotrophoblasts form and secrete HCG. Very high serum levels of HCG are characteristic of these tumors.

Elevated serum levels of many different substances can be useful in the diagnosis of germ cell tumors. To summarize briefly, markedly elevated levels of HCG are associated with choriocarcinoma, while elevated levels of AFP are most characteristic of yolk sac tumors and embryonal carcinoma. But there are many overlaps between tumors, and many tumors are composed of multiple types of germ cell malignancies. The only definitive statement that can be made is that elevated serum levels of AFP are not seen in a tumor that is a pure seminoma.

LEUKEMIA

Acute leukemia

- Acute lymphocytic leukemia (ALL)
- Acute myelocytic leukemia (AML)

Chronic leukemia

- Chronic lymphocytic leukemia (CLL)
- Chronic myelocytic leukemia (CML)

The leukemias are malignancies of white blood cells that are characterized by monoclonal proliferations of malignant cells in the bone marrow and the peripheral blood. The leukemias are subdivided into those with symptoms that develop rapidly, the acute leukemias, and those in which the symptoms develop more slowly, the chronic leukemias. Each of these two groups can be further divided into types that arise from lymphoid cells or nonlymphoid cells, the latter being myeloid cells. This produces two types of acute leukemias, namely, acute lymphocytic leukemia (ALL) and acute myelocytic leukemia (AML); and two types of chronic leukemias, namely, chronic lymphocytic leukemia (CLL) and chronic myelocytic leukemia (CML).

The acute leukemias result from neoplastic proliferations of immature cells called blasts. We say that these blasts look immature because their nuclei characteristically have nucleoli. These immature cells proliferate in the bone marrow and may spill over into the peripheral blood (leukemia). Although blasts are typically found in the peripheral blood of patients with acute leukemia, this is not always the case. Cases of acute leukemia where the blasts are not found in the peripheral blood are called aleukemic leukemia. The only way to diagnose acute leukemia definitively is to find numerous blasts within the bone marrow. By convention, the diagnosis of acute leukemia is made when the amount of blasts within the marrow is more than 30%.

The proliferating blasts may be either lymphoblasts (found in patients with ALL) or myeloblasts (found in patients with AML). Clinically it is not enough just to make the diagnosis of acute leukemia. We must further distinguish between ALL and AML, because the chemotherapy for each of these types of acute leukemia is different. Additionally there are important clinical and prognostic differences between these two types of acute leukemia. For example, ALL is more often associated with leukemic infiltration of the CNS. Since chemotherapeutic drugs don't penetrate the blood-brain barrier well, patients with ALL (but not AML) may be given prophylactic radiation to the head.

ACUTE LYMPHOCYTIC LEUKEMIA

FAB classification

- L1 → small, homogeneous blasts
- L2 → large, pleomorphic blasts with nuclear clefts
- L3 → cytoplasmic vacuoles

Immunologic classification

1. T cell lineage
2. B cell lineage
   - Mature B ALL
   - Pre-B ALL
   - Early pre-B ALL

In the past ALL was divided by the French-American-British classification (FAB classification) into three types: L1, L2, and L3. This classification was based upon the appearance of the lymphoblasts. L1 blasts, the most common subtype overall and the most common type in children, are small lymphoblasts that all look alike, that is, they are homogenous. L2 blasts, found more commonly in adults, are larger and have irregular nuclear borders. Finally, L3 blasts are characterized by cytoplasmic vacuoles that stain positively for lipid (oil red O stain).

An important concept to understand about the neoplastic hematologic disorders is that many times the same malignant cell can be found in either the peripheral blood (leukemia) or the lymph nodes (lymphoma). In fact, several of these neoplastic hematologic disorders characteristically have malignant cells in the peripheral blood and lymph nodes at the same time. To illustrate this idea, consider the following. If L3 blasts are found within the bone marrow and the peripheral blood, the diagnosis is L3-ALL. In contrast, if the same cells are found outside of the blood, such as within lymph nodes, the diagnosis is Burkitt's lymphoma.

The FAB classification of ALL was relatively simple, but unfortunately, it had little clinical correlation. Now, we further classify ALL based upon immunologic characteristics of the lymphoblasts (Fig. 19-1). This separates ALL into three types: T-cell ALL, B-cell precursor ALL, and B-cell ALL. The first two characteristically have positive nuclear staining for the enzyme terminal deoxytransferase (TdT), while the latter B-cell ALL is negative. It is important to realize that TdT is an enzyme marker for immature cells. Therefore, T-cell ALL and B-cell precursor ALL are forms of "immature" ALL, while B-cell ALL, in which the cells do not stain for TdT, is considered to be a "mature" form of ALL.

T-cell ALL is most often found in young male patients who present with a mediastinal mass. Think "T" for T-cell ALL and "T" for thymus, which is located within the mediastinum. In fact, many patients with T-ALL have malignant cells within their lymph nodes. If the disease predominantly affects the lymph node, it is called T-cell lymphoplastic lymphoma.

B-cell precursor ALL is further divided into three types: null cell, common, and pre-B types. Common B-cell precursor ALL is characterized by positive staining for the cell surface marker CD10. This particular marker is also called CALLA. The "C" in CALLA in fact stands for "common," as in the name "common" B-cell precursor ALL. Pre-B precursor ALL is characterized simply enough by the presence of cytoplasmic μ heavy chain. Recall that these same cells, pre-B cells with cytoplasmic μ heavy chains, accumulate in patients with Bruton agammaglobulinemia.

Finally, B-cell ALL is mature ALL and is characterized by the presence of surface immunoglobulin (sIg). In fact, B-cell ALL is identical to the L3 type of ALL, which is the leukemic form of Burkitt's lymphoma.

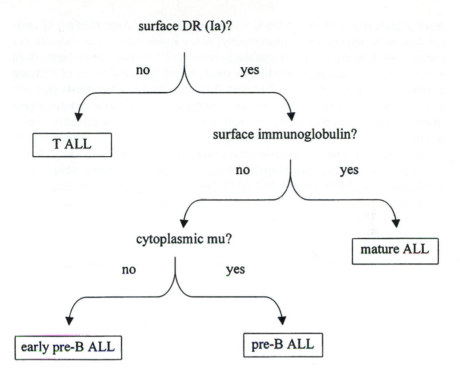

Figure 19-1 Immunologic Classification of ALL

FAB CLASSIFICATION OF ACUTE MYELOCYTIC LEUKEMIA

- M0 = undifferentiated leukemia
- M1 = myeloblastic leukemia without maturation
- M2 = myeloblastic leukemia with maturation
- M3 = hypergranular promyelocytic leukemia
- M4 = myelomonocytic leukemia
- M5 = monocytic leukemia
- M6 = erythroleukemia (di Guglielmo's disease)
- M7 = acute megakaryocytic leukemia

In contrast to ALL, AML is characterized by the proliferation of myelo-blasts. These immature cells may contain intracytoplasmic rod-shaped structures called Auer rods. These structures are abnormal aggregates of lysosomes (primary granules) and are never found within lymphoblasts. Auer rods are of critical diagnostic importance. Unfortunately, many times these Auer rods are not present and then there is no morphologic way to differentiate myeloblasts from lymphoblasts. Instead, special stains are used. Recall that some forms of ALL are characterized by the presence of nuclear TdT. In contrast, myeloblasts lack this enzyme and instead are characterized by the presence of cytoplasmic myeloperoxidase. This is an enzyme that is normally found within primary granules of neutrophils. A stain for myeloperoxidase is the myeloperoxidase stain (makes sense). Another stain for AML is the sudan black stain, which stains lipids.

Unfortunately, the FAB classifies AML into eight (!) different subdivisions, these being called M0 through M7 AML. Rather than learn each of these eight types, make a quick mental note of the fact that M5 AML is associated with monoblasts, M6 AML with erythroblasts, and M7 AML with megakaryoblasts. However, from a conceptual standpoint, it is worthwhile to understand in depth one particular type of AML, namely, M3 AML. This type of acute leukemia is the result of a neoplastic proliferation of promyelocytes, and is therefore also called acute promyelocytic leukemia.

There are two rather important facts to be aware of concerning acute promyelocytic leukemia. First, this type of leukemia is associated with a characteristic chromosomal translocation: t(15;17). This translocation involves the PML (promyelocytic) unit on chromosome 15 and the retinoic acid receptor α (RAR-α) on chromosome 17. One of the functions of vitamin A (associated with retinoic acid) concerns the maturation of epithelial structures. M3 AML, associated with an abnormal retinoic acid receptor, is essentially the result of defective maturation of myeloid cells, which are stopped in their maturation at the promyelocyte stage. In fact, therapy with all-*trans*-retinoic acid enables these neoplastic promyelocytes to mature to neutrophils. The other important clinical fact associated with M3 AML relates to the fact that normal promyelocytes have numerous cytoplasmic granules. In fact, these neoplastic promyelocytes have numerous granules and numerous intracytoplasmic Auer rods. These granules contain thromboplastic substances that can activate the coagulation cascade. Therefore M3 AML is associated with the formation of disseminated intravascular coagulation (DIC), especially if chemotherapy kills and ruptures the leukemic cells.

CHRONIC LYMPHOCYTIC LEUKEMIA

- Peripheral lymphocytosis with smudge cells
- Similar to small lymphocytic lymphoma
- Indolent clinically
- Most cases arise from B lymphocytes

Like the acute leukemias, the chronic leukemias can originate from lymphocytes or myelocytes. Therefore the two main types of chronic leukemias are chronic lymphocytic leukemia (CLL) and chronic myelocytic leukemia (CML). CLL is the most indolent of all the leukemias and typically occurs in older individuals. (The mean age at the time of diagnosis is 60.) The neoplastic lymphocytes, found within the bone marrow and in the peripheral blood, are small, mature-appearing lymphocytes. Because they are neoplastic and fragile, they characteristically rupture when peripheral blood is smeared into a glass slide. This produces many smudge cells ("parachute cells") in peripheral blood smears, which are characteristic of CLL. The neoplastic lymphocytes of CLL are very similar to the neoplastic lymphocytes of small lymphocytic lymphoma (SLL). If the neoplastic lymphocytes primarily involve the blood and bone marrow, the diagnosis is CLL. In contrast, if the same neoplastic cells primarily involve the lymph nodes, the diagnosis is SLL.

The neoplastic cells of CLL may originate from either B lymphocytes or T lymphocytes. Therefore, there are two immunophenotypic types of CLL, namely B-cell CLL and T-cell CLL. More than 95% of the cases of CLL are B-cell CLL. These cells are characterized by the presence of B-cell markers, such as surface immunoglobulin (either IgM or IgD), and CD markers specific for B cells, namely CD19, 20, and 21. Importantly and paradoxically, B-cell CLL is associated with one particular T-cell marker: CD5. This marker is thought to be responsible in some way for the high incidence of autoimmune hemolytic anemia (AIHA) in patients with CLL.

CHRONIC MYELOCYTIC LEUKEMIA

- Peripheral leukocytosis
- Myeloproliferative syndrome
- Associated with Philadelphia chromosome
- Decreased LAP
- Progressive disease

Chronic myelocytic leukemia (CML) is characterized by the neoplastic proliferation of relatively mature myeloid cells. The bone marrow of these patients is hypercellular because of a proliferation of all cell lines. In the peripheral blood, there is a marked increase in the number of neutrophils, bands, and metamyelocytes. The differential diagnosis of this peripheral blood leukocytosis includes a reactive, non-neoplastic proliferation of neutrophils, such as with an infection. Reactive, non-neoplastic, markedly increased numbers of leukocytes in the peripheral blood are called leukemoid reactions. In this type of reaction the enzymes within the granules of neutrophils, such as alkaline phosphatase, are increased. This increases the leukocyte alkaline phosphatase (LAP) score. In contrast, the neoplastic cells in patients with CML are abnormal, and these neutrophil enzymes are decreased. This results in a decreased LAP.

The other diagnostic finding in patients with CML is the presence of a characteristic chromosomal translocation: t(9;22). In this translocation, called the Philadelphia chromosome, the oncogene *c-abl* on chromosome 9 is translocated to the breakpoint cluster region (bcr) on chromosome 22. This forms a new gene that produces a new protein called P210. This enzyme has potent tyrosine kinase activity, which is thought to produce the abnormal cell growth of CML.

Although CML is classified as a chronic leukemia, most cases progress within five years to an accelerated phase that terminates as a blast crisis. This latter disease is characterized by a proliferation of blast cells which, unlike the acute leukemias, is generally unresponsive to chemotherapy. Interestingly, these blasts may be either myeloblasts or lymphoblasts. How can chronic myeloid leukemia terminate in a lymphoid blast crisis? The key to understanding this is to realize that CML is a clonal proliferation of pluripotential stem cells. Pluripotential means that these neoplastic cells have the potential to differentiate into other types of cells, such as lymphoblasts.

NON-HODGKIN'S LYMPHOMA

Nodular (follicular) lymphomas

- Older age group
- Present with widespread disease
- Better prognosis
- Less responsive to chemotherapy
- Arise from B lymphocytes

Diffuse lymphomas

- Younger age group (with exceptions)
- Present with localized disease
- Worse prognosis
- More responsive to chemotherapy
- Arise from either B lymphocytes or T lymphocytes

Generally speaking, the non-Hodgkin's lymphomas (NHL) can be divided histologically into nodular forms and diffuse forms. The nodular NHL are characterized by occurring in an older age group, presenting more often with widespread disease (higher stage), having a better prognosis, and responding less often to chemotherapy. All nodular NHL result from neoplastic proliferations of B lymphocytes. Histologically these nodules can resemble the germinal centers of lymphoid follicles, but features that are associated with neoplastic nodules include an increased number (crowding) of nodules of uniform size that are located in both the cortex and the medulla. These nodules are composed of a monotonous proliferation of cells.

WORKING FORMULATION OF NON-HODGKIN'S LYMPHOMAS

Low-grade lymphomas

- Small lymphocytic lymphoma (SLL)
- Follicular small cleaved cell lymphoma
- Follicular mixed small and large cell lymphoma

Intermediate-grade lymphomas

- Follicular large cell lymphoma
- Diffuse small cleaved cell lymphoma
- Diffuse mixed small cleaved and large cell lymphoma
- Diffuse large cell lymphoma

High-grade lymphomas

- Immunoblastic lymphoma
- Lymphoblastic lymphoma
- Small noncleaved cell lymphoma

The Working Formulation divides the non-Hodgkin's lymphomas into low grade, intermediate grade, and high grade lymphomas based on their prognosis. The low grade NHL include small lymphocytic lymphoma (SLL), follicular small cleaved NHL, and follicular mixed small cleaved and large cell NHL. The intermediate grade NHL include follicular large cell NHL, diffuse small cleaved NHL, diffuse mixed small cleaved and large cell NHL, and diffuse large cell NHL. The high grade NHL include immunoblastic lymphoma, lymphoblastic lymphoma, and small noncleaved NHL (Burkitt's lymphoma).

Rather than look at each of these subtypes in depth, a few important basics are worth mentioning. First, small lymphocytic lymphoma is clinically and histologically similar to CLL and has the best prognosis of any of the non-Hodgkin's lymphomas. Analogously, lymphoblastic lymphoma is similar clinically to T-cell ALL. Patients may have a mediastinal mass, because most lymphoblastic lymphomas are of T-cell origin and may involve the thymus. Histologically, lymphoblastic lymphoma is characterized by immature lymphocytes (lymphoblasts) with convoluted "chicken footprint" nuclei.

Finally, an important subtype of small noncleaved cell lymphoma is Burkitt's lymphoma. This type of lymphoma is common in Africa and typically involve the maxilla or mandible of children. In contrast, the American type of small noncleaved NHL commonly involve the abdomen (bowel, ovaries, or retroperitoneum). Histologically, Burkitt's lymphoma is characterized by a diffuse proliferation of small, noncleaved lymphocytes. A "starry-sky" appearance is typically present. This "starry-sky" appearance, which can be seen with any high-grade lymphoma, is due to macrophages phagocytizing the debris of rapidly proliferating malignant cells. (The "stars" are the macrophages, while the "sky" is the malignant cells.)

HODGKIN'S DISEASE

1. Malignant cell is Reed-Sternberg cell
2. Subtypes
   - Lymphocyte predominant HD
   - Mixed cellularity HD
   - Lymphocyte depleted HD
   - Nodular sclerosis HD

Hodgkin's disease (HD) is characterized by the proliferation of malignant Reed-Sternberg (RS) cells within the appropriate inflammation background. Hodgkin's lymphoma is separated from the NHL because of distinct clinical features. The clinical presentation of patients with HD frequently simulates an infectious process. In fact a significant amount of the tumor tissue consists of inflammatory cells. This immune response, rather than the neoplastic Reed-Sternberg cells, provides the basis for the classification of HD into four subtypes (quite different from the non-Hodgkin's lymphomas).

The diagnosis of HD is made by histologic examination of an involved lymph node. The largest lymph node of a group of enlarged nodes should be examined, because smaller lymph nodes may reveal only reactive changes and lack diagnostic features of Hodgkin's disease. The sine qua non for the histologic diagnosis of Hodgkin's disease is the Reed-Sternberg cell (RS cell). The RS cell usually has two mirror-image nuclei, each containing a large ("inclusion-like") acidophilic nucleolus surrounded by a clear area ("owl-eyed" appearance). There are several variants of RS cells, including mononuclear cells, L-H ("popcorn") cells, lacunar cells, and pleomorphic cells.

HD is subdivided into different types based on the number of RS cells and the type of inflammatory response that is present. Additionally, RS variants may be found within specific subtypes. In lymphocyte-predominant HD, there are numerous lymphocytes, but very few RS cells. The lymphocytic and histiocytic RS variant (L and H cell or popcorn cell) may be found in this type. The lymphocyte-depleted type of HD has few lymphocytes and numerous RS cells, many of which are pleomorphic in appearance (pleomorphic variants). In nodular sclerosis HD, varying numbers of RS cells may be found, but the presence of atypical cells surrounded by large, clear spaces (lacunar cells) is characteristic. The mixed cellularity type of HD has no specific RS variant, but numerous eosinophils and plasma cells are seen.

CARCINOMAS AND SARCOMAS

Carcinomas

- Arise from epithelial cells
- Lymphatic spread

Sarcomas

- Arise from mesenchymal tissue
- Hematogenous spread

Malignant tumors are named and subdivided based on their cell or origin, that is, either totipotential cells or differentiated cells. Malignant tumors that are derived from differential cells are divided into two general categories: carcinomas and sarcomas. Carcinomas are malignant tumors that arise from epithelial cells; sarcomas are malignant tumors that arise from mesenchymal tissue. There are several basic differences between these two types of malignancies. Carcinomas more commonly metastasize through lymphatic spread, which usually follows the natural lymphatic drainage. For example, breast carcinomas of the upper outer quadrant (the most common location) spread first to axillary lymph nodes. Carcinomas of the inner quadrant spread via the lymphatics along the internal mammary arteries. Carcinomas of the lung metastasize first to the peribronchial and hilar lymph nodes and then to the mediastinal lymph nodes. In contrast to the lymphatic spread of carcinomas, sarcomas more commonly metastasize through the blood vessels (hematogenous spread), but this is not a hard and fast rule. The liver and the lungs are the most common site for hematogenous spread (since the liver drains all portal blood, and the lungs drain all of the caval blood).

CARCINOMAS
Squamous cell carcinoma

- Skin cancer
- Lung cancer
- Esophageal cancer
- Cervical cancer

Adenocarcinoma

- Lung cancer
- Colon cancer
- Stomach cancer
- Prostate cancer
- Endometrial cancer

Transitional cell carcinoma

- Bladder cancer
- Renal cancer (pelvis)

Clear cell carcinoma

- Renal cancer (cortex)
- Vaginal cancer

Carcinomas are further classified according to their growth patterns and histologic characteristics. For example, adenocarcinomas form glandular structures, while squamous cell carcinomas form keratin. Furthermore, the growth pattern of carcinomas generally relates to their epithelial cell or tissue of origin. That is, tissue that forms glandular structures forms adenocarcinomas; tissue that has stratified squamous epithelium forms squamous cell carcinoma; and tissue that has transitional epithelium forms transitional cell carcinoma. A few specific examples will illustrate this concept.

CARCINOMAS OF THE LUNG

Small cells

- Small cell carcinoma

Nonsmall cells

- Squamous cell carcinoma
- Adenocarcinoma
- Bronchioloalveolar carcinoma
- Large cell carcinoma

Lung cancers are classified according to their histologic appearance. First they are divided into two groups based on the size of the tumor cells, namely, small cell carcinomas and nonsmall cell carcinomas. Small cell carcinomas (sometimes called "oat cell" carcinoma) have scant amounts of cytoplasm, and their nuclei are small, round, and rarely have nucleoli.

The nonsmall cell carcinomas are classified according to the differentiation of the tumor cells. Squamous cell carcinomas are characterized by keratin pearl formation, intracytoplasmic keratin, or the formation of intercellular bridges. Adenocarcinomas are characterized by the formation of glandular structures. They typically are found at the periphery of the lung (peripheral carcinomas) and sometimes may be found in an area of previous scar (scar carcinoma). Nonsmall cell carcinomas of the lung that do not form glands or have squamous differentiation are called undifferentiated large cell carcinomas.

One particular type of bronchogenic carcinoma (considered by some to be a form of adenocarcinoma) is bronchioloalveolar carcinoma (BAC). This tumor is characterized by well-differentiated, mucus-secreting, columnar epithelial cells that infiltrate along the alveolar walls and spread from alveolus to alveolus through the pores of Kohn. This pneumonic spread can be mistaken for pneumonia with a chest X-ray.

HORNER'S SYNDROME

- Ptosis (drooping of eyelid)
- Miosis (constriction of pupil)
- Anhidrosis (absence of sweating)

Localized manifestation of lung cancers of the upper lobes include pain in the arm in the distribution of the ulnar nerve (Pancoast tumor) or Horner's syndrome. Horner's syndrome results from interruption of the oculosympathetic pathway. Hypothalamic fibers project to the lateral horn of the spinal cord at T1 (these fibers are the hypothalamospinal tract). From there preganglionic sympathetic fibers travel to the superior cervical ganglion and pass by the apex of the lung. At this location lung cancers of the apex of the lung may disrupt this oculosympathetic path. Symptoms result from sites that are normally supplied by the superior cervical ganglion. These include the sweat glands of the face (anhidrosis), the dilation of the pupil via the long ciliary nerve (pupil constriction), and the Müller muscle of the eyelid (ptosis of the upper lid). Therefore, the symptoms of Horner's syndrome are ipsilateral ptosis, miosis, and anhidrosis.

CARCINOMAS OF THE GI TRACT

Esophagus

- Squamous cell carcinoma
- Adenocarcinoma

Stomach

- Adenocarcinoma
- Signet ring cell carcinoma

Small intestine

- Adenocarcinoma
- Carcinoid
- Lymphoma

Colon

- Adenocarcinoma

Most malignant tumors of the esophagus are squamous cell carcinomas (because the normal histology of the esophageal mucosa is stratified squamous epithelium). These tumors, which are usually moderately differentiated tumors having prominent keratin formation, are usually found in the middle third of the esophagus. Predisposing factors to the development of esophageal squamous cell carcinomas include alcohol consumption, tobacco (smoking or chewing), dietary factors (nitrosamines), and *achalasia* (abnormal dilation of the esophagus). The remainder of the malignancies of the esophagus are adenocarcinomas. These adenocarcinomas are typically found in the lower third of the esophagus, and like esophageal squamous carcinomas are associated with smoking and alcohol consumption. In contrast, however, is the important fact that esophageal adenocarcinomas are associated with chronic gastroesophageal reflux, which produces Barrett's esophagus.

The most common type of malignancy of the stomach is an adenocarcinoma. There are basically two types of gastric adenocarcinomas (disregarding adenocarcinomas found at the GE junction, which are generally associated with Barrett's mucosa): the intestinal type and the diffuse type. The intestinal type, which is decreasing in frequency in the United States, is thought to arise from gastric mucous cells that have undergone intestinal metaplasia. Histologically this type of malignant tumor consists of infiltrating groups of intestinal-type glands that are similar to colon adenocarcinomas. In contrast, the diffuse type of gastric carcinoma (the frequency of which is not changing of late in the United States) is thought to arise from native gastric mucous cells and histologically does not form glands. Instead these tumor cells infiltrate as individual mucin-secreting malignant cells (signet-ring cells). (One trivial fact: Krukenberg tumor refers to gastric signet ring carcinoma that has metastasized to the ovaries.)

Tumors of the small intestine are much rarer when compared to tumors at other sites of the gastrointestinal tract. The two most frequent malignant tumors of the small intestine are adenocarcinomas and carcinoids. Adenocarcinomas of the small intestine are similar grossly and microscopically to adenocarcinomas of the colon. They occur most often in the duodenum at the ampulla of Vater.

Carcinoid tumors arise from cells of the neuroendocrine system which, as part of the APUD (amine precursor uptake and decarboxylation) system, are capable of secreting many products. Grossly carcinoid tumors tend to be multiple when they occur in the intestines and characteristically have a yellow-tan color on sectioning. Histologically they are composed of nests of relatively bland-appearing monotonous cells. Carcinoid tumors are capable of secreting many products such as serotonin, gastrin, or ACTH. Serotonin, the most common product of carcinoid tumors, produces the carcinoid syndrome, which is characterized clinically by the combination of diarrhea, episodic flushing, bronchospasm, and skin lesions. Secretion of gastrin produces the Zollinger-Ellison syndrome, which is characterized clinically by recurrent duodenal peptic ulcers. Secretion of ACTH clinically produces Cushing's syndrome. Two important immunoperoxidase stains for the diagnosis of carcinoid tumors are the neuron-specific enolase (NSE) stain and the chromogranin stain. Electron microscopy reveals membrane-bound, dense-core neurosecretory granules in the cytoplasm of the tumor cells. It is important to realize that with carcinoid tumors (like almost all endocrine tumors) the only reliable criteria for the diagnosis of malignancy is the presence of metastasis (not histologic criteria like mitoses, necrosis, or vascular invasion). The risk of malignancy for carcinoid tumors varies with the location of the primary tumor and is as follows: appendix (less than 1%), ileum (60%), rectum (15%), colon (questionable high %), and stomach (questionable high %).

Colon cancer is a frequent type of cancer in adults of the United States. It may be found in the left side of the colon ("napkin ring" or "apple core" gross appearance) or the right side of the colon (polypoid mass). In either location, bleeding may produce an iron deficiency anemia. Histologically the vast majority of colon cancers are adenocarcinomas.

CARCINOMAS OF THE URINARY TRACT

Kidney

- Clear cell carcinoma
- Transitional cell carcinoma
- Wilms' tumor

Urinary bladder

- Transitional carcinoma
- Squamous cell carcinoma

Grossly renal carcinomas are greater than 3 cm in diameter and are yellow in color. This color is similar to tumors of the adrenal cortex, and thus another name for renal cell carcinoma is hypernephroma. Microscopically the majority of lesions are composed of fairly uniform cells with clear cytoplasm that stains positively for glycogen and lipid (an important diagnostic feature). These tumors arise from the renal epithelial cells and thus may be classified as adenocarcinomas, but tubular formation, not glandular formation may be present. Clinically these tumors can produce the combination of costovertebral pain, a palpable mass, and hematuria. This classic triad of symptoms, however, is only seen in a minority of patients.

Carcinomas originating in the renal pelvis (not the cortex) originate from transitional epithelial cells and microscopically are similar to tumors arising in the urinary bladder (transitional cell carcinomas). Malignant tumors of the kidney in children are called nephroblastomas (Wilms' tumor) and histologically reveal a combination of metanephric blastema, undifferentiated mesenchymal cells, and immature tubule or glomerular formation.

Malignant neoplasms of the bladder may be transitional cell carcinomas (and most common type), squamous cell carcinomas (which produce keratin), or adenocarcinomas (which form glandular structures). Transitional cell carcinomas (TCCs) may be either papillary or flat lesions. Papillary TCCs, which are the most common type of bladder cancer, may be either invasive or noninvasive.

Noninvasive papillary TCCs are not referred to as being in situ, as that term implies a noninvasive, nonpapillary lesion. Nonpapillary (flat) TCCs may also be invasive (into the lamina propria or muscularis) or noninvasive (in situ). Factors associated with the development of transitional cell carcinomas include industrial exposure to betanaphthylamine, cigarette smoking, and the long-term use of phenacetin.

Squamous cell carcinomas of the urinary bladder are quite rare except in Egypt and other areas of the Middle East where they are associated with infections with schistosomiasis. Similarly, adenocarcinomas of the urinary bladder are quite rare, except when they are associated with either urachal epithelial remnants located in the dome of the bladder, glandular metaplasia, or cystitis glandularis.

SARCOMAS

- Fibroblasts → fibrosarcoma
- Blood vessels → angiosarcoma
- Cartilage → chondrosarcoma
- Bone → osteogenic sarcoma and Ewing's sarcoma

Primary malignancies arising in or around bone include osteosarcomas (osteogenic sarcomas), chondosarcomas, and Ewing's sarcoma. Osteosarcomas are highly malignant tumors of bone. They are characterized histologically by the presence of anaplastic tumor cells that produce osteoid. Patients are usually young males between the ages of 10 and 20 who present with pain and swelling. X-rays reveal bone destruction with characteristic subperiosteal elevation that forms a triangular shadow between the bone cortex and the raised periosteum (Codman's triangle). Osteosarcomas in younger patients are associated with mutations of the retinoblastoma (Rb) gene. In older patients there is an association of osteogenic sarcomas with Paget's disease of bone and radiation exposure.

Ewing's sarcoma is an uncommon malignant bone tumor that primarily affects patients younger than 20 years of age. This tumor is usually located in the diaphysis or metaphysis of the long bones (not the epiphysis). Histologically the tumor is composed of small, uniform, round cells that are similar in appearance to lymphocytes. To differentiate this lesion from lymphoma and neuroblastoma, PAS staining of glycogen-positive, diastase-sensitive cytoplasmic granules within the tumor cells of Ewing's sarcoma is characteristic. Also useful in differentiation from neuroblastoma is the fact that Ewing's sarcoma is associated with the chromosomal translocation t(11;22).

NEOPLASIA—PART TWO: CARCINOGENESIS

·

- Carcinogenesis
- Oncogenes
- Retroviruses
- Chromosomes and Cancer
- Neuroblastoma
- Multistep Theory of Colon Cancer
- Colon Polyps
- Chemical Carcinogens
- Cancer of the Endometrium
- Cancer of the Breast
- Radiation

- Cancer of the Skin
- Viruses
- Cancer of the Liver
- Chromosome Instability Syndromes
- Cancer Incidence
- Geography
- Paraneoplastic Syndromes
- Multiple Endocrine Neoplasia
- Pheochromocytoma
- Tumor Markers

· · · · · · · · · · · ·

CARCINOGENESIS

Neoplastic proliferations

- Result from damage to the DNA of a cell
- Clonal proliferation

Non-neoplastic proliferations

- Polyclonal proliferations

Neoplasia results from the proliferation of a group of cells that all originate from a single cell. This point is basic and quite important. All neoplasms are monoclonal proliferations of cells (in contrast to non-neoplastic proliferations of cells that originate from many different cells, called polyclonal proliferation). The monoclonal proliferation of neoplastic cells was first described in women who are heterozygous for certain polymorphic X-linked markers, such as the enzyme glucose-6-phosphate dehydrogenase (G6PD). (Polymorphic means that at one locus there are several forms of a particular gene that produce different forms of the same enzyme, called isoenzymes.) Females have two X chromosomes in each cell, but one of these chromosomes is randomly inactivated in each cell early during embryogenesis. If a female inherited two different genes that code for two different G6PD isoenzymes (each gene on one of the X chromosomes), then the random inactivation of X chromosomes would result in a mixture of cells with these two different enzymes (called mosaicism). This is exactly the case if you examine the smooth muscle cells that form the wall of the uterus. If a woman had two different genes coding for G6PD (say, gene A and gene B), her uterus would reveal a mixture of smooth muscle cells, some with gene A and some with gene B. Now suppose a tumor originated from these smooth muscle of her uterus. If this tumor (a leiomyoma) was a polyclonal proliferation of cells, it would contain a mixture of cells, some with gene A and some with gene B, just like the normal smooth muscle wall. What happens instead is that all of the cells are the same and contain either gene A or gene B. There is no mixture of cell types. This indicates that neoplasms are monoclonal proliferations of cells.

ONCOGENES

- p-onc → genes that code for normal growth and differentiation proteins
- c-onc → genes that code for proteins associated with the development of cancer (oncogenes)
- v-onc → an oncogene that is present within a virus

How does DNA damage actually result in tumor cell proliferation? One way is by interfering with the genes that are associated with normal growth and differentiation, such as growth-promoting genes, growth-inhibiting genes, and apoptosis-controlling genes. Proto-oncogenes (p-oncs) are cellular genes that promote normal growth and differentiation, while oncogenes are genes that cause cancer. The products of these proto-oncogenes are many different proteins that have many different functions. We explored these functions in depth in the chapter dealing with cell growth. A normal cellular proto-oncogene may function as an abnormal cellular oncogene (c-onc gene) if it produces more of its protein product than it should.

RETROVIRUSES

Acute transforming viruses

• Transduction → contain viral oncogene (v-onc)
• Form tumors rapidly

Slow transforming viruses

• Do not contain viral oncogene
• Form tumors slowly → insertional mutagenesis

Why do these normally functioning genes start functioning abnormally? This can happen as the result of several mechanisms, such as mutations of genes, translocations of genes, amplification of genes, or interaction of genes with viruses. Increased production of protein by oncogenes can be the result of increased transcription of these genes. This can be the result when certain viral genes are inserted into the DNA of cells. This process is associated with a specific type of RNA virus that is called a retrovirus (Fig. 20-1). These viruses are capable of making DNA from RNA because they have the enzyme reverse transcriptase. Retroviruses have three special genes: *gag* (which codes for core protein), *pol* (which codes for the polymerase reverse transcriptase), and *env* (which codes for the envelope protein). In addition, these genes are flanked by long terminal repeat units (LTRs) which can turn on any gene that is located near these LTRs. If one of these long repeat units were located near a proto-oncogene, it could turn it on and make it oncogenic. LTRs can turn on p-oncs through either a slow process or a fast process. The fast way involves the incorporation of a proto-oncogene into the genome of retrovirus by a process called retroviral transduction. A proto-oncogene can be captured (transduced) by a virus through a chance recombination with the DNA of a host cell. Once this gene is within the retrovirus it is called a viral oncogene (v-onc). These viral oncogenes produce excess protein because they are located near a LTR. Viruses that carry a v-onc are called acute transforming retroviruses because they can rapidly form tumors, since the oncogene is located within the viral genome and is always located near the LTRs.

Proto-oncogenes may also become oncogenic by slow transforming viruses, which are retroviruses that do not have their own viral oncogene. Instead these

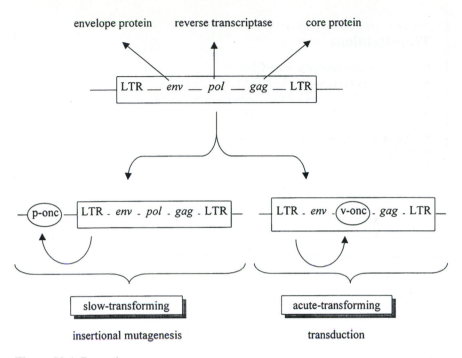

Figure 20-1 Retroviruses
Retroviruses contain the gene *pol* which codes for the enzyme reverse transcriptase. These viruses also contain long terminal repeats (LTRs) that activate nearby genes. A virus may incorporate an oncogene into its genome by a process called transduction. This type of virus is called an acute-transforming virus because its viral oncogen (v-onc) can rapidly cause abnormal tumor growth. A slow-transforming virus does not contain a v-onc and instead needs to be randomly inserted near an oncogene in the host DNA. This process is called insertional mutagenesis and produces tumors slowly.

viruses must be inserted near a proto-oncogene so that their viral LTRs can convert a p-onc into a cellular oncogene. This process is called insertional mutagenesis and is slow because the virus must be inserted near the p-onc by chance.

CHROMOSOMES AND CANCER
Point mutations

- *c-ras* → adenocarcinomas

Translocations

- *c-abl* on chromosome 9 → CML
- *c-myc* on chromosome 8 → Burkitt lymphoma
- *bcl-2* on chromosome 18 → nodular lymphoma

Gene amplification

- *N-myc* → neuroblastoma
- *c-neu* → breast cancer
- *c-erb B2* → breast cancer

A proto-oncogene can also be transformed into an oncogene either by changing the regulation of the gene or by changing the structure of the gene. These changes can be produced by point mutations within the proto-oncogene, by translocations involving the proto-oncogene, or by amplification of the proto-oncogene. Point mutations can change the structure of proto-oncogenes and change their functioning. An example is the *ras* oncogene whose normal product, p21, has GTPase activity (Fig. 7-3). This activity is amplified by binding to GAP and is inactivated by its own GTPase activity. Point mutations involving the *ras* oncogene can inhibit its binding to GAP and decrease its GTPase activity. This decreases its inactivation and prolongs its growth-promoting actions.

Chromosomal translocations may result in structural changes or overexpression of genes. One of the more important translocations associated with malignancy is a translocation that involves the oncogene *c-myc* on chromosome 9 and a portion on chromosome 22 called the breakpoint cluster region (bcr). This translocation, t(9;22), is so important that it has its own name. It's called the Philadelphia chromosome and is characteristic of chronic myeloid leukemia (CML).

Two other oncogenes that are associated with characteristic translocations are worth knowing: *c-myc* and *bcl-2*. Patients with Burkitt lymphoma, an unusual type of lymphoma, have chromosomal translocations that involve the oncogene *c-myc* located on chromosome 8. *c-myc* can be translocated to the heavy chain region on chromosome 14, the kappa light chain region on chromosome 2, or the lambda light chain region on chromosome 22. Therefore, the translocations that are associated with Burkitt lymphoma include (8;14), (8;2), and (8;22). Finally, the oncogene *bcl-2*, found on chromosome 18, is translocated to the immunoglobulin heavy chain gene region on chromosome 14 in many follicular (nodular) lymphomas. Normally some of the B lymphocytes that are produced within germinal centers are destroyed by the process of apoptosis. In nodular lymphomas expression of *bcl-2* prevents the apoptosis of these proliferating cells.

NEUROBLASTOMA

- Malignant tumor of adrenal medulla
- Abdominal mass in young child
- Increased urinary VMA
- Aggressiveness associated with amplifications of *N-myc*
- May de-differentiate into benign ganglioneuroma

Gene amplification is another mechanism by which oncogenes can be activated. Two patterns produced by gene amplification are the formation of multiple, small, chromosome-like structures (double minutes) and the formation of homogenous staining regions (HSRs). Examples of gene amplification are seen with *N-myc* (neuroblastoma), *c-neu* (breast cancer), and *c-erb B2* (breast cancer).

Neuroblastomas are malignant tumors of the adrenal medulla that occur in very young patients. This tumor causes the child to present with an abdominal mass. Histologically the tumor is composed of small cells forming groups of cells that are arranged in a ring around a central mass of pink neural filaments (Homer-Wright rosettes). Electron microscopy reveals neurosecretory granules, and immunohistochemical stains are positive for neuron-specific enolase (NSE). These highly aggressive tumors are special because some will spontaneously regress and some will de-differentiate into benign tumors, such as ganglioneuromas. The number of *N-myc* copies correlates with the aggressiveness of the tumor. De-differentiation into a ganglioneuroma is associated with a marked reduction in this gene amplification.

MULTISTEP THEORY OF COLON CANCER

1. Epithelial hyperplasia
   - Loss of APC gene
2. Formation of adenoma (dysplasia)
   - Loss of DNA methylation
   - Mutation of *ras* gene
   - Loss of DCC gene
3. Carcinoma
   - Loss of p53 gene

COLON POLYPS

Neoplastic polyps

- Tubular adenomas
- Mixed tubulovillous adenomas
- Villous adenomas

Non-neoplastic polyps

- Hyperplastic polyps
- Inflammatory polyps (pseudopolyps)
- Lymphoid polyps
- Juvenile polyps (retention polyps)

In the chapter dealing with cell growth we explored in depth the mechanisms through which oncogenes function to control growth, and we examined how these mechanisms could function abnormally to produce neoplasia. We also looked at the relationship of neoplasia to the decreased functioning of anti-oncogenes. Although we discussed the mechanisms of oncogenes and anti-oncogenes as separate, individual events, cancer is not simply the result of a single change in the DNA of a cell. It is generally believed that cancer results from a multistep process that involves multiple abnormalities of multiple oncogenes and cancer suppressor genes. The development of colon cancer illustrates this stepwise process. Cancer of the colon is preceded by a series of histologic abnormalities. Initial hyperplasia of the epithelium is followed by the formation of an adenoma, one type of colon polyp. There are several types of colon polyps, which can be classified as being non-neoplastic (no malignant potential) or neoplastic (precursors of cancer). Neoplastic polyps originate from proliferating dysplastic epithelium characterized histologically by stratification of cells that have plump, elongated nuclei. As a group these neoplastic colon polyps are called adenomatous polyps. Based on their architecture, these adenomatous polyps are classified as either tubular adenomas, villous adenomas, or mixed tubulovillous adenomas. The risk for malignancy is dependent upon the size of the polyp, the type, and the amount of dysplasia present. The risk of malignancy is greatest for large villous polyps.

It is important to realize, however, that most colon polyps are non-neoplastic and are the result of abnormal maturation or inflammation. Hyperplastic polyps histologically have a serrated "saw-tooth" appearance and essentially are thought to be an aging change. Inflammatory (pseudo-) polyps consist of inflamed regenerating epithelium, as seen in patients with Crohn's disease or ulcerative colitis. Lymphoid polyps contain intramucosal lymphoid tissue, while juvenile (retention) polyps contain abundant stroma and dilated glands filled with mucus. An interesting fact about juvenile polyps, which are typically seen in children or young adults, is that they are prone to self-amputation, and patients may find them floating in the toilet (a disturbing finding for the patient).

CHEMICAL CARCINOGENS
Initiators

- Tobacco smoke → many tumors
- Benzene → leukemias
- Vinyl chloride → angiosarcomas of the liver
- Beta-naphthylamine → cancer of the urinary bladder
- Azo dyes → tumors of the liver
- Aflatoxin → hepatoma
- Asbestos → mesotheliomas and lung tumors
- Arsenic → skin cancer

Promoters

- Saccharin → bladder cancer in rats
- Hormones (estrogen)

Many different chemicals have been associated with the development of cancer. Chemical carcinogenesis occurs in two stages: initiation and promotion. Initiation results from the exposure to an appropriate dose of a carcinogen (the initiator) that damages a cell. Initiation alone is not sufficient to cause tumor formation, but once the DNA is damaged, the damage is permanent (irreversible). If at any time following exposure to the initiator the cell is exposed to another type of chemical (the promoter), a cancer may form. A chemical that is just a promoter by itself will not cause cancer. Also, exposure to a promoter before exposure to an initiator has no effect. The cellular changes produced by promoters do not affect the DNA directly, so the effects of promoters are reversible. Additionally, if the time between doses of the promoter is too great, a tumor will not result. This implies that there is a threshold level for promoters.

Chemicals that are initiators are either direct-acting or indirect-acting compounds. A direct-acting agent is a carcinogen. An indirect-acting agent is a procarcinogen and requires metabolic conversion into an active carcinogen form. Chemicals that are direct-acting initiators include alkylating agents, such as cancer chemotherapeutic drugs (an example being cyclophosphamide).

Indirect-acting initiators include polycyclic aromatic hydrocarbons and lots of stuff that start with the letter A (aromatic amine, azo dyes, aflatoxin, asbestos, and arsenic). An example of an aromatic amine is beta-naphthylamine, which is associated with bladder tumors and tumors in industrial workers (aniline dye or rubber industry workers). Azo dyes, such as butter yellow and scarlet red, are associated with liver tumors. Aflatoxin is produced by *Aspergillus flavus* and is associated with the development of hepatocellular carcinoma. Asbestosis is associated with multiple malignancies including bronchogenic carcinoma and malignant mesothelioma. Arsenic is associated with the development of skin cancers.

Two examples of chemical promoters include saccharin (associated with bladder cancer in rats) and hormones, such as estrogen and DES (diethylstilbestrol).

CANCER OF THE ENDOMETRIUM

- Risk factor → prolonged unopposed estrogen stimulation
- Preceded by endometrial hyperplasia
- Histology → adenocarcinoma

Estrogen is very important in the pathogenesis of cancer of the endometrium (adenocarcinoma). Endometrial adenocarcinoma occurs primarily in perimenopausal and postmenopausal women and is related to prolonged, excess estrogen production (unopposed by progesterone). Risk factors for endometrial adenocarcinoma are states of relative hyperestrinism and include obesity, diabetes, hypertension, nulliparity (no pregnancies), early menarche, and late menopause. For example, in patients who are obese there is increased aromatization of androstenedione to estrone in adipose tissue. The absence of pregnancy (pregnancy being a progesterone state), like late menopause, increases the length of time to which the endometrium is stimulated by the ovarian production of estrogen. Interestingly, cigarette smoking, which interferes with the hepatic conversion of estrone to the active metabolite estriol, is associated with a decreased risk of endometrial cancer. Also, women with ovarian agenesis do not develop endometrial cancer unless there is an exogenous source of estrogen.

Endometrial adenocarcinomas grossly may present as a polypoid mass within the uterine cavity or a diffuse tumor that infiltrates into the endometrium or myometrium. Histologically they usually are composed of malignant, infiltrating glandular structures. If there are areas of nonmalignant squamous differentiation within these tumors, they are called adenoacanthomas. If there are areas of malignant squamous differentiation, they are called adenosquamous carcinoma.

CANCER OF THE BREAST

Ductal carcinoma

- Ductal carcinoma in situ (DCIS)
- Infiltrating ductal carcinoma

Lobular carcinoma

- Lobular carcinoma in situ (LCIS)
- Infiltrating lobular carcinoma

Histologic variants

- Medullary carcinoma
- Tubular carcinoma
- Mucinous (colloid) carcinoma
- Papillary carcinoma
- Paget disease

Prolonged estrogen stimulation (an imbalance between estrogen and progesterone) is also associated with cancer of the breast. This is illustrated by an association of breast cancer with early menarche (before age 12), late menopause (after age 50), nulliparous women (no pregnancies), and obesity (increased estrogen synthesis in fat depots). The exact pathogenesis of breast cancer is unknown, but many factors have been found to be associated with an increased risk for developing breast cancer. The strongest risk factor is the age of the patient. The incidence of breast cancer increases with age; it is markedly uncommon before the age of 25. The incidence also increases with a family history of breast cancer in first-degree relatives.

The most common type of breast cancer originates from the ducts of the breast and is called ductal carcinoma. It is important to compare this type of breast cancer with cancer arising from the lobules of the breast. Lobular carcinoma of the breast, both in situ and invasive, is important clinically because of its tendency to occur in multiple sites within the same breast or in the opposite breast. In situ lobular carcinoma is characterized histologically by a proliferation of cells of the terminal duct lobular unit that fill and expand the lobules. Unlike intraductal carcinoma, papillary and cribriform structures are not formed and neither is there central necrosis. Invasive lobular carcinoma is unique because of its tendency to infiltrate the stroma in a single file fashion. This pattern is not seen with invasive ductal carcinoma. Infiltrating lobular carcinomas also form concentric "targets" around ducts, and they have an increased frequency of being estrogen receptor positive.

There are several variant forms of breast cancer that are also quite important. For example, Paget disease is a form of ductal carcinoma that arises in the main excretory ducts of the breast and typically involves the overlying nipple and areola. Histologically the large tumor cells have clear cytoplasm and infiltrate the epidermis as single cells. The majority of cases are associated with an underlying intraductal carcinoma, or less commonly, an invasive ductal carcinoma.

Mucinous production is abundant in colloid carcinoma, while a peripheral lymphoid infiltrate is quite characteristic of medullary carcinoma. Both of these special types of breast cancer have a better prognosis than either ductal or lobular carcinoma. Tubular carcinomas, which are composed of small, irregular, comma-shaped or pointed glands, also have a better prognosis.

RADIATION

1. Ionizing radiation
   - Leukemia
   - Thyroid cancer
2. Ultraviolet (UV) radiation
   - Skin cancer

Electromagnetic radiation (X-rays and gamma rays) and particles (alpha particles, beta particles, protons, and neutrons) are all carcinogenic. Cancers closely associated with ionizing radiation include leukemias and thyroid cancers.

There are three types of UV radiation based on the wavelengths of the radiation: UVA (320–400 nm), UVB (280–320 nm), and UVC (200–280 nm). UVA is thought to be harmless (but this is debated), and UVC is blocked by the ozone layer. UVB is thought to be associated with the development of skin cancer. The pathogenesis of these skin cancers is related to the formation of pyrimidine dimers in DNA. UVB also causes mutations in oncogenes and tumor suppressor genes, particularly the *ras* and p53 genes.

CANCER OF THE SKIN
Basal cell carcinoma

- Classic type
- Superficial type
- Morphea-like type

Squamous cell carcinoma

- Sun-induced
- Immunosuppression
- Chronic scars

Melanoma

- Superficial spreading melanoma
- Nodular melanoma
- Acral lentiginous melanoma
- Lentigo maligna melanoma

Basal cell carcinoma, which originates from the pluripotential cells of the basal layer of the epidermis, is the most common tumor in individuals with pale skin. Basal cell carcinomas are locally invasive, but metastases are quite rare. The classic clinical appearance of a basal cell carcinoma is a pearly papule with raised margins and a central ulcer (rodent ulcer). Histologic examination reveals infiltrating groups of basophilic (blue colored) cells. Characteristically there is palisading (lining up of cells) at the periphery of groups of tumor cells and peritumoral clefting. Variants of basel cell carcinoma, which are not infrequent, include the superficial type (which may be multifocal), the morphea-like type, and the pigmented type. The latter may be mistaken clinically for malignant melanoma because of the pigmentation, while the morphea-like type has marked fibrosis and is difficult to eradicate locally.

Squamous cell carcinomas (SCC) are also a common type of skin cancer. They are usually found on sun-exposed skin of fair-skinned individuals and occur as a result of sun exposure and damage. DNA damage due to exposure to ultraviolet radiation is the most common etiology of SCC; however, they are also associated with other conditions such as immunosuppression or inherited defects in DNA repair. SCC can also develop in an area of chronic scarring, such as an osteomyelitis draining sinus tract or an old burn scar. Importantly, an SCC arising in the latter is more likely to metastasize than an SCC occurring in sun-damaged skin.

Melanomas are highly malignant tumors of the skin that arise from melanocytes of nevus cells. There are basically four types of invasive malignant melanoma. The most common type is superficial spreading melanoma, which is characterized by its lateral (radial) growth and upward infiltration of malignant cells within the epidermis having a "buckshot" appearance (Pagetoid cells). Nodular melanomas are characterized by their dermal (vertical) growth and their minimal lateral (radial) growth. Acral lentiginous melanoma is an uncommon type of melanoma that is characterized by its unique location on the palm, the sole, or the subungual area. Finally, lentigo maligna melanoma, which is found in older individuals (mean age of 70 years), arises from a preexisting, in situ lesion that is called a lentigo maligna (Hutchinson freckle). Lentigo malignas are found on sun-exposed skin and produce large, flat, irregularly pigmented lesions. Histologically lentigo malignas reveal atypical melanocytes scattered throughout the basal layer of an atrophic epidermis with sun damage to the dermis. Since the lesion is in situ, no dermal invasion (vertical phase) is seen. When dermal invasion is present the lesion is invasive and is called a lentigo maligna melanoma.

VIRUSES

RNA viruses

- Acute-transforming viruses
- Slow-transforming viruses
- HTLV-1 → adult T cell leukemia/lymphoma

DNA viruses

1. HPV
   - Cervical neoplasia
2. EBV
   - African Burkitt lymphoma
   - Carcinoma of the nasopharynx
   - B cell immunoblastic lymphoma
3. Hepatitis B and hepatitis C
   - Liver cancer

Both RNA viruses and DNA viruses have been implicated in the pathogenesis of cancer. Earlier we discussed several types of RNA viruses and the mechanisms by which they produce tumors. A third type of retrovirus that has been associated with malignancy is HTLV type 1 (HTLV-1), which has been associated with the development of adult T cell leukemia/lymphoma (ATLL). This disease, endemic in southern Japan and the Caribbean area, is associated with T cell leukemias and lymphomas in a minority of infected patients after a very long latent period. Infection of lymphocytes produces a characteristic clover-leaf appearance of these cells in the peripheral blood. Patients also develop characteristic skin lesions and hypercalcemia. HTLV-1 does not contain an oncogene (v-onc), but does contain the typical retroviral genes *gag*, *pol*, and *env*, along with LTRs (Fig. 20-1). HTLV-1, however, contains two additional genes, *tax* and *rex*. *Tax* turns on the LTRs, which in turn can activate nearby genes. If that gene is the gene for the T cell growth factor (IL-2), then uncontrolled proliferation of T lymphocytes can result.

Examples of DNA viruses that have been associated with neoplasia include papovaviruses, herpes viruses, and hepadnaviruses. Three types of papovavirus associated with cancers include polyoma virus, SV40, and human papillomavirus (HPV). Of these three, the one that is most important (by far) is HPV. More than 60 different types of HPV have been described, and each type is associated with different neoplastic processes. Most importantly, certain types of HPV are associated with the development of cervical cancer. Types 6 and 11 have a low risk and are more often associated with the production of a benign tumor (condyloma acuminata). Types 31, 33, 35, and 51 are associated with an intermediate risk, while types 16 and 18 are associated with a high risk.

Epstein-Barr virus (EBV) is a member of the herpes virus family and is associated with the development of the African type of Burkitt lymphoma, B cell lymphomas in immunocompromised individuals, and nasopharyngeal carcinoma (especially in southern China and Arctic Eskimos). EBV infects epithelial cells of the oropharynx and also B lymphocytes via a specific membrane receptor (CD21).

Finally, several types of hepadenaviruses (liver viruses) are associated with the development of malignant tumors of the liver (hepatocellular carcinoma). Both hepatitis B virus (HBV) and hepatitis C virus (HCV) are associated with the development of cirrhosis of the liver and the subsequent development of malignant tumors.

CANCER OF THE LIVER

1. Hepatocellular carcinoma
   - Cirrhosis
   - Hepatitis B and C
   - Aflatoxin
2. Cholangiocarcinoma
   - Thorotrast
   - *Clonorchis sinensis*
3. Angiosarcoma
   - Vinyl chloride
   - Thorotrast
   - Arsenic

The most common primary malignancy of the liver is hepatocellular carcinoma (hepatoma). In addition to being associated with certain viral infections (hepatitis B and hepatitis C viruses), they are also associated with aflatoxin and cirrhosis. Aflatoxin is produced by *Aspergillus flavus*, which can be found on improperly stored grains and nuts. Microscopic sections of these tumors reveal pleomorphic tumor cells that form trabecular patterns, which are similar to the normal architecture of the liver. Hepatomas may secrete alpha fetoprotein (AFP), a tumor marker that can also be seen in yolk-sac tumors and fetal neural tube defects. Clinically hepatocellular carcinomas have a tendency to grow into the portal vein or the inferior vena cava, and may be associated with several types of paraneoplastic syndromes (see below). There is a microscopic fibrolamellar variant of hepatocellular carcinoma that is seen more often in females, is not associated with AFP, is grossly encapsulated, and has a better prognosis.

It is important to compare the characteristics of hepatocellular carcinomas with another type of primary tumor of the liver, namely, cholangiocarcinoma, which is a malignancy of bile ducts. This tumor is associated with thorotrast and infection with the liver fluke (*Clonorchis sinensis*), but it is not associated with cirrhosis. Histologically the tumor cells have cytoplasmic mucin (not found in hepatomas).

Finally, angiosarcomas are malignant tumors that originate from blood vessels. Histologically they reveal infiltrating vessels that are lined by pleomorphic or atypical endothelial cells. Angiosarcomas of the liver are associated with exposure to vinyl chloride, thorotrast, and arsenic.

CHROMOSOME INSTABILITY SYNDROMES

- Xeroderma pigmentosa
- Ataxia-telangiectasia
- Fanconi syndrome
- Bloom syndrome

There are four autosomal recessive disorders characterized by defects in DNA repair (chromosome instability syndromes). Patients with xeroderma pigmentosum have a marked increased incidence of skin cancers because they cannot repair abnormal pyrimidine dimers that are induced by UVB light. Patients with ataxia-telangiectasia have defective repair of ionizing radiation and have an increased risk of developing lymphoid malignancies. Patients with Fanconi anemia have cells that are sensitive to DNA cross-linking. As a result, patients have an increased incidence of leukemia. Patients with Bloom syndrome are sensitive to many different DNA-damaging agents. They have an increased risk of many cancers, but patients with Bloom syndrome also suffer from severe immunodeficiency and growth retardation.

CANCER INCIDENCE

Males

- Prostate > lung (most common cause of death) > colon

Females

- Breast > lung (most common cause of death) > colon

Looking at statistics is always a tricky venture, and looking at cancer statistics is no exception. First of all, when examining cancer statistics pay particular attention to whether the cancer statistics are referring to incidence or cause of death. The statistics for these two are not the same. By far the most common tumor (incidence) is skin cancer. It is so common in fact, that skin cancer is usually left off cancer lists. After skin cancer, the most common cancer in males is prostate cancer followed by lung cancer and then colorectal cancer. In females, the most common form of cancer after skin cancer is breast cancer, followed by lung cancer and colorectal carcinoma. Lung cancer, however, is the most common cause of cancer deaths in both sexes. In males, the overall cancer death rate has increased, while in females, it has fallen slightly. In both sexes, the death rate from lung cancer has been rising, while the death rate for the majority of other cancers has stayed the same or fallen. Cancers with notably decreased rates include gastric cancer and uterine cancer.

The incidence of cancer generally increases with the age, and therefore cancers are particularly infrequent in children. Tumors that are found in both children and adults include certain types of leukemias, bone tumors (osteogenic sarcomas), and brain tumors, while tumors found in children but not adults include neuroblastomas (adrenal gland) and nephroblastomas (immature malignant tumor of the kidney).

GEOGRAPHY

- Central Africa → cancer of the liver
- India and China → cancer of the nasopharynx
- Japan → cancer of the stomach

There are geographic differences in the incidence of various types of cancer. Some parts of the world have cancer rates for certain malignancies that are far higher than in other parts of the world. Example of this include the following: Central Africa and cancer of the liver (due to hepatitis B and aflatoxin); India and cancer of the pharynx (due to betel nuts and Epstein-Barr virus); New Zealand and melanoma (due to lack of pigmentation and solar exposure); and Japan and cancer of the stomach (due to smoking of food).

PARANEOPLASTIC SYNDROMES

- Cushing syndrome → lung cancer
- Carcinoid syndrome → lung cancer or carcinoid tumor of the small intestine
- SIADH (syndrome of inappropriate ADH secretion) → lung cancer and intracranial neoplasms
- Hypercalcemia → lung cancer or multiple myeloma
- Hypocalcemia → medullary carcinoma of the thyroid
- Hypoglycemia → liver cancer and tumors of the mesothelium (mesotheliomas)
- Polycythemia → kidney tumors, liver tumors, and cerebellar vascular tumors

---

Collections of symptoms produced by tumors that are not the result of local mass effect or metastases are called paraneoplastic syndromes. Bronchogenic carcinomas are associated with many paraneoplastic syndromes such as Cushing syndrome (ectopic ACTH production), hyponatremia (ectopic antidiuretic hormone production), hypercalcemia (ectopic parathyroid hormone-like substance or prostaglandin E production), hypocalcemia (calcitonin), and gynecomastia (gonadotropins). Lung cancers (or pulmonary disease) can produce an abnormal rounded shape of the fingers called "clubbing" or "pulmonary hypertrophic osteoarthropathy." Lung cancers are also associated with multiple (migratory) venous thrombosis (migratory thrombophlebitis or Trousseau's sign), but this sign is more classically associated with carcinoma of the pancreas.

Increased numbers of red cells in the peripheral blood (erythrocytosis) is associated with increased erythropoietin production by some tumors, particularly tumors of the kidney (renal cell carcinoma), tumors of the liver (hepatocellular carcinoma), and a very strange tumor of the cerebellum (cerebellar hemangioblastoma).

MULTIPLE ENDOCRINE NEOPLASIA

MEN type I (Wermer's syndrome)

- Parathyroid
- Pituitary
- Pancreas

MEN type II (Sipple syndrome)

- Parathyroid
- Medullary carcinoma of thyroid
- Pheochromocytoma

MEN type III (MEN IIb)

- Medullary carcinoma of thyroid
- Pheochromocytoma
- Mucosal neuromas

PHEOCHROMOCYTOMA

1. Tumor of adrenal medulla
2. Secretes norepinephrine or epinephrine (secondary hypertension)
3. Increased urinary VMA
4. 10% tumor
   - 10% malignant
   - 10% bilatral
   - 10% extraadrenal
   - 10% familial

Combinations of neoplasms affecting different endocrine organs in the same patient are referred to as multiple endocrine neoplasia (MEN) syndromes. There are several types of MEN. Patients with type I MEN (Wermer's syndrome) have pituitary adenomas, parathyroid hyperplasia (or adenomas), and neoplasms of the pancreatic islets (most commonly gastrinomas, which produce the Zollinger-Ellison syndrome). Type IIa MEN (Sipple syndrome) is characterized by the combination of medullary carcinoma of the thyroid, pheochromocytoma of the adrenal medulla, and hyperparathyroidism. Finally, MEN type IIb (type III) is associated with medullary carcinoma of the thyroid, pheochromocytoma of the adrenal medulla and multiple mucocutaneous neuromas.

In contrast to MEN, combinations of autoimmune diseases affecting different endocrine organs are called polyglandular syndromes. There are several types of polyglandular syndromes. Patients with type I polyglandular autoimmune syndrome have at least two of the triad of Addison's disease, hypoparathyroidism, and mucocutaneous candidiasis. Type II, Schmidt's syndrome, is not associated with either hypoparathyroidism or mucocutaneous candidiasis, but instead is associated with autoimmune thyroid disease (Hashimoto's thyroiditis) and insulin-dependent diabetes.

TUMOR MARKERS

Beta-HCG (human chorionic gonadotropin)

- Choriocarcinoma
- Hydatidiform mole
- Dysgerminoma
- Seminoma (minority of cases)

AFP (α-fetoprotein)

- Liver cancer
- Yolk sac tumors
- Embryonal carcinoma

Alpha1-antitrypsin

- Liver cancer
- Yolk sac tumors

PSA (prostate-specific antigen)

- Adenocarcinoma of prostate

CEA (carcinoembryonic antigen)

- Adenocarcinomas of colon, pancreas, stomach, and breast (nonspecific marker)

CA-125

• Ovarian cancer

S-100

• Melanoma
• Neural tumors

Tumor markers are a diverse group of biochemical substances that are associated with certain tumors. These markers include hormones, oncofetal antigens, proteins, mucins, and glycoproteins. Human chorionic gonadotropin (HCG) is a hormone that is associated with trophoblastic tumors, especially choriocarcinoma. Alpha-fetoprotein (AFP) is a glycoprotein that is synthesized by the yolk sac and the fetal liver and is associated with yolk sac tumors of the testes and liver cell carcinomas. Prostate-specific antigen (PSA) and prostatic acid phosphatase (PAP) are associated with cancer of the prostate. Carcinoembryonic antigen (CEA) is a glycoprotein that is associated with many cancers including adenocarcinomas of the colon, pancreas, lung, stomach, and breast. It is fairly nonspecific and may even be increased in benign disorders.

Abscess. A localized collection of neutrophils and necrotic debris.

Acanthocytes. Red blood cells with numerous irregularly shaped spikes on their surface. Acanthocytes can be found in patients with abetalipoproteinemia or liver disease.

Acantholysis. Separation of the keratinocytes within the epidermis, which results in intraepidermal (suprabasal) bullae. Acantholysis is seen in patients with pemphigus vulgaris.

Acanthosis. Increased thickness of the epidermis of the skin.

Achalasia. Absence of normal relaxation of the lower esophageal sphincter (LES) that is due to decreased or absent ganglion cells in the myenteric plexus of the body of the esophagus. The increased LES pressure and the absence of peristaltic waves in the lower esophagus cause the esophagus to become dilated above the level of the LES. Patients with achalasia have an increased risk of developing aspiration pneumonia and squamous cell carcinoma.

Agenesis. Complete failure of an organ to develop. In contrast to aplasia no anlage is present.

Alcoholic hyaline. Eosinophilic intracytoplasmic inclusions within liver cells that are composed predominately of prekeratin intermediate filaments. Alcoholic hyaline, also called Mallory bodies, is a nonspecific finding found in several liver diseases.

Amenorrhea. Lack of menstruation. Amenorrhea may be primary or secondary. The most common cause of secondary amenorrhea in premenopausal females is pregnancy.

Amyloid. Any fibrillar protein with a "beta-pleated sheet" configuration that stains brown with iodine, pink with hematoxylin and eosin stain, and dark red with the congo red stain. When viewed under polarized light, amyloid stained with the congo red stain displays an apple-green birefringence.

Anaphylaxis. Signs and symptoms produced by type I hypersensitivity reactions. Anaphylactic reactions can be localized or systemic.

Anasarca. Generalized accumulation of edema fluid in the body.

Anergy. Failure of immune cells to react to normal antigens. Anergy is one of the signs of sarcoidosis.

Aneurysm. Abnormal dilatation of a blood vessel. Aneurysms can be classified based on their cause, their shape, or their location.

Angina. Chest pain that is caused by decreased blood flow to the heart. Nitrous oxide is a substance that causes dilation of blood vessels. Substances that are metabolized to nitrous oxide (nitroglycerin) are beneficial in the treatment of angina.

Angioedema. Vascular-induced nonpitting edema of soft tissue. Inherited deficiencies of C1 esterase inhibitor can produce recurrent angioedema of the face. A deficiency of C1 esterase inhibitor leads to excess production of bradykinin, which causes increased vascular permeability and angioedema.

Anlage. Primitive mass of cells.

Anthracosis. Deposition of carbon particles within macrophages in and around the lungs.

Anti-oncogenes. Genes that normally function to regulate and prevent growth. Anti-oncogenes are also called tumor suppressor genes. Examples of these suppressor genes include *NF-1*, *Rb*, and *p53*.

Aplasia. Complete failure of an organ to develop. In contrast to agenesis an anlage is present.

Apocrine metaplasia. Epithelial cells with abundant eosinophilic cytoplasm and apical cytoplasmic "snouts" in breast tissue with fibrocystic changes.

Apoptosis. An active form of cell death characterized by the synthesis of self-destructive enzymes, condensation of nuclear chromatin, formation of apoptotic bodies, and lack of an inflammatory infiltrate. In contrast to necrosis, apoptosis usually involves the death of single cells or small clusters of cells.

Arteriosclerosis. A general term that refers to sclerosis and rigidity of arteries. Three vascular diseases that are characterized by arteriosclerosis are atherosclerosis, arteriolosclerosis, and Mönckeberg's arteriosclerosis.

Ascites. Excess fluid in the peritoneal cavity. The pathogenesis of ascites involves increased pressure in the sinusoids causing increased flow into the lymphatic vessels. This excess lymphatic flow results in leakage of lymphatic fluid into the peritoneal space.

Atelectasis. Collapse of the alveoli in the lungs.

Atheromas. Fibrous plaques in medium to large sized arteries produced by atherosclerosis. Atheromas have a cholesterol-laden core with an overlying fibrous cap. The cells within an atheroma include smooth muscle cells, macrophages, and leukocytes. Both smooth muscle cells and macrophages can ingest lipid to form foam cells. The extracellular matrix material within atheromas include collagen, elastic fibers, and proteoglycans. Intracellular and extracellular lipid is also present. Fatty streaks are thought to be precursors of atheromatous plaques.

Athetosis. Slow, writhing movements that are characteristic of lesions of the basal ganglia.

Atresia. Hypoplasia or aplasia of a segment of a tubular structure, such as blood vessels, bile ducts, the esophagus, or the intestines.

Atrophy. A reversible decrease in the size of an organ or tissue that is due to a decrease in the size of preexisting cells and not a decrease in the number of cells. Atrophy may be a physiologic or pathologic process. Most commonly pathologic atrophy is the result of decreased blood flow.

Atypical lymphocytes. Lymphocytes with abundant cytoplasm that are characteristic of viral infections, particularly infectious mononucleosis. The cytoplasm may be indented by adjacent erythrocytes, and sometimes is described as having a "ballerina-skirt" appearance.

Autocrine effects. Actions of a chemical on the cell that produced that chemical.

Autophagy. The digestion of intracellular material by the formation of autophagolysosomes. Autophagy is analogous to the process of heterophagy.

Azotemia. Increased blood urea nitrogen (BUN) and creatinine levels in the blood that is usually the result of decreased glomerular filtration rate. Azotemia can be classified according to prerenal, renal, and postrenal causes.

Bradykinesia. Slowness of voluntary movements seen in patients with Parkinson's disease.

Bronchiectasis. Abnormal dilatation of bronchi, usually the result of repeated bacterial infections.

CD. Membrane target regions that are recognized by groups of similar antibodies. CD stands for "cluster designation." Peripheral blood T lymphocytes have the surface markers CD2, CD3, CD5, and CD7. T lymphocytes can also be divided into two subtypes based on their surface CD markers. Helper T lymphocytes are CD4 positive, while cytotoxic T lymphocytes are CD8 positive. B lymphocytes have the surface markers CD19, CD20, CD21, and CD22.

Chemotaxis. The process by which white blood cells are attracted to certain areas. The most significant chemotactic agents for neutrophils include bacterial products, complement components (C5a), products of the lipoxygenase pathway (5-HETE and leukotriene B4), and cytokines. These chemotactic factors function through the Gq second messenger system.

Cholestasis. Accumulation of bile pigment within hepatocytes. Bile may be deposited within bile ductules and form bile plugs, or it may be deposited outside of bile ducts and form bile lakes.

Chorea. Sudden, purposeless jerky movements that are characteristic of lesions of the basal ganglia.

Claudication. Muscle pain. An important cause of claudication is decreased blood flow to muscles.

Coagulative necrosis. A type of necrosis that is usually produced by decreased blood flow or infarction. Histologically the nuclei of the necrotic cells are gone, but the outlines of the cells remain.

Congestion. Impaired blood flow that results from impaired venous drainage. Congestion is also called passive hyperemia and produces a blue-red color grossly.

Cor pulmonale. Right ventricular hypertrophy that is the result of intrinsic disease of the lungs. Pulmonary diseases that can cause cor pulmonale include COPD, interstitial fibrosis, multiple pulmonary emboli, and pulmonary hypertension.

Crescents. Characteristic proliferation of epithelial cells within the Bowmann space of the glomerulus in patients with rapidly progressive glomeru-lonephritis.

Crypt abscesses. Aggregates of neutrophils within the lumens of the crypts of the colon. Crypt abscesses are characteristic of the inflammatory bowel dis-eases (ulcerative colitis and Crohn's disease).

Cyanosis. A blue color of the skin that is caused by an increase in the amount of unoxygenated hemoglobin in the blood.

Cytokines. Products of cells that affect the function of other cells. Mono-cytes release monokines, and lymphocytes release lymphokines. Two of the most important categories of cytokines are the interleukins and the in-terferons.

Diapedesis. Migration of neutrophils across the wall of blood and into the inter-stitial tissue. Diapedesis occurs mainly within venules.

Dysplasia. Non-neoplastic disorganized abnormal growth patterns. The degree of dysplasia is usually determined by the thickness of the epithelium having these abnormal changes. Degrees of dysplasia include mild dysplasia, mod-erate dysplasia, and severe dysplasia.

Dyspnea. Subjective feeling of shortness of breath usually associated with car-diac disease.

Dystrophin. A protein found on the inner surface on the sarcolemma that is absent in patients with Duchenne muscular dystrophy.

Dysuria. Pain and burning with urination. Dysuria can be a symptom of an infection of the urinary bladder or prostate.

Ecchymoses. Larger hemorrhages that are greater than 1 cm in diameter.

Edema. Excess fluid in the interstitial tissue or serous cavities. There are two types of edema. One is the result of inflammation (inflammatory edema) and the other is the result of abnormalities of pressure (noninflammatory edema). Inflammatory edema is called an exudate and is characterized by extravascular fluid having a high protein content, cellular debris, and a spe-cific gravity of >1.020. Noninflammatory edema is called a transudate and is characterized by a lack of protein and cells and a low specific gravity.

Embolus. A intravascular mass that is carried by the flow of blood to another site within the vascular system. Most emboli are formed from thrombi, and most originate in veins.

Endocrine effects. Systemic actions of chemicals irrespective of the location of the cell that produced that chemical.

Enterotoxins. Exotoxins produced by bacteria that act upon intestinal mucosal cells. The enterotoxins produced by *Escherichia coli* and *vibrio cholera* are ADP-ribosyl transferases that transfer NAD to membrane Gαs-proteins and inhibit them.

Epithelioid cells. Activated tissue macrophages that have abundant cytoplasm. Aggregates of epithelioid cells are called granulomas.

Erosions. Loss of the most superficial portion of the mucosa. Erosions are different from mucosal ulcers, which involve the full thickness of the mucosa.

Exophthalmus. Protrusion of the eyes that is characteristically seen in patients with Graves' disease.

Fibrillin. A glycoprotein produced by fibroblasts that provides the scaffolding for elastin in the connective tissue. Defective synthesis of fibrillin is associated with Marfan syndrome.

Fibrinoid necrosis. A type of necrosis that is characterized by the deposition of immune complexes and necrotic material within blood vessels. Fibrinoid necrosis is characteristic of type III hypersensitivity disorders.

Flocculent densities. Amorphous densities in mitochondria that are characteristic of irreversible cellular injury.

Free radicals. Unstable, reactive molecules that have a single, unpaired electron in their outer orbit. Examples of free radicals include superoxide, the hydroxyl radical, and carbon tetrachloride.

Frequency. A urinary tract symptom that refers to voiding small amounts of urine at frequent intervals.

Gangrene. A type of necrosis of the extremities that is the result of arterial obstruction. Dry gangrene consists of mainly of coagulative necrosis, while wet gangrene has liquefactive necrosis due to superimposed bacterial infection.

GAP. GTPase-activating protein that catalyzes the hydrolysis of GTP bound to G proteins. This is a major mechanism for the inactivation of the *ras* protein product p21.

Ghon complex. A characteristic lesion of primary tuberculosis that consists of a subpleural lesion near the fissure between the upper and lower lobes and enlarged caseous lymph nodes that drain the pulmonary lesion.

Gowers maneuver. A clinical finding in children with muscular dystrophy in which the child uses the stronger arm and shoulder muscles to rise up from the floor because of weakness of the pelvic girdle muscles.

G proteins. Substances that are active when bound to GTP and inactive when bound to GDP. A chemical messenger binds to the inactive G protein and GTP is exchanged for GDP. This causes the G protein to become active. Active GTP-bound G proteins have inherent GTPase activity that converts the GTP back to GDP. This reaction inactivates the G protein.

Grade. Histologic estimation of the degree of differentiation of a tumor. The better (lower) the grade, the better the prognosis.

Granulation tissue. Tissue composed of proliferating capillaries and fibroblasts that is produced during the process of tissue repair. Histologic examination of granulation tissue reveals numerous endothelial cells and fibroblasts with large nuclei and prominent nuclei.

Granulomas. Aggregates of activated macrophages. These cells are called epithelioid cells because they have abundant cytoplasm that is somewhat similar to the abundant cytoplasm of epithelial cells. Other cells that may be present in granulomas include lymphocytes, plasma cells, and giant cells. Giant cells, which are formed by the fusion of epithelioid cells, are large cells with abundant cytoplasm and many nuclei. Granulomas with a unique type of central necrosis are called caseating granulomas and are characteristic of tuberculosis. Granulomas that lack the central necrosis of caseating granulomas are called noncaseating granulomas. Examples of diseases characterized by noncaseating granulomatous inflammation include sarcoidosis, fungal infections, and foreign body reactions.

Hematoma. A localized area of hemorrhage within tissue.

Hemiballismus. Sudden, wild flailing of one arm that is characteristic of lesions of the subthalamic nuclei.

Hemochromatosis. Systemic deposition of hemosiderin within macrophages and parenchymal cells that is associated with organ dysfunction. Hemochromatosis may be a primary (idiopathic) disease, or it may be secondary to some other abnormality. Secondary hemochromatosis is most common in patients with chronic hemolytic anemias.

Hemolysis. Destruction of red blood cells. Hemolysis can be intravascular or extravascular. Intravascular hemolysis releases hemoglobin into the blood (hemoglobinemia) which binds to haptoglobin. When haptoglobin levels are depleted, free hemoglobin is oxidized to methemoglobin, and then both hemoglobin and methemoglobin are secreted into the urine (hemoglobinuria and methemoglobinuria). Within the renal tubular epithelial cells, hemoglobin is reabsorbed, hemosiderin is formed, and when these cells are shed into the urine, hemosiderinuria results. Since extravascular hemolysis does not occur within the vascular compartment, hemoglobinemia, hemoglobinuria, methemoglobinuria, and hemosiderinuria do not occur. Unlike intravascular hemolysis, extravascular hemolysis causes hypertrophy and hyperplasia of the mononuclear phagocytic system which, if it takes place in the spleen, may lead to splenomegaly.

Hemoptysis. Coughing up blood.

Hemorrhage. The leakage of blood from a blood vessel (bleeding).

Hemosiderosis. Systemic deposition of hemosiderin within macrophages that is not associated with organ dysfunction.

Heterophagy. The uptake and digestion of extracellular material via phagocytosis or pinocytosis. Heterophagy involves the formation of a secondary lysosome and is analogous to the process of autophagia.

Heteroplasm. The combination of different DNA sequences at a particular locus in a single cell. Heteroplasty often refers to the combination of normal and abnormal mitochondrial genes.

Heterozygous. An individual who has two different alleles at a particular gene site (locus).

Homozygous. An individual who has two identical alleles at a particular gene site.

Hyaline. A nonspecific term that describes any material, inside or outside of the cell, that stains a homogenous red color with the routine hematoxylin and eosin stain.

Hydrocephalus. Enlargement of the ventricles. Hydrocephalus may result from increased cerebrospinal fluid (CSF) secretion, decreased CSF absorption, or obstruction. Hydrocephalus is most often caused by blockage of the normal flow of CSF. This blockage may be located along the ventricular system or along the subarachnoid path. The former causes focal enlargement of a protein of the ventricular system that does not communicate with the subarachnoid space and is called a noncommunicating hydrocephalus. The latter causes a diffuse enlargement of the ventricular system and is called a communicating hydrocephalus.

Hydropic degeneration. Excess accumulation of water in a cell causing it to swell. Hydropic degeneration is a sign of reversible cellular injury.

Hyperemia. Increased capillary blood flow caused by arteriolar dilatation. Hyperemia is also called active hyperemia and produces a reddish color grossly. Conditions associated with hyperemia include blushing, exercise, and inflammation.

Hyperplasia. Increased numbers of cells in a tissue or organ.

Hypertrophy. Increased size of the cells in a tissue or organ. Hypertrophy usually occurs in tissue composed of permanent (nondividing) cells, such as skeletal muscle, cardiac muscle, and smooth muscle.

Hyphae. The filamentous structure of molds. A mass of hyphae form a mycelium. True hyphae have cross-walls that divide the hyphae into multiple cells (septate hyphae).

Hypoplasia. A reduction in the size of an organ due to a developmental abnormality that produces a decrease in the number of cells. Hypoplastic organs tend to be normal in structure but small in size.

Hypoxia. Decreased oxygenation of tissue. Hypoxia may be the result of disease processes that affect the normal transport of oxygen from the lungs to the tissue. Examples of these abnormalities include decreased blood flow, diseases of the lungs, diseases of the blood vessels, or diseases of the blood itself.

Infarction. An area of ischemic necrosis that results from decreased arterial or venous blood flow. Infarcts can be classified on the basis of their color or by the presence of bacteria. Infarcts may be anemic (white) or hemorrhagic (red). White infarcts occur with arterial occlusion in solid tissues. Red infarcts occur with venous occlusion, congested tissues, or organs with a double or collateral blood supply.

Ischemia. Decreased blood flow.

Jaundice. A descriptive clinical term for a yellow discoloration of skin and sclerae due to the accumulation of bilirubin in tissues.

Karyotype. A picture composed of the chromosomes of a cell sorted by length.

Colchicine is used to prepare karyotypes because it blocks mitosis at metaphase by disrupting microtubules.

Kernicterus. Deposits of unconjugated bilirubin in the brain of neonates and premature infants with unconjugated hyperbilirubinemia due to the immaturity of the blood-brain barrier. This deposition can severely damage the brain and produce mental retardation or death.

Koilocytosis. The cytopathic viral effect produced by human papilloma virus (HPV). This change is seen as enlarged squamous epithelial cells that have shrunken nuclei ("raisin-oid") and large cytoplasmic vacuoles around the nucleus. The change is most often seen in dysplasia of the cervix and condyloma.

Kwashiorkor. A disease of malnourishment in children that is characterized by a lack of protein intake with barely adequate caloric intake.

Langerhans cells. Dendritic antigen-processing cells found within the epidermis. Langerhans cells have large amounts of class II antigens on their surface and are characterized by cytoplasmic Birbeck granules, which by EM examination appear shaped like tennis rackets.

Langhans giant cell. A type of giant cell that is found within the caseating granulomas of tuberculosis. Langhans giant cells have nuclei that are arranged at the periphery of the cytoplasm (creating a horseshoe pattern).

Lentigo. A pigmented skin lesion that results from melanocytic hyperplasia in the basal layers of the epidermis along with elongation and thinning of the rete ridges.

Leukoerythroblastosis. Immature white cells (myelocytes) and immature red cells (nucleated red blood cells) in the peripheral blood. The combination of teardrop red blood cells, leukoerythroblastosis, and abnormal platelets in the peripheral smear are highly suggestive of myeloid metaplasia with myelofibrosis.

Lines of Zahn. Characteristic laminations found in arterial pre-mortem thrombi that are formed by layers having abundant platelets separated by layers having abundant white cells.

Lipofuscin. A fine granular, golden-brown pigment that is formed from indigestible material within lysosomes. Lipofuscin is a "wear and tear" pigment that is most commonly found within the hearts of elderly individuals or patients with severe malnutrition.

Liquefactive necrosis. A type of necrosis that is the result of tissue digestion of lysosomal enzymes. Liquefactive necrosis is seen with bacterial infections and infarction of the brain.

Lower motor neuron (LMN) signs. Muscle atrophy, flaccid paralysis, absent deep tendon reflexes.

Malaise. A generalized "not well" feeling.

Marasmus. A disease of malnourishment in children that is characterized by a total lack of calories (starvation).

Megacolon. A dilated portion of the large intestines. Megacolon may be seen in young children or adults. In young children megacolon is usually associated with Hirschsprung disease (congenital aganglionic megacolon) which is caused by a failure of the neural crest cells to migrate all the way to the anus. In adults megacolon may be associated with ulcerative colitis.

Megaloblastic anemia. A type of anemia characterized by abnormally maturing red blood cell precursors called megaloblasts. Histologically these cells are characterized by delayed maturation of the nucleus. Megaloblastic anemia is produced by a deficiency of vitamin B12 or folate.

Menorrhagia. Excessive bleeding during menstruation.

Metaplasia. Replacement of one cell type by another.

Monoclonal. A proliferation of cells that all originated from a single cell. Monoclonal proliferations are usually neoplastic proliferations.

Monocytoid B cells. A type of B lymphocyte that superficially resembles a monocyte and is found within the lymph nodes of a few disorders, such as toxoplasmosis.

Monokines. Cytokines that are secreted by monocytes.

Myelodysplastic syndromes. A group of disorders that are characterized by abnormal changes in the developing cells in the bone marrow. These disorders are usually associated with an increase in the number of blasts in the marrow and have an increased risk for the subsequent development of an acute leukemia. In the past these disorders were called preleukemia syndromes.

Myeloproliferative syndromes. A group of clonal disorders that are characterized by an increase in the number of proliferating cells in the bone marrow. In contrast to the myelodysplastic syndromes, the myeloproliferative syndromes lack dysplastic features. The four myeloproliferative disorders are polycythemia rubra vera, chronic myelocytic leukemia, myelofibrosis, and essential thrombocytopenia.

Necrosis. Death of large sheets of cells, usually associated with an inflammatory infiltrate. The cytoplasm of necrotic cells becomes eosinophilic, while the nuclei become small and basophilic. This latter change is called pyknosis. The pyknotic nuclei can break up into multiple small fragments, or they can fade away. The former change is called karyorrhexis, while the latter is called karyolysis.

Neurofibrillary tangles. Bundles of filaments in the cytoplasm of neurons that contain an abnormal form of a microtubule-associated protein. Neurofibrillary tangles are found in the brain of patients with Alzheimer's disease.

Nystagmus. Characteristic jerky, back-and-forth movements of the eyes.

Oligohydramnios. Too little amniotic fluid. Causes of oligohydramnios include agenesis of the kidneys and urinary obstruction. Bilateral agenesis of the kidneys can produce Potter's syndrome.

Oncocytes. Epithelial cells that have numerous mitochondria which impart a distinctive pink appearance to the cytoplasm. Oncocytic cells can be found lining the papillary projections of a Warthin's tumor or in the thyroid gland of a patient with Hashimoto's thyroiditis.

Opsonins. Substances that bind to foreign material and cause them to become phagocytized by white blood cells. Most microorganisms are not recognized by leukocytes until they are coated with opsonins. Two of the most important opsonins are the Fc portion of immunoglobulin and complement factors C3b and iC3b.

Orthopnea. Dyspnea that occurs upon lying down.

Osteophytes. New bone formation at the edges of bone in patients with osteoarthritis due to the loss of cartilage. Osteophytes located over the distal interphalangeal (DIP) joints are called Heberden's nodes, while osteophytes located at the proximal interphalangeal (PIP) joints are called Bouchard's nodes.

Pallor. A pale color.

Pancytopenia. A decrease of all cell lines in the peripheral blood. Pancytopenia produces anemia (decreased numbers of red cells), leukopenia (decreased numbers of white cells), and thrombocytopenia (decreased numbers of platelets). Important causes of pancytopenia include aplastic anemia and the myelodysplastic syndromes.

Papilloma. A benign glandular neoplasm that has fingerlike projections and a central fibrovascular core.

Paracrine effects. Actions of a chemical on cells in the vicinity of the cell that produced that chemical.

Parakeratosis. Retention of the nuclei of squamous epidermal cells into the normally anucleate keratin layer.

Penetrance. The percent of individuals with the abnormal gene who express the abnormal trait. Penetrance is an "all or none" phenomenon. A reduced penetrance of 50% indicates that 50% of those having the abnormal gene will express the abnormal trait.

Petechiae. Very small, pinpoint hemorrhages.

Phagocytosis. The uptake and ingestion of large substances like bacteria.

Pinocytosis. The uptake and ingestion of small macromolecules like LDL.

Polyclonal. A proliferation of cells that originated from multiple cells and not a single cell. Polyclonal proliferations of cells are usually reactive and not neoplastic.

Polycythemia. Increased numbers of red blood cells in the peripheral blood. Polycythemia may be a relative polycythemia due to a decrease in the plasma volume, or it may be an absolute polycythemia due to a real increase in the total red cell mass. Primary polycythemia is due to a defect in myeloid stem cells and is called polycythemia rubra vera.

Polyhydramnios. Too much amniotic fluid. Developmental abnormalities that impair fetal swallowing of amniotic fluid will lead to polyhydramnios. Causes include esophageal atresia and severe anomalies of the CNS.

Primary lysosomes. Clathrin-coated intracellular vesicles that contain many types of enzymes, such as acid hydrolases. Primary lysosomes combine with phagocytic vesicles to form secondary lysosomes (phagolysosomes).

Pronto-oncogenes. Cellular genes that promote normal growth and differentiation.

Pruritus. Itching of the skin.

Psammoma bodies. Small laminated calcified bodies seen histologically in papillary tumors of the ovary, papillary carcinoma of the thyroid, meningiomas, or mesotheliomas.

Purpura. Small hemorrhages that are up to 1 cm in diameter.

Secondary lysosomes. Phagolysosomes that are formed by the fusion of primary lysosomes and phagocytic vesicles. Defective formation of secondary lysosomes in neutrophils is characteristic of Chediak-Higashi syndrome.

Senile plaques. Focal collections of neuritic processes surrounding a central amyloid core that are found in the brain of patients with Alzheimer's disease.

Sideroblasts. Red cell precursors in the normal bone marrow that contain ferritin granules.

Smudge cells. Fragile lymphocytes that are seen in peripheral smears of patients with chronic lymphocytic leukemia. The term "smudge cells" also refers to the cytopathic effect of adenovirus on the epithelial cells in the lung.

Spike and dome pattern. Characteristic microscopic changes produced by expansion of the glomerular basement membrane between and over electron-dense subepithelial deposits seen in patients with membranous glomerulopathy.

Spina bifida. A general term that refers to abnormal fusion of the vertebral arches of the lowest vertebral arches. There are several disorders in the group of developmental abnormalities that have varying degrees of severity.

Spongiosis. Edema within the epidermis that is characteristic of acute (eczematous) dermatitis.

Stage. Clinical estimation of the size and the extent of the spread of a tumor. The system generally used to stage malignant tumors is the TNM classification. Staging has proved to be of greater clinical value than grading to predict the prognosis of malignant tumors.

Steatorrhea. Greasy, bulky, light-colored stools. Steatorrhea is a sign of malabsorption and can be seen in patients with chronic pancreatitis due to the absence of lipase, which is essential for the digestion of fat.

Steatosis. Accumulation of triglycerides within cells. Steatosis is also called fatty change. Liver steatosis serves as the model of cellular fatty change. Microvesicular steatosis refers to the accumulation of small lipid droplets that do not displace the nucleus and is associated with acute toxic hepatocellular injury. Macrovesicular steatosis refers to the accumulation of large lipid droplets that cause the nucleus to be displaced to the side of the cell and is associated with chronic hepatocellular injury, such as malnutrition or chronic alcohol abuse.

Superantigen. A special type of antigen that is capable of binding to both class II MHC and the TCR outside of the normal antigen binding area. Superantigens are capable of causing massive activation of T cells in the peripheral blood. An example of this is the TSST-1 toxin, which is associated with the toxic shock syndrome (TSS) and is secreted by some strains of *Staph aureus.*

Surfactant. A lipid produced by type II pneumocytes that reduces the surface tension between air and fluid interfaces in the alveoli of the lung. Synthesis of surfactant increases throughout fetal development, but is maximal at about 35 weeks. A deficiency of surfactant causes the lungs to collapse with expiration and is associated with hyaline membrane disease.

Tetany. Spontaneous tonic muscular contractions. Tetany can be produced by hypocalcemia. Two clinical tests to demonstrate tetany are Chvostek's sign (tapping on the facial nerve produces twitching of the ipsilateral facial muscles) and Trousseau's sign (inflating a blood pressure cuff for several minutes produces painful carpal muscle contractions).

Thrombosis. Formation of a solid mass of blood within the blood vessels of the heart.

Tingible-body macrophages. Macrophages within reactive germinal centers that have phagocytized cellular debris. The presence of tingible-body macrophages are useful in the histologic differentiation between reactive follicular hyperplasia and follicular lymphomas.

Tram-track pattern. Characteristic histologic change seen in patients with membranoproliferative glomerulonephritis due to the splitting of the glomerular basement membrane by proliferating mesangial cells and mesangial material.

Upper motor neuron (UMN) signs. Spastic paralysis, hyperactive deep tendon reflexes, positive Babinski reflex.

Urgency. The feeling of having to urinate immediately.

Urticaria. Prurtic edematous areas of the skin caused by the local release of substances from mast cells due to a type I hypersensitivity reaction. The common term for urticaria is "hives."

Xanthelasmas. Yellow fatty deposits typically located around the eyelids. Xanthelasmas may be seen in patients with hyperlipidemia.

Xanthomas. Lipid tumors of skin. Xanthomas may be associated with hyperlipidemias or liver diseases.

• I N D E X •

Page numbers in italic indicate illustrations. Page numbers followed by *t* indicate tables.

ISBN 0-07-008321-5

90000

9 780070 083219

BROWN: BASIC CONCEPTS/PATH